DRUG ACTION AND DESIGN:
Mechanism-Based Enzyme Inhibitors

DEVELOPMENTS IN BIOCHEMISTRY

DRUG ACTION AND DESIGN:
Mechanism-Based Enzyme Inhibitors

Proceedings of The Twentieth Annual Medicinal Chemistry Symposium, Amherst, New York, U.S.A., on May 21-23, 1979

Editor:

THOMAS I. KALMAN
Department of Medicinal Chemistry, State University of New York at Buffalo, Amherst, New York, U.S.A.

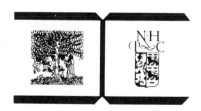

ELSEVIER/NORTH-HOLLAND
NEW YORK • AMSTERDAM • OXFORD

© 1979 by Elsevier North Holland, Inc.

with the exception of those articles lacking a copyright line on their opening chapter
pages whose copyrights reside with the individual authors.

Published by:

Elsevier North Holland, Inc.
52 Vanderbilt Avenue, New York, New York 10017

Sole distributors outside U.S.A. and Canada:

Elsevier/North-Holland Biomedical Press
335 Jan van Galenstraat, P.O. Box 211
Amsterdam, The Netherlands

Library of Congress in Cataloging in Publication Data

Medicinal Chemistry Symposium, 20th, Amherst, N.Y.,
    1979.
    Drug action and design: mechanism-based enzyme inhibitors
    (Developments in biochemistry; v. 6 ISSN 0165-1714

    Bibliography: p.
    Includes index.
    1. Enzyme inhibitors—Congresses. 2. Drugs—Physiological effect—
    Congresses. I. Kalman, Thomas I. II. Title. III. Series. [DNLM: 1. Chemistry,
    Pharmaceutical—Congresses. 2. Enzyme inhibitors—Congresses. W1
    DE997VG v. 6 / QU143 M489 1979d]
QP601.5.M4   1979   615'.7   79-17370
ISBN 0-444-00345-2

Manufactured in the United States of America

Contents

Preface

The 1979 Medicinal Chemistry Symposium was the 20th of a series of annual symposia held by the Department of Medicinal Chemistry in the School of Pharmacy of the University of Buffalo. In addition to the fulfillment of their primary educational function, these conferences have contributed to the promotion of free exchange of ideas and information between scientists from the pharmaceutical industry, research institutions and the academia in a variety of subject areas over the past two decades. The proceedings of previous symposia have not been published, in spite of the excellent presentations of all the distinguished speakers.

The topic of this year's symposium was chosen in recognition of a rapidly developing interdisciplinary field and also as a tribute to the late B.R. Baker who was one of the founders of these Symposia. Dr. Baker's pioneering contributions to the rational design of enzyme inhibitors (Baker, B.R., Design of Active-Site-Directed Irreversible Enzyme Inhibitors - The Organic Chemistry of the Enzymic Active-Site, Wiley, New York, 1967), paved the way for the current exciting advances reflected on the pages of this volume.

I would like to thank my collegues, Chairman A.J. Solo and the members of the Department of Medicinal Chemistry for serving as discussion leaders and Professor T.J. Bardos, whose memorable 20th Anniversary Address highlighted the program of the Symposium. I would also like to recognize Dean D.H. Murray's enthusiastic support of the idea of the publication of these Proceedings. The devoted and expert help of librarian Mrs. P.G. Kobelski in the preparation of the subject index was invaluable and is greatly appreciated. It is a pleasure to acknowledge the helpful cooperation and understanding of Ms. S. Koscielniak of Elsevier North-Holland, Inc. Last, but not least, thanks are due to the active participants, who made this year's symposium a success.

Amherst, New York   T.I. Kalman
August, 1979

To the members of my family
who missed me on too many nights

Acknowledgments

Financial support for this Symposium has been generously provided by:

Conferences in the Disciplines, Presidential Endowment Fund
(State University of New York at Buffalo)

Predoctoral Training Grant GM07145 from the National Institute
of General Medical Sciences, National Institutes of Health,
United States Public Health Service

Merck and Co., Inc.

Pfizer, Inc.

Richardson-Merrel, Inc.

A.M. Robins Co., Inc.

Schering Corporation

The Upjohn Co.

List of Participants

Abushanab, E.	University of Rhode Island, Kingston
Albrecht, H.	Hoffman-La Roche, Inc. Nutley, NJ
Alks, V.	Roswell Park Memorial Inst., Buffalo, NY
Anderson, W.K.*	State University of New York, Buffalo
Andrulis, P.J.	Andrulis Research Corp., Bethesda, MD
Angelino, N.	Roswell Park Memoiral Inst., Buffalo, NY
Ashton, W.T.	Merck Sharp & Dohme Res. Labs., Rahway, NJ
Baldoni, J.	Penn. State University, University Park
Bambury, R.	Diamond Shamrock Corp., Painesville, OH
Barash, L.	Merck Sharp & Dohme Res. Labs., Rahway, NJ
Bardos, T.J.*	State University of New York, Buffalo
Bartlett, D.L.	Johns Hopkins University, Baltimore, MD
Bartlett, P.A.	University of California, Berkeley
Bayless, A.	Norwich-Eaton Pharmaceuticals, Norwich, NY
Blanchard, J.	University of Wisconsin, Madison
Blessing, R.	The Medical Foundation of Buffalo, NY
Blum, M.	University of Toronto, Ontario, Canada
Bobek, M.	Roswell Park Memorial Inst., Buffalo, NY
Boger, J.S.	Merck Sharp & Dohme Res. Labs., West Point, PA
Boots, M.R.	Medical College of Virginia/VCU, Richmond
Bosies, E.	Boehringer Mannheim GMBH, Mannheim, West Germany
Breiner, R.	State University of New York, Buffalo
Bronstein, R.E.	Roswell Park Memorial Inst., Buffalo, NY
Capps, T.M.	FMC Corporation, Middleport, NY
Cassady, J.M.	Purdue University, W. Lafayette, IN
Cavanaugh, P.F., Jr.	State University of New York, Buffalo
Chan, K.	Hoffmann-La Roche, Inc., Nutley, NJ
Chang, C.P.	State University of New York, Buffalo
Chheda, G.B.	Roswell Park Memorial Inst., Buffalo, NY
Chmielewicz, Z.F.	State University of New York, Buffalo
Chowdhry, V.	E.I. du Pont & Co., Wilmington, DE
Chu, D.	Abbott Laboratories, North Chicago, IL
Chwang, L.	St. Jude Children's Research Hospital, Memphis, TN
Clark, R.	Syntex Corp., Palo Alto, California
Clarke, F.H.	CIBA-GEIGY, Ardsley, NY
Coatsworth, M.J.	State University of New York, Buffalo
Coburn, R.A.*	State University of New York, Buffalo
Coleman, H.D.	State University of New York, Buffalo
Conway, W.D.*	State University of New York, Buffalo
Cook, P.D.	Warner-Lambert/Parke Davis, Ann Arbor, MI
Cook, P.F.	University of Wisconsin, Madison
CORY, M.*	Wellcome Research Labs., Research Triangle Park, NC
COWARD, J.K.*	Yale University School of Medicine, New Haven, CT
Damon, R.	Sandoz, Inc., E. Hanover, NJ
De, N.C.	Roswell Park Memorial Inst., Buffalo, NY
Delecki, D.	Whyeth Labs., Philadelphia, PA
DeTitta, G.	The Medical Foundation of Buffalo, Inc., NY
Dinan, F.J.*	State University of New York, Buffalo
Doherty, J.B.	Merck Sharp & Dohme, Res. Labs., Rahway, NJ
Doldouras, G.	Merck Sharp & Dohme, Res. Labs., Rahway, NJ
Dolle, R.E.	State University of New York, Buffalo
Domagala, J.	Warner-Lambert/Parke Davis, Ann Arbor, MI

Draper, R.W.	Schering Corp., Bloomfield, NJ
Duax, W.*	The Medical Foundation of Buffalo, Inc., NY
Dubas, L.	E.I. du Pont & Co., Wilmington, DE
Dubicki, H.	Starks Associates, Inc., Buffalo, NY
Dunn, J.A.	State University of New York, Buffalo
Dutta, S.P.	Roswell Park Memorial Inst., Buffalo, NY
Evans, B.E.	Merck Sharp & Dohme Res. Labs., West Point, PA
Fame, T.	State University of New York, Buffalo
Fedor, L.*	State University of New York, Buffalo
Finnegan, R.A.*	State University of New York, Buffalo
FISHER, J.F.*	Harvard University, Cambridge, MA
FLASHNER, M.*	SUNY College of Env. Sci. & Forestry, Syracuse, NY
Fogt, S.W.	Diamond Shamrock Corp., Painesville, OH
Franck, R.W.	Fordham University, Bronx, NY
Gaeta, F.C.A.	Bristol-Myers Laboratories, Syracuse, NY
Gala, D.	State University of New York, Buffalo
Gangjee, A.	State University of New York, Buffalo
Garmaise, D.L.	Abbott Laboratories, North Chicago, IL
Gawron, O.	Duquesne University, Pittsburg, PA
Gill, R.	University of Wisconsin, Madison
Glennon, R.A.	Medical College of Virginia/VCU, Richmond
Goldman, D.	State University of New York, Buffalo
Gordon, E.M.	Squibb Institute of Medical Research, Princeton, NJ
Graham, D.W.	Merck Sharpe & Dohme Res. Labs., Rahway, NJ
Griffith, R.K.	University of Michigan, Ann Arbor
Haber, S.B.	E.I. du Pont & Co., Wilmington, DE
Harrison, E.A., Jr.	Penn. State University, York, PA
Hartzell, S.	Roswell Park Memorial Inst., Buffalo, NY
Harvison, P.	State University of New York, Buffalo
Heck, J.V.	Merck Sharpe & Dohme Res. Labs., Rahway, NJ
Hedrich, L.W.	Gulf Oil Chemicals Co., Shawnee Mission, KS
Heindel, N.	Lehigh University, Bethlehem, PA
Hibit, J.	State University of New York, Buffalo
Ho, J.	State University of New York, Buffalo
Ho, W.	McNeil Laboratories, Ft. Washington, PA
Ho, Yau-Kwan*	State University of New York, Buffalo
Ho, Yee-Kin	State University of New York, Buffalo
HOLDEN, K.G.*	Smith Kline & French Labs., Philadelphia, PA
Holtwick, J.	University of Illinois
Holyoke, C.W.	E.I. du Pont & Co., Wilmington, DE
Hong, C.	Roswell Park Memorial Inst., Buffalo, NY
Hsiao, L.	Starks Associates, Inc., Buffalo, NY
Hsiao, M.	State University of New York, Buffalo
Hupe, D.J.	University of Michigan, Ann Arbor
Ibok, I.S.U.	State University of New York, Buffalo
Jain, V.K.	Cooper Laboratories, Inc., Cedar Knoll, NJ
Jaworski, R.	University of Wisconsin, Madison
Johnson, R.B.	University of Wisconsin, Madison
Jones, A.N.	State University of New York, Buffalo
Jones, G.H.	Syntex Research, Palo Alto, California
JUNG, M.*	Merrell International Research Center, Strasbourg, France
Kalman, T.I.*	State University of New York, Buffalo
Kaminski, J.J.	Schering Corp., Bloomfield, NJ
Kavai, I.	Roswell Park Memorial Inst., Buffalo, NY
Keller, J.W.	University of Wisconsin, Madison

Kellog, M.S.	Pfizer Central Research, Groton, CT
Kessler, J.	SUNY College of Env. Sci. & Forestry, Syracuse, NY
Kisliuk, R.L.	Tufts University School of Medicine, Boston, MA
Kompis, I.	Hoffmann-La Roche, Inc., Nutley, NJ
Korytnyk, W.	Roswell Park Memorial Inst., Buffalo, NY
Kramer, D.L.	Roswell Park Memorial Inst., Buffalo, NY
KRANTZ, A.*	State University of New York, Stony Brook
Ku, H.S.	Diamond Shamrock Corporation, Painesville, OH
Kulinski, R.F.	State University of New York, Buffalo
Kung, H.F.	State University of New York, Buffalo
Kung, M.P.	State University of New York, Buffalo
Landesman, P.	State University of New York, Buffalo
Lang, S.A., Jr.	Lederle Labs., Pearl River, NY
Lawson, W.B.	New York State Dept. of Health, Albany, NY
Lee, M.L.	Sandoz, Inc., E. Hanover, NJ
Lever, O.W., Jr.	Burroughs Wellcome Co., Res. Triangle Park, NC
Liebowitz, S.	Medical College of Virginia/VCU, Richmond
Lippert, B.	Merrell Research Center, Cincinnati, OH
Lovsted, E.	Duquesne University, Pittsburg, PA
MacNintch, J.E.	Bristol Labs., Syracuse, NY
McCombie, S.W.	Schering Corp., Bloomfield, NJ
McPherson, H.	State University of New York, Buffalo
Magee, T.A.	Diamond Shamrock Corp., Painesville, OH
Manhas, M.S.	Stevens Inst. of Technology, Hoboken, NJ
Matz, S.	Diamond Shamrock Corp., Painesville, OH
Marquez, V.E.	National Institutes of Health, Bethesda, MD
MAYCOCK, A.L.*	Merck Sharp & Dohme Res. Labs., Rahway, NJ
Mazur, R.H.	G.D. Searle & Co., Chicago, IL
Meloche, H.P.	PAP Institute, Miami, FL
Menon, G.K.	Smith Kline Animal Health Prods., West Chester, PA
METCALF, B.W.*	Merrell Research Center, Cincinnati, OH
Miyano, M.	G.D. Searle & Co., Chicago, IL
Moore, G.G.I.	Riker-3M, St. Paul, MN
Morin, R.B.	Bristol-Myers Co., Syracuse, NY
Morrison, R.	Burroughs Wellcome Co., Res. Triangle Park, NC
Mullen, G.B.	Wyeth Laboratories, Inc., Philadelphia, PA
Mulumba, B.	State University of New York, Buffalo
Murray, D.H.*	State University of New York, Buffalo
Nadelson, J.	Sandoz, Inc., E. Hanover, NJ
Nadkarni, M.V.	National Cancer Institute, Silver Spring, MD
Naff, M.B.	National Cancer Institute, Silver Spring, MD
Nemec, J.	St. Jude Children's Res. Hosp., Memphis, TN
New, J.S.	State University of New York, Buffalo
Novotny, J.	Starks Associates, Inc., Buffalo, NY
Numazawa, M.	Medical Foundation of Buffalo, Inc., NY
O'Brien, T.A.	Harvard University, Cambridge, MA
ONDETTI, M.A.*	Squibb Institute for Medical Res., Princeton, NJ
Osawa, Y.	Medical Foundation of Buffalo, Inc., NY
Panzica, R.P.	University of Rhode Island, Kingston
Parham, J.C.	Sloan-Kettering Institute, Rye, NY
Parker, A.M.	State University of New York, Buffalo
Parsons, J.	Starks Associates, Inc., Buffalo, NY
Partyka, R.A.	Bristol Laboratories, Syracuse, NY
Pattison, I.C.	Warner-Lambert/Parke-Davis, Ann Arbor, MI
Paul, B.	Roswell Park Memorial Inst., Buffalo, NY

Perchonock, C.D.	Smith Kline & French Labs., Philadelphia, PA
Perlman, M.	State University of New York, Buffalo
Person, N.B.	State University of New York, Buffalo
Petrie, C.R.	Roswell Park Memorial Inst., Buffalo, NY
Pruess, D.L.	Hoffmann-La Roche, Nutley, NJ
Putt, S.R.	Warner-Lambert/Parke Davis, Ann Arbor, MI
RANDO, R.R. *	Harvard Medical School, Boston, MA
Redl, G.	Westwood Pharmaceuticals, Inc., Buffalo, NY
Rittle, K.E.	Merck Sharp & Dohme Res. Labs., West Point, PA
Robinson, R.A.	FMC Corp., Middleport, NY
Rogers, M.E.	Medical College of Virginia/VCU, Richmond
Russell, P.	Roswell Park Memorial Inst., Buffalo, NY
Rutigliano, E.	State University of New York, Buffalo
Ryu, E.K.	Argonne National Lab., Argonne, IL
Sambor, D.H.	State University of New York, Buffalo
Sanders, W.J.	Smith Kline Animal Health Prods., West Chester, PA
SANTI, D.V.*	University of California, San Francisco
Schaeffer, H.J.	Burroughs Wellcome Co., Res. Triangle Park, NC
Schinazi, R.	Emory University School of Medicine, Atlanta, GA
Schloss, J.V.	University of Wisconsin, Madison
Schroeder, A.C.	Roswell Park Memorial Inst., Buffalo, NY
Schulenberg, J.W.	Sterling-Winthrop Research Inst., Rensselaer, NY
Schwab, L.S.	University of Rochester Medical Center, Rochester, NY
Schwender, C.F.	Warner-Lambert/Parke Davis, Ann Arbor, MI
Scott, M.E.	SUNY College of Env. Sci. & Forestry, Syracuse, NY
Scozzie, J.A.	Diamond Shamrock Corp., Painesville, OH
Semler, J.R.	State University of New York, Buffalo
Shah, R.	State University of New York, Buffalo
Sharma, M.	Roswell Park Memorial Inst., Buffalo, NY
Sharma, R.A.	Roswell Park Memorial Inst., Buffalo, NY
Sheridan, R.	Princeton University, Princeton, NJ
Shih, H.C.	State University of New York, Buffalo
Showalter, H.D.H.	Warner-Lambert/Parke-Davis, Ann Arbor, MI
Silver, M.S.	Amherst College, Amherst, MA
SILVERMAN, R.B.*	Northwestern University, Evanston, IL
Simcox, P.D.	Diamond Shamrock Corp., Painesville, OH
Smith, J.	State University of New York, Buffalo
Smithwick, E.L., Jr.	Eli Lilly & Co., Indianapolis, IN
Solo, A.J.*	State University of New York, Buffalo
Starks, D.	Starks Associates, Inc., Buffalo, NY
Starks, F.	Starks Associates, Inc., Buffalo, NY
Steffens, J.J.	Mobil Chemical Co., Edison, NJ
Stephani, R.A.	St. John's University, Mamaroneck, NY
Strube, R.E.	Walter Reed Army Inst. of Res., Washington, DC
Stubbe, J.	Yale University, New Haven, CT
Stubbins, J.F.	Medical College of Virginia/VCU, Richmond
Suto, M.	State University of New York, Buffalo
Sweatlock, J.	State University of New York, Buffalo
Sweeney, T.R.	Walter Reed Army Inst. of Res., Washington, DC
Tanenbaum, S.W.	SUNY College of Env. Sci. & Forestry, Syracuse, NY
Taylor, M.D.	State University of New York, Buffalo
Tecle, H.	Warner-Lambert/Parke-Davis, Ann Arbor, MI
Thedford, R.	Clark College, Atlanta, GA
Thomas, A.M.	Abbott Laboratories, N. Chicago, IL
Thorsett, E.D.	Merck Sharp & Dohme Res. Labs., Rahway, NJ
Thress, D.	State University of New York, Buffalo

Tieckelmann, H.   State University of New York, Buffalo
Tobes, M.C.   University of Michigan, Ann Arbor
TOMASZ, A.*   The Rockefeller University, New York, NY
Tomesch, J.   Sandoz, Inc., E. Hanover, NJ
Tramposch, K.M.   State University of New York, Buffalo
Triggle, D.   State University of New York, Buffalo
Tullman, R.H.   University of Kansas, Lawrence, KS
Upeslacis, J.   Lederle Laboratories, Pearl River, NY
Verderame, M.   Albany College of Pharmacy, Albany, NY
Viola, R.E.   University of Wisconsin, Madison
Wailand, J.   State University of New York, Buffalo
WALSH, C.T.*   Mass. Inst. of Technology, Cambridge
Wattanabe, S.   Roswell Park Memorial Inst., Buffalo NY
Wedler, F.C.   Penn. State University, University Park
Wei, C.C.   Hoffmann-La Roche, Inc., Nutley, NJ
White, R.L.   Norwich-Eaton Pharmaceuticals, Norwich, NY
Wiseman, J.S.   Merrell Research Center, Cincinnati, OH
WOLFENDEN, R.V.*   University of North Carolina, Chapel Hill
Wright, J.   Schering Corp., Bloomfield, NJ
Yalowich, J.C.   State University of New York, Buffalo
Young, R.N.   Merck Frosst Labs., Pointe Claire/Dorval, Que., Canada
Zusi, F.C.   Westwood Pharmaceuticals, Buffalo, NY

---

*
INVITED SPEAKERS' and discussion leaders' names are marked with an asterisk.

I
Transition State Analogs

Published 1979 by Elsevier North Holland, Inc.

Kalman, ed. Drug Action and Design: Mechanism-Based Enzyme Inhibitors

TRANSITION STATE AFFINITY AND DRUG DESIGN: THE ROLE OF SOLVENT WATER

RICHARD WOLFENDEN

Department of Biochemistry, University of North Carolina,

Chapel Hill, North Carolina 27514, USA

Most enzyme reactions take place very rapidly, occurring with a half-time that may be in the neighborhood of a millisecond, as compared with perhaps a year for the same reaction in the absence of enzyme. The path of the enzyme reaction can thus be said to follow a deep cleft in what would otherwise be a high-energy landscape for the conversion of reactant to product. Because the cleft is narrow and deep, the pathway of the enzyme reaction can in principle be described very exactly, as compared with the nonenzymatic reaction that may proceed by a variety of paths that resemble each other in energy. The very depth of the cleft raises experimental difficulties, since events occur very rapidly in an inaccessible environment. Because of the delicacy of protein structures, and the very close fit of the active site to substrates and inter-mediates, one cannot vary the composition of the solvent, the substrate or the enzyme and be sure that one understands the basis for any effects that may be observed.

In trying to get around this problem, we can take advantage of a special feature of catalytic systems, their ability to lower the free energy of the transition state for conversion of reactant to product. Enzymes have, or can easily adopt, a structure complementary to that of the altered substrate in the transition state; in fact they are templates designed through natural selection for this purpose.[1] Transition state analogs are stable compounds, designed to resemble fleeting intermediates in substrate transformation. Because of this resemblance, they are bound by the enzyme very much more tightly than sub-strates are bound. Because they are chemically stable and cannot collapse to form products, their affinity for the enzyme persists and they are exception-ally potent metabolic inhibitors. Because their complexes are formed in a mockery of the normal catalytic process, examination of their exact structures may reveal the answers to questions about the catalytic process itself and suggest possible directions for improvements in drug design. I'd like to discuss one of these cases in detail, and go on to consider some new develop-ments in thinking about these questions.

The first enzyme, for which a deliberate attempts was made to prepare a transition state analog, was triosephosphate isomerase, which is believed to act through a general base mechanism as shown in Fig. 1. Seeking an analog of the ene-diolate intermediate that is formed by proton abstraction from substrates, we hit upon a carboxylic acid as having the right configuration and electrostatic properties.[2] Hydroxamic acids also share some of these properties[3], and when they were tested as potential inhibitors, they were found to exhibit K_i values very much lower than K_m values of the anhydrous substrates. Similar reasoning was used in the later devlopment of inhibitors of glucose phosphate isomerase [4] and ribose phosphate isomerase[5].

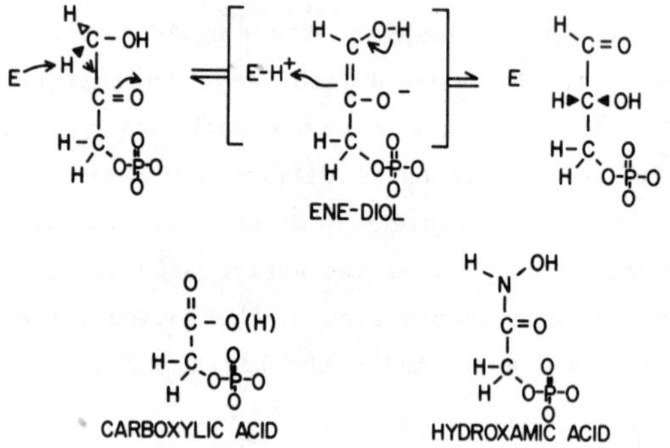

Fig. 1: Isomerase Inhibitors

These inhibitors show several distinguishing characteristics, documented in most detail for 2-phosphoglycollic acid. Changing pH affects the affinity of the enzyme for this inhibitor in the same way that it affects the rate enhancement produced by the enzyme as a catalyst[6]. The inhibitor also brings about major, reversible, contractions of the unit cell of the crystalline enzyme under appropriate conditions.[7] Although these changes are interesting, they tend to interfere with the determination of the structure of the complexes, since the inhibited crystals are no longer isomorphous with the native enzyme crystals. Efforts to solve the structure are continuing in David Phillips' laboratory at Oxford. A promising development is the crystallization of the enzyme from yeast by Dr. Fred Hartman; Dr. Gregory Petsko (personal communication) finds that these crystals seem to be ideal for refinement of the structures in question.

If the detailed structure of the enzyme-inhibitor complex is, for the moment, inaccessible, we could at least hope to learn something about the form of the inhibitor that is actually bound. When Dr. Yasuko Tomozawa examined the K_i of phosphoglycollate as a function of changing pH, she found that its binding varied in a manner consistent with exclusive uptake of inhibitor with 2 negative charges[6]. There are two possible di-anions shown below:

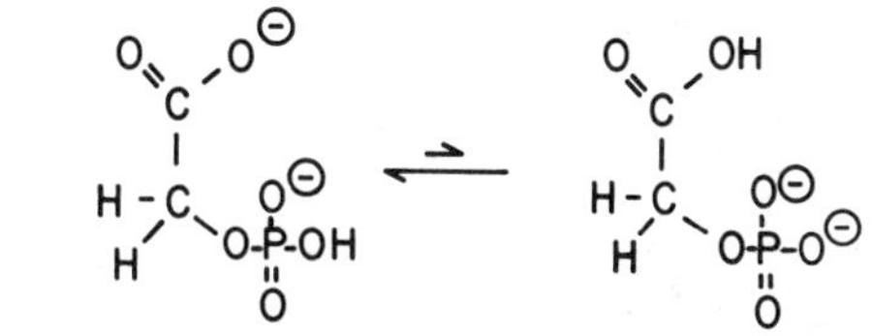

MAJOR DI-ANION   MINOR DI-ANION

From the known pK_a values of typical carboxylic and phosphoric acid derivatives, one would expect the tautomer with separated charges to be the more populous species. Using a procedure analogous to that used for determining the abundance of the uncharged versus the zwitterionic forms of amino acids, we can estimate the major di-anion shown above to be favored by a factor of about 300, based on the observed pK_a values of 2-phosphoglycollic acid and its carboxylic acid esters and amides. Although the tautomer with separated charges is the more abundant, Tomozawa also established that the enzyme binds substrates productively only in forms in which the phosphoryl group is doubly ionized. It therefore seemed not unlikely that the minor tautomer of the inhibitor might be the form bound by the enzyme. When we prepared carboxyl-^{13}C-labelled inhibitor, and examined its carbon and phosphorus magnetic resonance shifts as a function of changing pH, in free solution and when bound to the enzyme, the results indicated that the bound inhibitor was not in either of the two di-anionic forms we had confidently expected, but was tri-anionic instead. The results force us to conclude that the enzyme, in binding the tri-anionic inhibitor, takes up a proton at a separate site[8]. The site of proton uptake is probably glu-165, the essential residue that is thought to serve as the general base catalyst for proton transfer. The pK_a of this group is 3.9, at least in the enzyme from yeast[6], and we can estimate that the affinity of the protonated enzyme for tri-anionic phosphoglycollate corresponds to a K_d of 6 x 10^{10} $\underline{M}$, some 5 orders of magnitude lower than the limiting values of K_m for anhydrous

substrates. This makes sense if the catalytic function of the enzyme is largely associated with its ability to stabilize ene-diolate intermediates in catalysis, since the complex containing the tri-anionic inhibitor closely resembles
such an intermediate complex, even in the detailed location of the proton that
is "in transit" in the normal catalyzed reaction (Fig. 2).

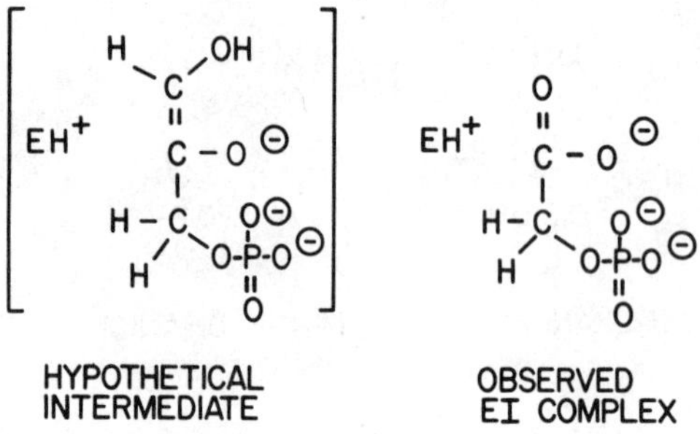

HYPOTHETICAL
INTERMEDIATE

OBSERVED
EI COMPLEX

Fig. 2: Ene-diolate intermediate and PGA tri-anion

Studies of this kind have begun to show how transition state analogs are
bound by enzymes. Their ultimate object is to explain, in terms acceptable to
a physical organic chemist, how such a very large increase in affinity is
possible in passing from the ES complex to the enzyme-substrate complex in the
transition state. Paradoxically, we do not wish so much to explain the fit of
the substrate to the active site, as the absence of fit, or of structural
complementarity. The very tight binding expected of ideal transition state
analogs would be pointless if the active site were not able to discriminate so
effectively against the substrate in the ground state. This is a problem far
more complex than that usually faced by an antibody, a hormone receptor or an
olfactory membrane.

In considering how much is really understood about "fit", one realizes
that these games are being played in a watery environment. Regardless of the
detailed mechanism of action of an enzyme, a constant requirement for its
inhibition is that water must usually be stripped away from interacting portions of the inhibitor and the site at which it is bound. In considering the
relative affinities of enzymes for substrate analogs, it is therefore of interest to inquire how easily they can be removed from solvent water into a featureless cavity of unit dielectric constant, that neither attracts nor repels

ligands, in which neither attractive nor repulsive interactions are present; it might then be possible to infer the presence of specific attractive or repulsive interactions that may be at work in the sites where inhibitors are bound.

For this purpose, the dilute vapor phase provides the most suitable frame of reference. Early measurements[9] of partial pressures of organic compounds over water established that free energies of water-to-vapor transfer of complex organic molecules approximately are an additive function of their constituent groups, as may be seen by comparison of the entries in Fig. 3. Using methods of greater sensitivity[10], we have extended these measurements to include polar molecules of biological interest (Fig. 4). Among this collection of uncharged molecules, it will be noted that the range of values is extensive, spanning some 11 kilocalories of solvation energy difference between hydrocarbons and amides of similar size. The extreme position of the peptide bond is noteworthy. These figures show that the strongly exergonic aminolysis of esters, fundamental to protein biosynthesis, is actually "driven" thermodynamically by solvation differences between reactants and products; in the vapor phase the

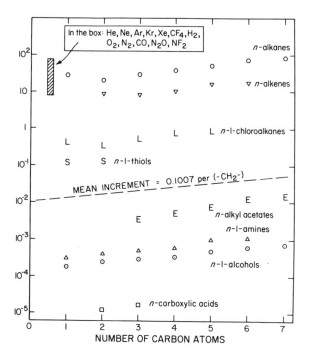

Fig. 3

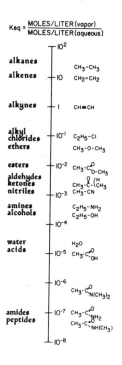

Fig. 4

reaction is actually endergonic. Because of the very great solvation energy of the peptide bond, we might guess that the binding of some peptides at anhydrous active sites of enzymes and other receptors would be enchanced by replacement of the -CO-NH- group by something less hydrophilic, whose removal from water would be less costly from a thermodynamic standpoint. Efforts to test this prediction are in progress.

If the affinity of an enzyme for an inhibitor were understandable in terms of its low hydrophilic character, this need not mean that the inhibitor is tighly bound for reasons unrelated to the mechanism of action of the enzyme. The action of enzymes, regardless of their mechanism of action, can be said to require a preferential affinity of the active site for activated intermediates in substrate transformation in water, as compared with its affinity for the substrates themselves in water. The work of A. J. Parker and other physical organic chemists has shown that there are many reaction that are strongly retarded by solvent water. Halide exchange into alkyl halides, for example, frequently proceeds 4 or 5 orders of magnitude more rapidly in an aprotic solvent such as DMF than it does in water, and there have been many similar observations for other S_N2 reactions and for the Hofmann elimination reaction. It seems reasonable to speculate, with Saul Cohen[11] and others, that enzymes might speed up reaction that proceed through relatively nonpolar intermediates, simply by dragging the reactants out of a watery environment, resulting in destabilization of the starting materials relative to the transition state. Much work has been done on "catalysis by desolvation" (Fig. 5) in mixed solvents, micelles and clathrate compounds.

We can even imagine, in some impossible world, an enzyme in which reacting portions of the substrate were effectively introduced into a vacuum, and ask what their reactivity would then be. With the advent of new techniques in mass spectrometry, it has become possible to measure and compare rates of reaction in water with rates of reaction in nothing at all, that is the vapor phase. The results are startling in magnitude. By simply removing solvent water, rates of reaction of alkyl halides with oxyanions can be increased by factors in the neighborhood of 10^{17}.[12] Thus, if an enzyme were to enhance the reactivity of a substrate by removing it from a watery environment, we might guess that an inhibitor that was hydrophobic, and saved the enzyme the trouble of stripping away water, might be very tightly bound indeed. A nice example of this is provided by the work of Gutowski and Lienhard, who find that pyruvate dehydrogenase is strongly inhibited by uncharged analogs of thiamine pyrophosphate.[13] Desolvation provides a plausible mechanism of action for this enzyme, since the uncatalyzed reaction was earlier shown to proceed very much more rapidly in nonpolar solvents than in water.[14]

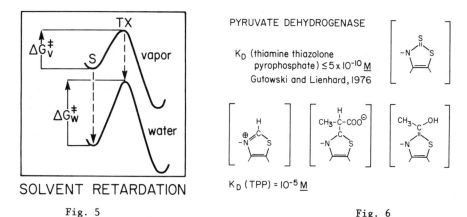

SOLVENT RETARDATION

Fig. 5

PYRUVATE DEHYDROGENASE

K_D (thiamine thiazolone pyrophosphate) $\leq 5 \times 10^{-10}$ $\underline{M}$
Gutowski and Lienhard, 1976

K_D (TPP) = 10^{-5} $\underline{M}$

Fig. 6

What are we to think of the more common group of reactions that proceed, in aqueous solution, through intermediates that are more polar in character than the starting materials, and are therefore subject to "water catalysis"? All the arguments given above work in reverse, and desolvation by itself would be counterproductive as a device for producing rate enhancement. Many S_N1 reactions, the ionization of sulfonates, and the quaternization of amines, proceed more rapidly in water than in less polar solvents, and nothing useful would be accomplished by merely taking the reactants into a waterless cavity.

To enhance the rate of reactions of this kind, there seem to be two alternative strategies that may not be mutually exclusive. One is to change the mechanism so that, on the enzyme, no intermediate more polar than the starting material is actually generated. This could be accomplished by allowing the reaction catalyzed by a glycosidase, for example, to pass through a covalent glycosyl-enzyme intermediate rather than the carbonium ion intermediate that would normally be generated during the acid-catalyzed reaction in solution; and β-galactosidase appears to act in this way[15]. Another strategy is to find a means of stabilizing charges that <u>are</u> generated, even more effectively than does solvent water. In a formal sense, catalysis of this kind requires extraction of an ion from aqueous solution, in preference to a neutral molecule closely related to it in structure. A catalyst, operating on these principles, would have to be a "super"-chelating agent, and it is quite clear from the behavior of ionophores and apo-heme proteins that this problem can be solved. It is also a striking fact that many enzymes show unusual affinities for small inhibitors such as oxalate, nitrate or phosphoglycollate (Fig. 1) that are at the same time transition state analogs and "beehives" of negative charge. It is of interest that the binding of such analogs often seems to be accompanied by changes in enzyme shape[16], just as valinomycin changes shape with the binding of potassium ion.[17]

Let me conclude with the suggestion that for many biochemical reactions in aqueous solution, the solvent makes overwhelmingly important contributions not only to the overall equilibrium of reaction, but also to the stabilization of the transition state. In considering the design of metabolic inhibitors, we need to investigate and exploit these effects, which are probably at least as important as the steric and electronic factors to which so much attention has been devoted.

References

1. Wolfenden, R., Accounts of Chemical Research 5, 10 (1972); Lienhard, G. E., Science 180, 149 (1973).

2. Wolfenden, R., Nature 223, 704 (1969).

3. Collins, K. D., J. Biol. Chem. 249, 136 (1974).

4. Chirgwin, J. M. and Noltmann, E. A., J. Biol. Chem. 250, 7272 (1975).

5. Woodruff, W. W. and Wolfeden, R., J. Biol.Chem. in press (1979).

6. Hartman, F. C., LaMuraglia, G. M., Tomozawa, Y. and Wolfenden, R., Biochemistry 14, 5274 (1975).

7. Johnson, L. N. and Wolfenden, R., J. Molec. Biol. 47, 93 (1970).

8. Campbell, I. D., Jones, R. B., Kiener, P. A., Richards, E., Waley, S. G., and Wolfenden, R., Biochem. Biophys. Res. Comm. 83, 347 (1978).

9. Butler, J. A. V., Trans. Faraday Soc. 33, 229 (1937); Hine, J. and Mookerjee, P. K., J. Org. Chem. 40, 292 (1975).

10. Wolfenden, R., Biochemistry 17, 201 (1978).

11. Cohen, S. G., Vaidya, V. M., and Schultz, R. M., Proc. Natl. Acad. Sci. 66, 249 (1970).

12. Olmstead, W. N. and Brauman, J. I., J. Amer. Chem. Soc. 92, 4219 (1977).

13. Gutowski, M. and Lienhard, G. E., J. Biol. Chem. 76, 4448, (1976).

14. Crosby, J. and Lienhard, G., J. Amer. Chem. Soc. 92, 5707 (1970).

15. Wentworth, D. F. and Wolfenden, R., Biochemistry 13, 4715 (1974).

16. Wolfenden, R., Ann. Rev. Biophys. Bioeng. 5, 271 (1976).

17. Duax, E. A., Science 176, 912 (1972).

DISCUSSION

ONDETTI: I wonder, if in the studies on the transfer from the liquid to the vapor phase, do you think that you can actually eliminate all the possible interactions between the water molecules in the vapor phase? Do you think that what you are measuring in the vapor phase is the isolated molecule?

WOLFENDEN: The question Dr. Ondetti raises is a good one. How do we know whether, for example, acetamide may retain bound water molecules when it goes into the vapor phase? The approach that we are using is to use infrared with cuvets of long light paths which allow one to look at the detailed vapor phase spectrum. We have also used ultraviolet in the case of some recent studies on indole. Because of the fine structure of the vapor phase spectra, I think we can say that indole, (not one of the molecules that I described), in the vapor phase is as naked as it would be, if it were coming out of liquid indole. We would like to extend that certificate of "nonhydration" to amides as well, but have not performed the infrared experiments yet.

CHOWDHRY: You seem to have looked at almost all acyl compounds that may be of interest. Did you also look at thioesters, since they obviously are important?

WOLFENDEN: We have looked at thioesters, but the numbers are still somewhat approximate. Thioesters appear to be very slightly less hydrophilic, than ordinary oxygen esters. A point raised by your question is whether the high energy character of thioesters is based on changing hydration during hydrolysis. I think that that is not true for thioesters, that the higher group transfer potential is an intrinsic property and the same is true of anhydrides. Acetic anhydride is a very high energy compound both in the vapor phase and in aqueous solution and one knows that it is fairly volatile. We would love to know about phosphate anhydrides but unfortunately, to this moment, we have not been able to get a phosphorous compound into the vapor phase. We have high hopes for the long light path measurements - we may have to go to the ultimate limit, which was achieved by the physicist Herzberg in 1948 when he made a spectrophotometric cuvet with 4 kilometer light path[1].

McCOMBIE: Could I ask, if your results differ from several numbers obtained by the normal distribution between two solvents? In other words, are you actually seeing some different values?

WOLFENDEN: There are quite a few differences, but we have not studied them methodically yet. One thing that does seem clear is that the range of values is greater, if one uses the vapor phase as a frame of reference. That is not unreasonable, because most of the solvents that have been used for reference have a dielectric constant higher than one. In recent studies, we have been measuring water-to-vapor distributions of the side chains of the amino acids. The distribution values are very different from the ones that were previously observed in a number of laboratories for water to alcohol distribution of free amino acids. It turns out though that this is not so much a question of the solvent that was looked at, as the fact that free amino acids are zwitterionic. The presence of a zwitterionic group disrupts the local solvation around the side chains associated with the amino acids to such an extraordinary extent that one sees inversions, order of magnitude changes in the relative distribution coefficients of amino acids between water and the nonpolar environment.

LAWSON: I wonder that in determining the hydrophobicity of compounds by this method, to what extent the results might be effected by the tendency of compounds to form organized aggregates? I am thinking *e.g.*, of the dimer of acetic acid and so forth.

WOLFENDEN: Yes. One of the important controls that one has to run is to eliminate the possibility (and it is a very real one in the case of compounds as polar as acetic acid and acetamide) that one is seeing dimers or higher aggregates. In the case of acetic acid and acetamide, at the concentrations at which we were doing these experiments, it has been clearly shown that one is dealing with a monomeric compound in aqueous solution. As to the possibility of aggregation in the vapor phase: that seems to be ruled out by our finding that the equilibrium constant for distribution from water to the vapor phase is unaffected by the absolute concentration of the compound that is present in water. If one were seeing aggregation, I think one would expect a non-linear relationship, a square or higher order effect of concentration on the apparent distribution coefficient. We have deliberately elevated the concentrations in the aqueous solution to quite high levels using cold solutes, in order to test for just this possibility.

COWARD: I have a comment regarding the S_N2 reactions that you mentioned. In looking at sulfonium and ammonium systems we have confirmed what is a sort of classical work by Hughes and Ingold[2]. They observed very large solvent effects in this type of reactions going from water to nonpolar low dielectric media; these cover 4 or 5 orders of magnitude over a small range of dielectric. In other words, if you look at structures which are involved in biological alkyl transfer reactions, namely sulfoniums and protonated amines (ammoniums), you also see the type of solvent effects described with alkyl halides.

REFERENCES

1. Bernstein, H.J., and Herzberg, G. (1948) J. Chem. Phys. 16, 30.
2. Ingold, C.K. (1969) Structure and Mechanism in Organic Chemistry, 2nd Ed., Cornell University Press, New York, p 457.

THE SYNTHESIS OF TRANSITION STATE ANALOGS AS POTENTIAL SPECIFIC INHIBITORS OF

GROUP TRANSFER ENZYMES

JAMES K. COWARD*
Department of Pharmacology
Yale University School of Medicine
New Haven, CT 06510

The reactions of S-adenosylmethionine (SAM) and 5-methyltetrahydrofolate

are many and varied (1-3). Of particular interest are the reactions of

SAM and decarboxylated SAM in enzyme-catalyzed methyl transfer and aminopropyl

transfer reactions, respectively. Similarly the ATP-dependent biosynthesis

of the folate polyglutamates (4,5) appears to be required for cell growth

(6). Thus, it would be of interest to be able to inhibit these group transfer

reactions in vitro and in vivo. This paper will be concerned primarily with

some preliminary results recently obtained in our laboratory on the syntheses

of transition-state analogs (multisubstrate adducts) as potential specific,

tight-binding inhibitors of the enzymes which catalyze these reactions.

Over the past several years, we have synthesized several metabolically

stable analogs as potential inhibitors of methylation and polyamine biosynthe-

sis (7,8). The two compounds of most interest are the 7-deaza analogs of

S-adenosylhomocysteine (SAH) and 5'-deoxy-5'-methylthioadenosine (MTA).

The SAH analog, S-tubercidinylhomocysteine (STH) has been shown to be a potent

inhibitor of methylation, both in vitro and in vivo (9). STH was designed

to resist metabolic degradation, and this has been demonstrated recently in

murine neuroblastoma cells (10). Similarly, 5'-deoxy-5'-methylthiotubercidin

(MTT), a known inhibitor of MTA phosphorylase (8) and aminopropyltransferase

(11), is effective as a MTA antagonist in whole cells (12,13). While these

*Present Address: Department of Chemistry, Rensselaer Polytechnic Institute,
Troy, NY 12181.

biological results are encouraging in terms of being able to design effective new drugs, the lack of specificity observed with these compounds suggested the synthesis of a new generation of inhibitors, designed to introduce the desired specificity. We have chosen to investigate the use of transition-state analogs (14) for this purpose, based on the proven ability of this type of analog to act as extremely potent and specific inhibitors of many single substrate enzyme reactions (ignoring, for this discussion, the second reactant in most cases, water). Our own interest in this approach has been stimulated by the ability of similar analogs to act as potent inhibitors of several enzymes which catalyze the reaction of two substrates (14-17); i.e., multisubstrate adducts (16).

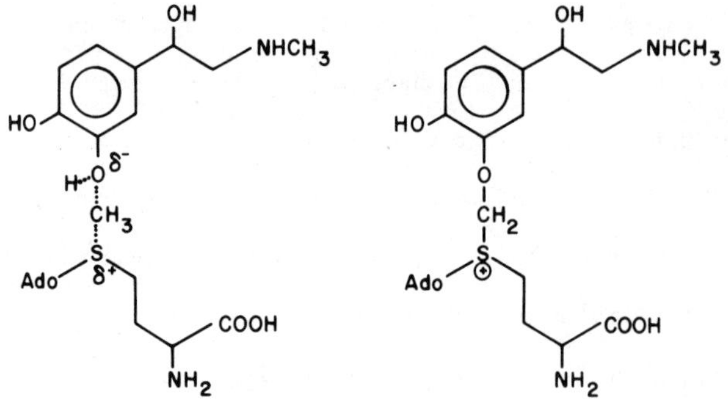

Figure 1: Transition-state and adduct proposed for COMT.

We have studied methylation of RNA and catecholamines using both steady-state kinetic analysis of the catechol-O-methyltransferase (COMT) reaction (18), stereochemistry of the COMT reaction (19), and kinetics of related model reactions (20,21). From these studies we have concluded that enzyme-catalyzed methylation reactions involve a direct displacement of the methyl groups by one of the catechol hydroxyls, with possible general-base catalysis of proton removal. These data suggested synthesis of the adduct shown in Figure 1. The syntheses were effected by the general routes shown in Figure 2, the details of which will be published separately (22). As indicated in Figure 3, only the substituted phenethyl sulfonium compounds ($X=CH_2$) are sufficiently stable for use in biological studies. This is not surprising if one considers that the sulfoniums where X=0, or X=S are similar to protonated thioacetals, which are unstable in aqueous media. Thus far, only methyl sulfonium derivatives have been prepared, and although the aminoacids have only very poor inhibitory activity against COMT, the adenosines are competitive inhibitors with K_i's = 200-500 µM. We are presently working on the synthesis of the fully substituted sulfonium, containing all three desired ligands, namely adenosine, catecholamine and homocysteine.

The biosynthesis of the polyamines, spermidine and spermine, involve transfer of an intact aminopropyl group from decarboxylated SAM to the nucleo-philic primary amine of putrescine and spermidine, respectively. The reaction is shown in Figure 4, together with the desired adduct. Although detailed mechanistic studies with purified spermidine or spermine synthase (aminopro-pyltransferase), similar to those discussed above for the COMT reaction have not been carried out, our experience in synthesizing the methylsulfoniums in Figure 3 led us to synthesize the methylsulfonium shown in Figure 4 as a potential inhibitor of polyamine biosynthesis. Our synthetic approach in this work has been to couple a suitably blocked 3-substituted-1,8-diamino-octane either to 5'-deoxy-5'-mercaptoadenosine (generated in situ from the

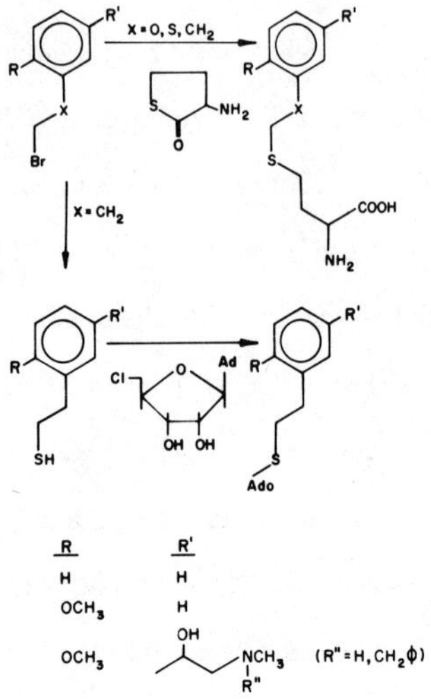

Figure 2: General routes of syntheses of COMT adducts.

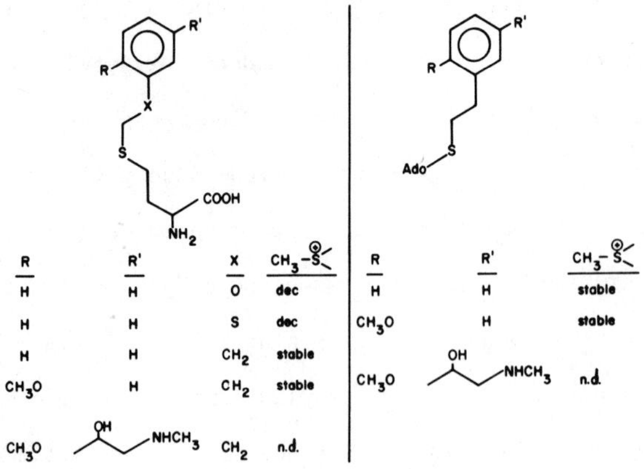

Figure 3: Stability of selected methylsulfoniums; n.d.: not determined.

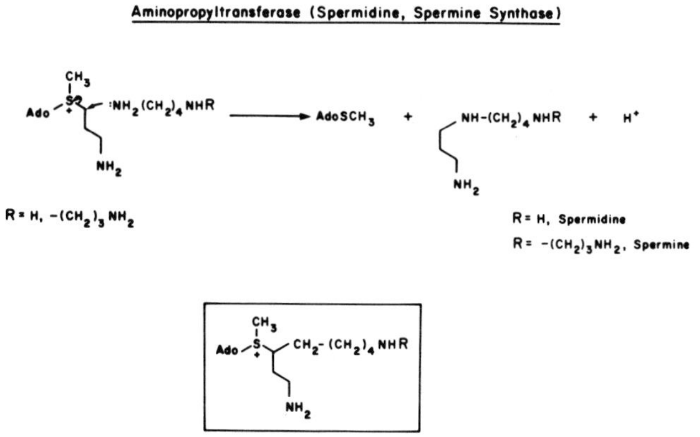
Aminopropyltransferase (Spermidine, Spermine Synthase)
Ado
AdoSCH3
R = H, Spermidine
R = -(CH2)3NH2, Spermine

Figure 4: General reaction and adduct for aminopropyltransferase.

corresponding 5'-thioacetyl derivatve (8)), or to 5'-deoxy-5'-chloroadenosine. The latter route is preferred, as the free 5'-thiol is very readily oxidized to the disulfide (8). The totally blocked thioether precursor of the methyl-sulfonium in Figure 4 has been prepared (23), and deblocking, followed by methylation should yield the desired compound.

The folate polyglutamates have been known for many years (3), but only recently has it been shown that these so-called folate conjugates are not simply "storage forms", but effective co-factors as such (24). The require-ment for folate polyglutamate synthesis in cell growth (6) suggested to us

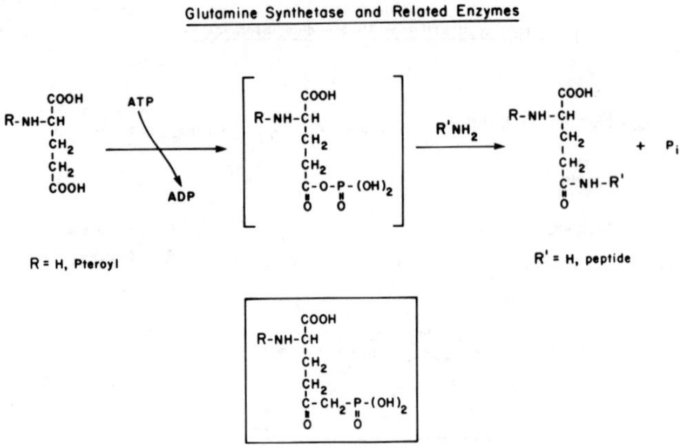

18

Glutamine Synthetase and Related Enzymes

Figure 5: General reaction and adduct for folate polyglutamate synthetase.

that characterization and inhibition of the polyglutamate synthesizing enzyme would be a valuable investigation. We have recently completed an initial study in which partial purification, and extensive characterization of the enzyme has been accomplished (25). Since all folates tested required ATP for the synthesis of their polyglutamate conjugates, the enzyme is a synthetase, and has been called folate polyglutamate synthetase. These data suggest the intermediacy of an acyl phosphate, analogous to that formed in the well-studied glutamine synthetase. The enzyme reaction of interest, and the desired adduct are shown in Figure 5. Our approach to the synthesis of this adduct has been to synthesize a suitably blocked β-glutamyl methanephosphonic acid, which could then be coupled to a pteroic acid derivative, as previously described for the simple folate conjugates (26). We have recently completed the synthesis of the blocked phosphonate as shown in Figure 6 (27). The inability to use

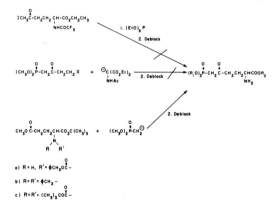

Figure 6: Routes of synthesis for γ-glutamylmethanephosphonic acid derivatives

the Arbuzov reaction to prepare complex acyl phosphonates has been reported previously (28). It should be noted that the carbobenzyloxy (Cbz) blocking group proved to be unsuitable in the coupling reaction with dimethyl methanephosphonic acid due to facile cyclization via pyroglutamate-type intermediates. Use of the di-t-butoxycarbonyl (di-boc) blocking group was effective in overcoming this problem.

We have taken advantage of some of the chemistry learned from the gluta-
myl phosphonate work to prepare similar derivatives of aspartate. These

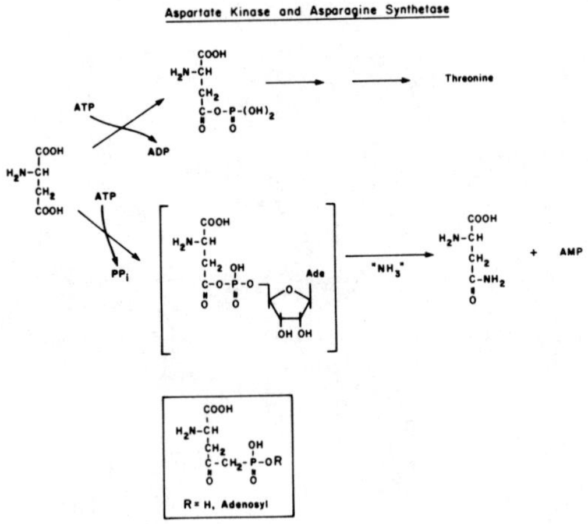

Figure 7: General reaction and adduct for aspartate kinase and asparagine
synthetase.

compounds are designed to inhibit reactions which involve β-aspartyl phosphate
derivatives as either a product (aspartate kinase), or an intermediate (asparagine synthetase (29)). The reactions and the proposed adduct are shown in
Figure 7. The synthesis of this type of adduct is not complicated by facile
cyclization, as in the glutamate case discussed above. Therefore, the Cbz
blocking could be used as shown. Coupling of a blocked (aspartyl) phosphonate

to adenosine leads to the desired AMP derivative.

The work described in this brief paper is an initial attempt to synthesize a new series of potent, specific inhibitors of certain group-transfer enzymes. The new chemistry developed should allow facile entry into these types of compounds in our future work.

REFERENCES

1. Salvatore, F., Borek, E., Zappia, V., Williams-Ashman, H.G. and Schlenk, F., ed., "The Biochemistry of Adenosylmethionine", Columbia University Press, New York.

2. Usdin, E., Borchardt, R.T., and Creveling, C.R., ed. (1979) "Transmethylation", Elsevier/North Holland, New York.

3. Blakley, R.L. (1969) "The Biochemistry of Folic Acid and Related Pteridines", North Holland, Amsterdam.

4. McGuire, J.J., Kitamoto, Y., Hsieh, P., Coward, J.K. and Bertino, J.R. (1979) in "Chemistry and Biology of Pteridines", Kisliuk, R.L., and Brown, G.M., ed., Elsevier/North Holland, New York, pp. 471-476.

5. Taylor, R.T., and Hanna, L.M. (1977) Arch. Biochem. Biophys., 181, 331-344.

6. McBurney, M.W. and Whitmore, G.F. (1974) Cell, 2, 173-182.

7. Coward, J.K., Bussolotti, D.L. and Chang, C.-D., (1974) J. Med. Chem., 17, 1286-1289.

8. Coward, J.K., Motola, N.C., and Moyer, J.D., (1977) J. Med. Chem., 20, 500-505.

9. Coward, J.K. and Crooks, P.A., in ref. 2, pp. 215-224.

10. Crooks, P.A., Dreyer, R.N., and Coward, J.K. (1979) Biochemistry, 18, 2601-2609.

11. Hibasami, H., Borchardt, R.T., Coward, J.K., and Pegg, A.E. (1979), manuscript submitted.

12. Ferro, A.J., in ref. 2, pp. 117-126.

13. Willis, R., personal communication.

14. Wolfenden, R., Ann. Rev. Biophys. Bioeng. (1976) 5, 271-306.

15. Cassio, D., Lemoine, F., Waller, J.P., Sandrin, E., and Boissonnas, R.A. (1967) Biochemistry, 6, 827-835.

16. Heller, J.S., Canellakis, E.S., Bussolotti, D.L., and Coward, J.K. (1975) Biochim. Biophys. Acta, 403, 197-207.

17. Ondetti, M.A., Rubin, B., and Cushman, D.W. (1977) Science, 196, 441-443; Ondetti, M.A., Condon, M.E., Reid, J., Sabo, E.F., Cheung, H.S., and Cushman, D.W. (1979) Biochemistry, 18, 1427-1430.

18. Coward, J.K., Slisz, E.P., and Wu, F.Y.-H. (1973) Biochemistry, 12, 2291-2297.

19. Woodard, R.W., Crooks, P.A., Coward, J.K., and Floss, H.G. (1979), manuscript in preparation; c.f. ref. 2, pp. 135-141.

20. Knipe, J.O. and Coward, J.K. (1979) J. Amer. Chem. Soc., 101, 4339-4348.

21. Coward, J.K. (1979) in "Low Molecular Weight Sulfur-Containing Natural Products", Zappia, V., Cavallini, D., and Gaull, G.E., ed., Plenum, in press.

22. Anderson, G.L., Bussolotti, D.L., Mariuzza, R., and Coward, J.K. (1979), manuscript in preparation.

23. Tang, K.C., Mariuzza, R., Anderson, G.L., and Coward, J.K. (1979) manuscript in preparation.

24. See, for example, Coward, J.K., Chello, P.L., Cashmore, A.R., Parameswaren, K.N., DeAngelis, L.M., and Bertino, J.R. (1975) Biochemistry, 14, 1548-1552.

25. McGuire, J.J., Hsieh, P., Coward, J.K., and Bertino, J.R. (1979) manuscript in preparation.

26. Coward, J.K., Parameswaren, K.N., Cashmore, A.R., and Bertino, J.R. (1974) Biochemistry, 13, 3899-3903.

27. Tang, K.C., Osber, M.P., and Coward, J.K. (1979) manuscript in preparation.

28. Corey, E.J. and Kwiatkowski, (1966) J. Amer. Chem. Soc., 88, 5654-5655; Arbuzov, B.A. (1964) Pure Appl. Chem., 9, 307-335.

29. Horowitz, B., and Meister, A. (1972) J. Biol. Chem., 247, 6708-6719.

DISCUSSION

KISLIUK: Is my understanding correct that the homofolate derivative is not a substrate for folate polyglutamate synthetase?

COWARD: That is correct.

KISLIUK: In connection with the inverse proportionality of tetrahydrofolate concentration with polyglutamate chain length in the synthesis, what concentration of tetrahydrofolate do you have to have, before you begin to see a lowering of the chain length? Are you proposing that as a physiological control?

COWARD: No, we have not gone that far. These types of analyses are fairly lengthy. We have analyzed the products at only the two concentrations, which I indicated, namely 5 and 35 μM tetrahydrofolate. We run the products through HPLC, which analyzes for the various oligoglutamates. What we have done is to look at the time course of formation of the oligoglutamates over about 10 hours. As it goes from 0 to 10 hrs, the chain length either continually increases to the tetra- or pentaglutamate derivative with 5 μM tetrahydrofolate or proceeds only to the diglutamate in the case of 35 μM concentration. We don't have data on anything in between, but we certainly plan to do that. Whether it is physiologically significant, we don't know. I just propose it as a speculation.

WOLFENDEN: There has been some work on phosphonate analogs of amino acid adenylates, as inhibitors of the activating enzymes for amino acids[1]. One wonders whether there might be some better bridging group than the methylene group - I wonder if you thought about that?

COWARD: There are three pertinent studies in this area. The earliest is by Cassio *et al.*[2] with aminoalcohol esters of AMP. These compounds are effective against isolated enzymes, and even seem to be effective in whole cells[3], although they have not been prepared with a radiochemical label and shown to get into the cells intact. These alcohol adenylates are phosphate esters, and presumably are suseptible to enzymic or non-enzymic hydrolysis. That is why we selected the more stable phosphonates. A paper from Cramer's lab[4] reported the synthesis of some phosphonate analogs of phenylalanyl adenylate. It was stated that some of these compounds inhibited the appropriate aminoacyl tRNA synthetase, but no details were given. A more recent study from Dixon's lab[1] indicated that a series of phosphonate analogs of glycyl and valyl adenylates were much less effective as inhibitors of valyl tRNA synthetase. There have been numerous reports of the successful use of phosphonates and related compounds in other systems[5,6], and we feel that they warrant further study.

FRANCK: I'm back on the adenosyl compounds. The trivalent sulfur is chiral. I am sure the S-adenosylmethionine is a single diastereoisomer, but in your analogs you could have two diastereoisomers. I wonder if you separated them and if you found out which one is more active?

COWARD: No, we have not dealt with that. You are certainly right; the sterochemistry of that sulfur of SAM is known and it is (-). The (+) isomer is an inhibitor of several methylases[7]. It is not clear whether we would inhibit these enzymes with both diastereoisomers of our adducts, but the only way to find that out is to make them and see what they do. I must say too, in line with what Dick Wolfenden said in his talk, we are certainly not

24

committed to the sulfonium linkage as the best. What we try to do is make
something that mimics as closely as possible (in the adduct), the atoms and
stereochemistry involved in the transition state. One could envision putting
some nonpolar moiety in place of the sulfonium, and one could get the correct
stereochemistry. Unfortunately, the data available with S-adenosylhomocysteine
analogs indicate that if you change that sulfur to a nonpolar residue or a less
polar one, such as methine, you see very poor inhibition of most methylases,
with the exception of the capping methylase of messenger RNA. More needs to
be done with these types of changes. Our work and work of others indicated
that sulfur is not a very productive place to make changes, so we are sticking
with the sulfonium and we will see what happens.

MARQUEZ: I would like to know, if you have tested some of your phosphonates
against glutamate synthetase and I want to know, if you have some figures as
to how potent they are and I wonder how they compare with carbamylphosphate,
which is a good inhibitor of that enzyme?

COWARD: I think Fred Wedler may want to answer this question.

WEDLER: The tightness of binding is very dependent upon the source of the
enzyme – the bacterial enzyme does not bind the phosphonate very tightly,
the mammalian enzyme does pretty well and the plant enzyme binds it very
tightly.

KALMAN: Could you comment on the antifungal antibiotics containing
aminomethine in place of the methylsulfonium group of S-adenosylmethione and
in particular, how these ammonium derivatives fit into the transition state
analog concept, with respect to the methyltransferases?

COWARD: Yes. A naturally occuring material that was isolated by the
people at Lilly[8] is called sinefungin, has an adenosine with an amino acid
moiety, which instead of having a sulfur, as in S-adenosylhomocysteine, has
an aminomethine:

$$NH_3^+$$

$$ADO \quad COO^-$$

$$NH_3^+$$

This molecule is not a very good inhibitor of most of the small molecule
methylases such as catechol O-methyltransferase, phenethanolamine N-methyl-
transferase and the like. It is also not a very good inhibitor of methyl
transferases of tRNA[9]. This goes along with the activity that we saw with
the corresponding amine, where we have a nitrogen in the place of sulfur[10]:

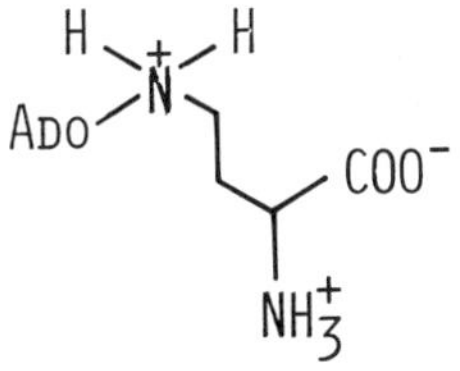

Sinefungin is very active against the methylase involved in the capping of messenger RNA[11], and it is also active against histamine N-methyl transferase[12]. My feeling is that sinefungin is active against these two enzymes because an imidazole moiety is methylated in both cases, and a charge is being developed on the N-atom of either the guanosine or the histidine, in addition to the methyl group. So, I feel that the reason for this activity of the amino-methine molecule may be due to its similarity to this transition state structure, although the kinetic data are not complete enough to support such a rationalization of this activity. The facts are that sinefungin is not very active with most small molecule methyl transferases and the most potent activity is seen in the methylation of the cap of mRNA.

STEFFANI: As you pointed out, the acylphosphates in case of glutamic acid are very prone to cyclization, in fact glutamic acid is easily cyclized under mild conditions. I was wondering, in the case of the keto phosphonates, *i.e.*, the keto phosphonate analog of glutamate, do you see evidence of amino carbinol or Schiff base formation due to cyclization with the carbonyl group?

COWARD: I would certainly think there is some equilibrium. The proton NMR spectrum of acyl phosphonates has a very nice characteristic doublet at about 3 ppm due to the methylene protons, which are split by phosphorous of the phosphonyl with a coupling constant about 20 hz. You see this all the way through the synthesis; it is a very nice characteristic of this type of molecule. At the last step, when you deblock to get the free amine, you begin to lose the nice splitting; it seems to be spread out. Also, there seems to be some exchange there. We have not looked at this in any detail, but it certainly would be in accord with some sort of equilibrium between free amino phosphonate and the cyclic imine or amino carbinol.

REFERENCES

1. Southgate, C.C.B. and Dixon, H.B.F. (1978) Biochem. J. 175, 461.
2. Cassio, D., Lemoine, F., Waller, J.P., Sandrin, E. and Boissonnas, R.A. (1967) Biochemistry 6, 827.

3. Robert-Gero, M., Lawrence, F. and Vigier, P. (1975) Cancer Res. 35, 3571
4. Goring, G. and Cramer, F. (1973) Chem. Ber. 106, 2460
5. Yount, R.G. (1975) Adv. Enzymol. 43, 1.
6. Engel, R. (1977) Chem. Rev. 77, 349.
7. Borchardt, R.T. and Wu, Y.S. (1976) J. Med. Chem. 19, 1099.
8. Fuller, R.W. and Nagarajan, R. (1978) Biochem. Pharmacol. 27, 1981.
9. Borchardt, R.T., personal communication.
10. Chang, C-D. and Coward, J.K. (1976) J. Med. Chem. 19, 684.
11. Pugh, C.S.G., Borchardt, R.T. and Stone, H.O. (1978) J. Biol. Chem. 253, 4075.
12. Fuller, R.W. loc. cit.

Kalman, ed. Drug Action and Design: Mechanism-Based Enzyme Inhibitors

THE INTERACTION OF N-ACETYLNEURAMINIC ACID AND ITS ANALOGS WITH NEURAMINIDASE

MICHAEL FLASHNER, JACK KESSLER AND STUART W. TANENBAUM
State University of New York, College of Environmental Science and Forestry,
Department of Chemistry, Syracuse Campus, Syracuse, New York 13210

INTRODUCTION

Neuraminidases (sialidases; E.C. 3.2.1.18) represent isofunctional enzymes

which hydrolyse α-ketosidically-linked sialic acids from a wide variety of low-

and high-molecular weight oligosaccharides or glycoproteins. Their importance

in pathobiological, immunobiological and molecular biological processes is

attested by the number of review articles which have dealt, in the past decade,

with their general properties, substrate specificities, potential clinical

applications, and use as analytical biochemical reagents in macromolecular

modifications[1-4].

Perhaps most striking is the presumed role of neuraminidases in the replica-

tion of influenza virus and in related diseases caused by other myxo- and para-

myxoviruses[5], as well as in the pathology of a variety of bacterial infec-

tions[6,7]. For this reason, a large number of natural and synthetic substances

have been screened for more than a quarter-century for their potential in

inhibiting the activities of such neuraminidases. The compounds delineated in

Fig. 1 are representative of those which have exhibited anti-enzyme action when

tested in vitro or acted as inhibitors of viral multiplication[8-11]. There is

little apparent structural or biochemical relationship among these empirically

developed inhibitors except for their aromaticity or their possession of hetero-

cyclic moieties with regions of conformational planarity. However, it should

be recognized that other glycohydrolases, e.g., β-D-galactosidase, also have

nonspecific avidities for aromatic structures either at their active regions

or at subsites[12].

A more rational insight into neuraminidase inhibition was the discovery by

1. THIOACRYLIC ACIDS

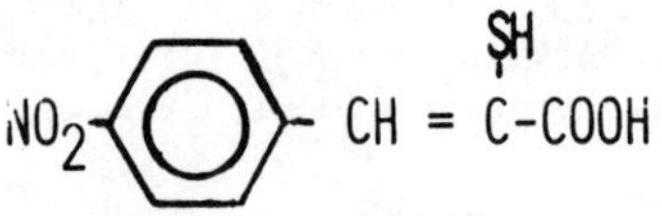

$$NO_2 - \bigcirc - CH = \overset{\overset{\displaystyle SH}{|}}{C} - COOH$$

2. AMINOPHENYLBENZIMIDAZOLES

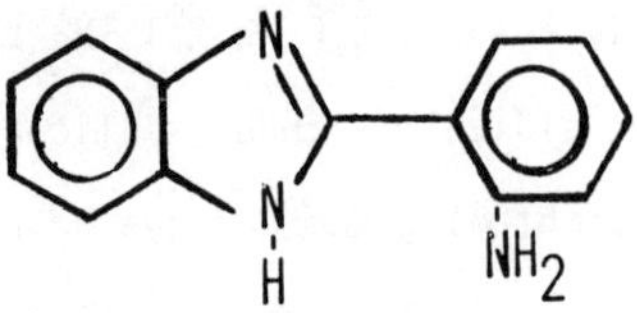

3. PHENYLOXAMIC ACIDS

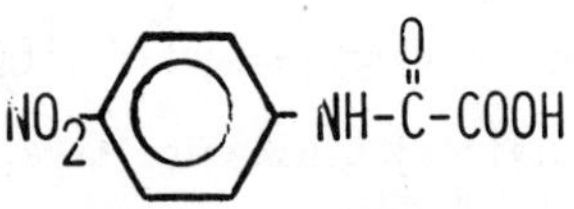

$$NO_2 - \bigcirc - NH - \overset{\overset{\displaystyle O}{\|}}{C} - COOH$$

4. REDUCED ISOQUINOLINES

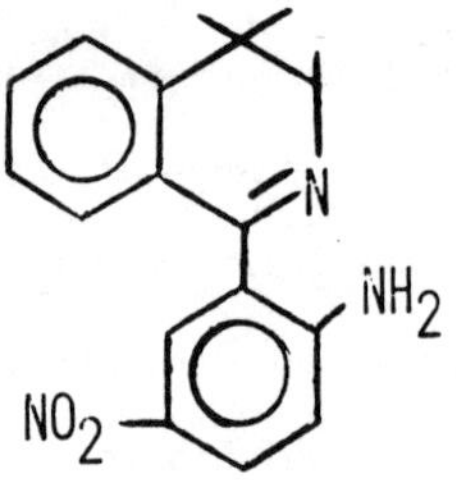

Fig. 1. Inhibitors of Neuraminidases.

Meindl, Tuppy and coworkers[13] that 2,3-dehydrosialic acids (but not their esters) are potent competitive inhibitors of *Vibrio cholera* neuraminidase; and following this, of a number of acyl derivatives tested, that 2,3-dehydro-N-trifluoro-acetylneuramic acid at $10^{-6}\underline{M}$ effectively inhibited influenza virus replication in tissue culture[14-16]. Taking these observations as a point of departure, we have begun in our laboratory a more detailed study of the mode of interaction of these compounds with another bacterial neuraminidase on the

assumption that better knowledge of the structure-function biochemistry of
this enzyme may lead to the design of mechanism-based inhibitors.

In order to carry out the foregoing objectives, it became necessary to
have at hand a replenishable supply of homogeneous neuraminidase. The viral
enzymes are multimeric as well as closely associated with the hemaglutinin;
while pathogenic bacterial neuraminidases, even after purification by sophis-
ticated biochemical technics, still remain contaminated by a variety of unwanted
proteins[17-19]. We therefore undertook to find by way of the elective culture
technic, a saprophytic microorganism which would produce, in relatively high
yield, an inducible, extracellular neuraminidase.

These experiments culminated in the isolation of a soil microorganism
designated *Arthrobacter sialophilus*[20] from which a homogeneous monomeric
glycoprotein of molecular weight *ca.* 88,000 was readily obtained[21]. In this
paper, we present further evidence[22] that 2-deoxy-2,3-dehydro-N-acetylneuraminic
acid (2,3-dehydroAcNeu) and its methyl ester are in point of fact transition-
state analogs and substrates for *Arthrobacter* neuraminidase. Based upon these
findings, it has now become possible to examine alternative enzyme reaction
mechanisms which are in analogy with those proposed for other glycohydrolases.
The fact that 2,3-dehydroAcNeu is a glycal derivative also lends itself toward
the plausible design of specific enzyme inactivators of either the suicide or
site affinity-labeling types[23].

MATERIALS AND METHODS

The ability to induce *A. sialophilus* (ATCC #31253) under well defined
conditions resulted in obtaining filtrates in which neither α-mannosidase,
α- and β-galactosidase, α- and β-fucosidase, N-acetyl-β-glucosamidase, N-acetyl-
β-glucosamidase, N-acetyl-β-glucosamidase nor protease activities were detected.
Under these protocols, neuraminidase from *A. sialophilus* was purified to
homogeneity by conventional procedures in yields approximating 1 mg/liter of

induction filtrate. The enzyme was judged to be homogeneous by SDS polyacryl-amide disc gel electrophoresis. This preparation was also examined by gel electrofocusing, which revealed one major band (85-90%), pI 5.35 ± 0.05 and 6 minor bands, pI's 5.25-5.70. Each band had catalytic activity. The essential properties of this enzyme are reviewed in Table 1[21,24].

TABLE 1

PROPERTIES OF *A. SIALOPHILUS* NEURAMINIDASE

Molecular weight	88,000
Number of subunits	single polypeptide chain
Carbohydrate content	2%
pH optimum	broad optimum between pH 5-6
pI	5.35 (major band)
Cation effects	Ca^{++}, Mg^{++}, Mn^{++}, and Co^{++} are without effect on activity
EDTA	no inhibition on enzyme activity
Linkage specificity	hydrolyses α-2,3; α-2,6; and α-2,8 linkages

Neuraminidase activity was assayed as described previously[21] with either N-acetylneuraminlactose (Boehringer Mannheim) or Collocalia mucoid[25] as substrates. In most cases, the Warren assay was employed, but for those experiments involving 2,3-dehydroAcNeu as substrate, the fluorimetric adaptation of Hammond and Papermaster[26] was used. Initial reaction rates were determined for all substrate concentrations either in the absence or presence of inhibitors. K_i's were determined by the graphic procedures recommended by Segel[27].

N-acetylneuraminic acid (AcNeu) was isolated from "edible bird's nest" as detailed earlier[28]. The anomeric methylketosides of AcNeu and their respective methyl esters were prepared according to published procedures[29,30]. 2,3-DehydroAcNeu and its methyl ester were synthesized according to Meindl and Tuppy[31].

RESULTS AND DISCUSSION

Comparative Biochemistry of Several Neuraminidases. The biochemical properties for the *Arthrobacter* neuraminidase resemble those described for the
Diplococcus pneumoniae and *Clostridium perfringens* enzymes, but are remarkably
different from the *V. cholerae* enzyme. While AcNeu and simple aromatic derivatives[11] inhibit the action of the latter preparation, they have no effect on
the *Arthrobacter* enzyme. Furthermore, the *Arthrobacter* enzyme is inhibited
(see below) by 2,3-dehydroAcNeu methyl ester whereas *V. cholerae* neuraminidase
is not. The *Vibrio* enzyme also has a metal requirement, namely Ca^{++} ions.
These observations would suggest that there are significant structural
differences in the active sites of these two neuraminidases.

Comparison of Enzyme Induction vs. Activity. We have initiated a study on
the factors controlling the induction and regulation of neuraminidase synthesis
in bacteria[32]. Since AcNeu is itself an inducer[32], we were able to test the
efficacy of a series of AcNeu analogs in order to determine which chemical
substituents are critical for enzyme induction, and to compare these results to
those already established for neuraminidase catalysis. The principal difference
appears to be the role played by the free carboxylate group of AcNeu. This
functionality is absolutely essential for catalysis. In contrast, AcNeu methyl
ester and the AcNeu-α-methyl glycoside methyl ester are each enzyme inducers.
Furthermore, since 2,3-dehydroAcNeu and its methyl ester also potentiate enzyme
synthesis, it would appear that the hydroxyl group at C-2 is not required.
Whether these latter compounds are actual inducers and are thus recognized by
proteins involved in the induction process, or are transformed by basal level
of neuraminidase by hydration (see below) is as yet unknown. In summary, it
would appear that the proteins involved in enzyme induction with *Arthrobacter*
have a broader specificity for AcNeu than that exhibited by its neuraminidase
for catalysis.

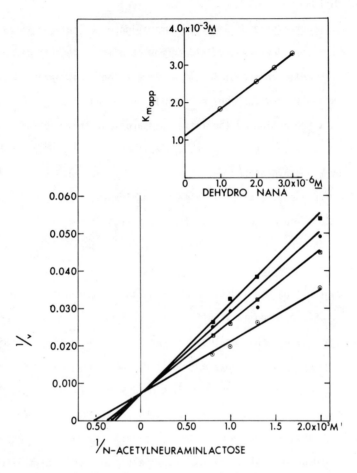

Fig. 2.   Inhibition of *A. sialophilus* neuraminidase by dehydro-NANA is 0.10 $\underline{M}$ citrate-phosphate buffer, pH 6.0, at 37°C. The concentration of N-acetylneura-minlactose is expressed in molarity and the velocities are expressed in enzyme units per milligram of protein. (0) 1.0 x 10^{-6} $\underline{M}$ inhibitor (□) 2.0 x 10^{-6} $\underline{M}$ inhibitor; (●) 2.5 x 10^{-6} $\underline{M}$ inhibitor; (■) 3.0 x 10^{-6} $\underline{M}$ inhibitor. Insert - plot of K_{mapp} vs inhibitor concentration.

<u>Kinetic Studies with 2,3-dehydroAcNeu and its Ester</u>. We have previously examined [22] a series of AcNeu analogs as potential substrates for the enzyme. At 10^{-3} $\underline{M}$, N-acetylneuraminly-α-methyl ketoside methyl ester and the N-acetyl-neuraminly-β-methyl ketoside or its methyl ester were neither substrates nor inhibitors of the *A. sialophilus* neuraminidase. 2,3-DehydroAcNeu and its methyl

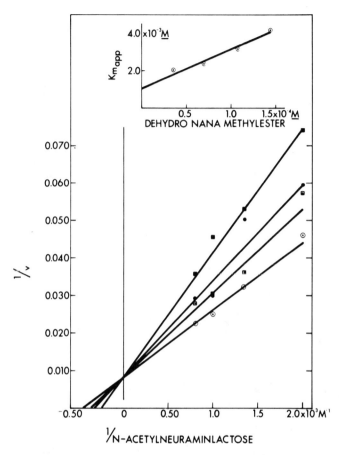

Fig. 3. Inhibition of *A. sialophilus* neuraminidase by dehydro-NANA methyl ester in 0.10 $\underline{M}$ citrate-phosphate buffer, pH 6.0, at 37°C. The concentration of N-acetylneuraminlactose is expressed in molarity and the velocities are expressed in enzyme units per milligram of protein (0) 3.6 x 10^{-5} M inhibitor; (☐) 7.2 x 10^{-5} $\underline{M}$ inhibitor; (●) 1.1 x 10^{-4} $\underline{M}$ inhibitor; (■) 1.4 x $\overline{10}^{-4}$ $\underline{M}$ inhibitor. Insert - plot of K_{mapp} vs inhibitor concentration.

esters are competitive inhibitors of the *Arthrobacter* neuraminidase exhibiting K_i's of 1.8 x 10^{-6} $\underline{M}$ and 4.8 x 10^{-5} $\underline{M}$, respectively (Figs. 2 and 3). The app K_m for the substrate, N-acetylneuraminlactose, is 1.0 x 10^{-3} $\underline{M}$. Assuming that this K_m value reflects the affinity of the substrate for the enzyme, these data indicate minimally that 2,3-dehydroAcNeu binds 714 times tighter to the enzyme than does this substrate while its esterified analog binds 20 times more tightly.

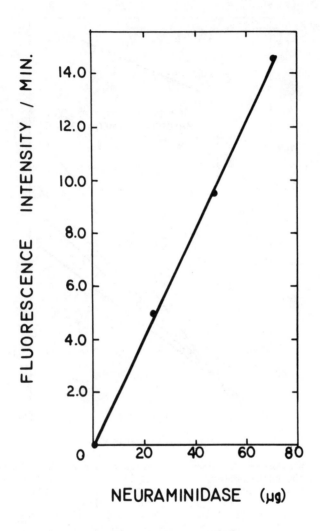

Fig. 4. Activity of neuraminidase as function of enzyme concentration. The concentration of dehydro NANA methyl ester was 7.86 x 10^{-3} M.

It has been demonstrated with several different glycosidases that structur-ally analogous glycals can also be substrates[33,34]. This finding also appears to hold for the *Arthrobacter* neuraminidase, since we now present evidence that 2,3-dehydroAcNeu and its methyl ester are each enzyme substrates. Enzyme activity for the hydration of 2,3-dehydroAcNeu methyl ester increased linearly

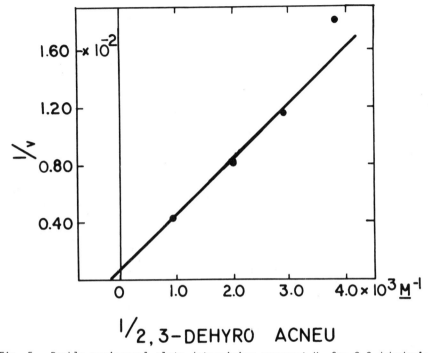

¹/₂,₃-DEHYRO ACNEU

Fig. 5. Double reciprocal plots determining apparent K_m for 2,3-dehydroAcNeu methyl ester. The concentration of substrate is expressed as molarity and velocities as enzyme units per mg of protein.

TABLE 2

COMPARISON BETWEEN HYDROLYSIS AND HYDRATION

Substrate	V_{max}	K_m ($\underline{M}$)	K_i ($\underline{M}$)	$\dfrac{k_{cat}}{k_{off}}$*
N-acetylneuraminlactose	54	1.0×10^{-3}	-	-
2,3-dehydroAcNeu methyl ester	0.018	6.0×10^{-3}	4.8×10^{-5}	124

$$*E + I \xleftarrow{\quad k_{off} \quad} \quad EI \quad \xrightarrow{\quad k_{cat} \quad} \quad E + P$$
$$\xrightarrow{\quad k_{on} \quad}$$

with concentrations up to 70 μg/0.5 ml protein, as shown in Fig. 4. From this, it can be inferred that the production of the Warren chromaphore is not a spontaneous (i.e., acid-catalyzed) interaction. Preliminary results would suggest that the hydroxyl group is added to the C-2 position generating AcNeu as the product. This conclusion is based upon the observation that periodate oxidation of either the hydration product or AcNeu yields chromaphores with identical fluorescent spectra (max. 579 mμ). The K_m value for 2,3-dehydroAcNeu methyl ester in the hydration reaction was determined from inverse plots as given in Fig. 5 and summarized in Table 2. The glycal is a very poor substrate, with V_{max} being some 3000 times less than the V_{max} for glycoside hydrolysis. The K_m for its hydration is 6.0×10^{-3} $\underline{M}$. Since the K_i is 4.8×10^{-5} $\underline{M}$, we can calculate the ratio of k_{cat}/k_{off} for this analog (Table 2). It should be noted that this ratio represents a minimum value, since the K_i (see above) appears to be a kinetic rather than thermodynamic constant. Following Wentworth and Wolfenden, who studied the interaction of D-galactal with β-galactosidase[33], we infer that the foregoing ratio of 124 indicates that the 2,3-dehydroAcNeu methyl ester is released from neuraminidase as the hydrated product rather than in unmodified form.

Mechanism of Enzyme Action. The criteria for defining a competitor inhibitor as a transition-state analog of the enzyme are first, the inhibitor must bind more tightly to the enzyme than does the substrate; and, second, that the conformation of the inhibitor is consistent with the structure of the transition-state postulated for the enzyme-catalyzed reaction. The original suggestion that glycals are effective glycohydrolase inhibitors because of their resemblance to the half-chair conformation of oxocarbonium ions generated during acid-catalyzed glycoside hydrolysis has been challenged[35], since the position of their unsaturation differs such that ring substitutents are misoriented with respect to the coplanar atoms. Alternative mechanisms for glycohydrolases have been proposed such as the S_N1-like mechanism for egg white lysozyme[36] and the S_N2 mechanism for almond β-glucosidase[37]. Intermediate between these two models is the proposed mechanism for β-galactosidase in which the initial formation of the oxocarbonium ion collapses to the galactosyl-enzyme intermediate[38].

Our current working model to explain the inhibition of glycoside hydrolysis by 2,3-dehydroAcNeu follows the extensive work by Wentworth and Wolfenden[33] with β-galactosidase, in which it was proposed that D-galactal undergoes an enzymatic addition-displacement reaction. Thus, neuraminidase could attack the double bond of 2,3-dehydroAcNeu generating an N-acetylneuraminyl-enzyme intermediate which would then be displaced by H_2O to yield AcNeu and regenerate the free enzyme. Regardless of succeeding refinements in reaction mechanism, the geometry at C-2 of AcNeu must pass through planarity sometime during the course of this reaction. Since 2,3-dehydroAcNeu has a planar conformation and also binds about 700 times more tightly to the enzyme than does N-acetyl-neuraminlactose, we have postulated that 2,3-dehydroAcNeu is a transition-state analog for neuraminidase[22].

As mentioned earlier, chemical modifications of the carboxylate group of AcNeu-α-ketosides, such as reduction to the alcohol or conversion to the ester or amide[1-3], have definitely established that the acid is essential for sub-strate binding. The finding that 2,3-dehydroAcNeu methyl ester is both a competitive inhibitor of sialic-α-ketosides as well as a substrate for neura-minidase has provided insight into defining the role played by the carboxylate group in glycoside hydrolysis[22]. All of these observations may be rationalized by assuming that a salt bridge between the substrate carboxylate and a catonic amino acid residue on the enzyme is required for the distortion of the sub-strate as envisioned in Fig. 6. Glycoside substrates for neuraminidase exist in the $^2C_5$ conformation and will therefore fit into the binding region only after assuming a planar-like structure. However, the methyl ester of 2,3-dehydroAcNeu already possesses a conformation resembling that of the distorted

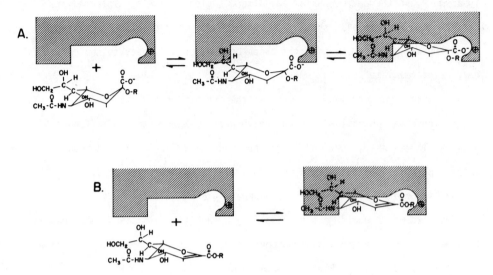

Fig. 6. Binding of substrates and transition-state analogs to *A. sialophilus* neuraminidase. In Fig. 3B, R = H or -CH$_3$.

enzyme-bound substrate, and therefore becomes bound with high affinity. The extensive work with egg white lysozyme establishes a precedent for this model since for substrate binding to occur, the C-6 hydroxymethyl group of N-acetyl-glucosamine undergoes distortion because of steric hindrance at subsite D[36].

Although the substrate and linkage specificity of viral and bacterial neuraminidases have been thoroughly examined[1-3] little is known concerning the role played by their amino acid residues in catalysis. In order to identify such essential residues, we have utilized "group specific" reagents as potential modifying agents[21]. At inhibitor to enzyme ratios of from 1000 to 10,000:1, the *Arthrobacter* neuraminidase was insensitive to a wide range of modifying reagents known to react with sulfhydryl, argininyl, lysyl, histidinyl, and carboxyl residues. From these data the active region appears to be inaccessible to these reagents. As Bachmayer[39] earlier reported for the *V. cholera* neuraminidase, we found N-bromosuccinimide (molar ratio of inhibitor to enzyme of 60:1) to completely inactivated the *Arthrobacter* neuraminidase. The kinetics of this inactivation were pseudo-first order with respect to enzyme. Complete protection of our enzyme against inactivation by N-bromosuccinimide was obtained when the assay was carried out in the presence of 9.0×10^{-5} $\underline{M}$ 2,3-dehydroAcNeu or its methyl ester. This finding reinforces the notion that the normal sequence of transitional events in the ultimate conversion of AcNeu derivatives to products involves stages which resemble these analogs spatially and electronically. These data also suggest that a tryptophan residue may be essential for the catalytic process, presumably by was of facilitating binding and hence distortion to postulated planar intermediates.

Prospectus. Many questions remain to be answered concerning the structure-function biochemistry of neuraminidases. With the eventual aim of designing mechanism-based inhibitors, we intend to continue endeavors to characterize the interaction of 2,3-dehydroAcNeu with the homogeneous *Arthrobacter* enzyme in order to better unravel the reaction mechanism for glycoside hydrolysis. The extensive and indeed almost explosive increase in knowledge concerning the chemistry of glycals[23,40,41] should provide a basis for the preparation of reagents of either the suicide or site-affinity labeling type for this enzyme. The application of such analogs should help to provide a more direct identification of those amino acid residues which are involved in enzymatic substrate binding and catalysis.

ACKNOWLEDGMENTS

The authors are grateful to Drs. Carl A. Miller and Philip Wang for carrying out some of these experiments. This work was supported by Public Health Service grant AI-12532 from the National Institute of Allergy and Infectious Diseases.

40

REFERENCES

1. Drzeniek, R. (1972) in Current Topics in Microbiology and Immunology, Arber, W. *et al.*, ed., Springer-Verlag, New York, Vol. 59, pp. 35-75.
2. Heide, K., Seiler, F. and Schwicks, H.G. (1974) Symposium on Neuraminidase, Behring Institute Mitteilungen, No. 55, Behringwerke A.G., Marburg, pp. 1-373.
3. Rosenberg, A. and Shengrund, C. (1976) Biological Role of Sialic Acids, Plenum Press, New York, pp. 1-375.
4. Bekesi, J.G., Roboz, J.P. and Holland, J.P. (1976) Ann. N.Y. Acad. Sci., 277, 313-331.
5. Kilbourn, E. (1975) The Influenza Virus and Influenza, Academic Press, New York, pp. 1-573.
6. Müller, H.E. (1974) in Symposium on Neuraminidase, Heide, K., Seiler, F. and Schwicks, H.G., ed., Behring Institute Mitteilunger, No. 55, Behring-werke A.G., Marburg, pp. 150-151.
7. Kelly, R.T., Grieff, D. and Farmer, S. (1966) J. Bacteriol., 91, 601-603.
8. Edmond, J.D., Johnston, R.G., Kidd, D., Rylance, H.J. and Sommerville, R.G. (1966) Br. J. Pharmac. Chemother., 27, 415-426.
9. Tute, M.S., Brammer, K.W., Kayne, B. and Broadbent, R.W. (1970) J. Med. Chem., 13, 44-51.
10. Haskell, T.H., Peterson, F.E., Watson, D., Plessas, N.R. and Culbertson, T. (1970) J. Med. Chem., 13, 697-704.
11. Brossmer, R., Ziegler, D. and Keilich, G. (1977) Hoppe-Seyler's Z. Physiol. Chem., 358, 391-400.
12. Nishikawa, A.H. and Bailon, P. (1975) Arch. Biochem. Biophys., 168, 576-584.
13. Meindl, P. and Tuppy, H. (1969) Hoppe-Seyler's Z. Physiol. Chem., 350, 1088-1094.
14. Meindl, P., Bodo, G., Palese, P., Schulman, J. and Tuppy, H. (1974) Virology, 58, 457-463.
15. Palese, P., Schulman, J.L., Bodo, G. and Meindl, P. (1974) Virology, 59, 490-498.
16. Palese, P. and Compans, R.W. (1976) J. Gen. Virol., 33, 159-163.
17. Den, H., Malinzak, D.A. and Rosenberg, A. (1975) J. Chromat., 111, 217-222.
18. Hatten, M.W.C. and Regoeczi, E. (1973) Biochim. Biophys. Acta, 327, 114-120.
19. Rood, J.J. and Wilkenson, R.G. (1974) Biochim. Biophys. Acta, 334, 168-170.
20. Tanenbaum, S.W. and Flashner, M. (1978) Can. J. Microbiol., 23, 1568-1572.
21. Wang, P., Tanenbaum, S.W. and Flashner, M. (1978) Biochim. Biophys. Acta, 523, 170-180.
22. Miller, C.A., Wang, P. and Flashner, M. (1978) Biochem. Biophys. Res. Comm., 83, 1479-1487.
23. Ferrier, R.J. (1969) Adv. Carbohydrate Chem., 24, 198-266.
24. Flashner, M., Wang, P., Hurley, J.B. and Tanenbaum, S.W. (1977) J. Bacteriol., 129, 1457-1465.
25. Howe, C., Lee, L.T. and Rose, H.M. (1961) Arch. Biochem. Biophys., 95, 512-520.
26. Hammond, K.S. and Papermaster, D.S. (1976) Anal. Biochem., 74, 292-297.
27. Segel, I.H. (1975) Enzyme Kinetics, Wiley Interscience, New York, pp. 107-111.
28. Martin, J., Tanenbaum, S.W. and Flashner, M. (1977) Carbohydrate Res., 56, 423-425.
29. Kuhn, R., Lutz, P. and MacDonald, D.L. (1966) Chem. Ber., 99, 611-617.
30. Yu, R.K. and Ledeen, R. (1969) J. Biol. Chem., 244, 1306-1313.
31. Meindl, P. and Tuppy, H. (1969) Mh. Chem., 100, 1295-1306.
32. Wang, P., Schafer, D., Miller, C.A., Tanenbaum, S.W. and Flashner, M. (1978) J. Bacteriol., 136, 874-879.

33. Wentworth, D.F. and Wolfenden, R. (1974) Biochem., 13, 4715-4720.
34. Hehre, E.J., Genghof, D.S., Sternlicht, H. and Brewer, C.F. (1977) Biochem., 16, 1780-1787.
35. Levvy, G.A. and Snaith, S.M. (1972) Advan. Enzymol. Relat. Areas Mol. Biol., 36, 151-181.
36. Imoto, T., Johnson, L.N., North, A.C.T., Phillips, D.C. and Rupley, J.A. (1972) The Enzymes, 7, 665-868.
37. Lai, H.L., Butler, L.G. and Axelrod, B. (1974) Biochem. Biophys. Res. Comm., 60, 635-640.
38. Sinnott, K.L. (1978) FEBS Lett., 94, 1-9.
39. Bachmayer, H. (1972) FEBS Lett., 23, 217-219.
40. Blackburne, I.D., Burfitt, A.I.R., Fredericks, P.F. and Guthrie, R.D. (1979) in Synthetic Methods for Carbohydrates, Khadem, H., ed., American Chemical Society, Washington, D.C., pp. 116-133.
41. Fraser-Reid, B. (1975) Acct. Chem. Res., 8, 192-201.

DISCUSSION

KORYTNYK: I would like to ask a question regarding the activities of the 2,3-dehydroAcNeu derivatives with respect to its affect on different neuraminidases. These analogs did not inhibit the *Vibrio cholerae* neuraminidase whereas the *Arthrobacter* enzyme was inhibited. Do these observations imply a completely different mechanism of hydrolysis, or what are your interpretations of these results?

FLASHNER: It is an excellent question. Let me re-emphasize that the 2,3-dehydroAcNeu inhibits both preparations. It is only the *Vibrio* neuraminidase which is not inhibited by the methyl ester of 2,3-dehydroAcNeu. There are also differences in the enzyme preparation that are worth noting. The *Arthrobacter* neuraminidase is a well characterized homogeneous enzyme, whereas the *V. cholerae* neuraminidase is a crude enzyme preparation, which has undoubtedly undergone significant proteolysis. As a result, some binding specificity towards the methyl ester may have been lost. We really have insufficient information available to adequately answer the second part of your question. The Ca^{++} -ion requirement for *V. cholerae* neuraminidase may suggest that different reaction mechanisms do exist.

BARASH: Do you have any evidence for the incorporation of your 2,3-dehydro-AcNeu derivatives into peptidoglycan?

FLASHNER: No, we do not.

WOLFENDEN: I am wondering about the situation in which you have a reversibly bound inhibitor also acting as a substrate. The bound inhibitor has two possible fates, one which is to be released back to the solution and the other is to be converted to product. I think that the K_i that is measured includes both off-rates so you get in fact only an upper limit on the true dissociation constant of the reversibly bound inhibitor. In your case, do you think that the K_i's for the 2,3-dehydroAcNeu derivatives represent an upper limit?

FLASHNER: Yes, the K_i's which we report do represent an upper limit. Since we now know that 2,3-dehydroAcNeu methyl ester is also a substrate for the enzyme, the true K_i may be significantly less than the value determined. This would mean that these derivatives would bind even more tightly to the enzyme than does the substrate. We are in the process of determining the individual rate constants in order to calculate a true dissociation constant for both 2,3-dehydroAcNeu and its methyl ester.

WOLFENDEN: So, at the moment, it is up in the air?

FLASHNER: Yes, it is.

WOLFENDEN: The induction of the enzyme by 2,3-dehydroAcNeu, I think is a very interesting observation. We tried to do the same thing with β-galacto-sidase. It is quite clear that the repressor protein has very few properties in common with the enzyme itself. In your case it seems to be an open possibility.

FLASHNER: The observation that 2,3-dehydroAcNeu is an inducer of neurami-nidase synthesis is indeed very interesting. I think the differences you just mentioned may be related to the fact that β-galactosidase is an intracellular enzyme, while neuraminidase is an extracellular enzyme under product induction by AcNeu. If enzymes have evolved to bind transition-states as you have described in your presentation, then the question arises as to why transport or repressor proteins, which do not alter their substrates, would effectively bind a presumed transition-state analog of the enzyme. This raises the possibility that the binding site for AcNeu in these proteins resemble in some way the binding site of the enzyme. I just want to re-emphasize that the 2,3-dehydroAcNeu may be hydrated by basal levels of neuraminidase so the actual inducer in these experiments is, in fact, AcNeu. However, since the methyl ester of 2,3-dehydroAcNeu is an effective inducer and a poor substate argues against catalytic transformation to product. This still remains to be established and we are planning to use labeled 2,3-dehydroAcNeu to further investigate the question as to whether transition-state analogs are actual inducers.

MELOCHE: I see two stereochemical events in your hydration reaction: a proton goes on C-3 and an OH- goes on C-2. It would be very interesting to find out whether the proton and the OH-group come into the same face at the C-2-3 trigonals of this system.

FLASHNER: We are in the process of doing experiments to answer these questions.

MELOCHE: Does hydrogen isotope go in during hydration?

FLASHNER: We are also planning on looking at isotope effects in the hydration reaction.

MELOCHE: I see resolving of configuration of C-3 of AcNeu to be rather easy, but I am not too sure about the configuration at C-2.

FLASHNER: Well, one way in which we anticipate determining the anomeric configuration at C-2 of AcNeu, as it is released from the enzyme, is by substrate catalysis. We are in the process of working out conditions for using alternate nucleophiles such as methanol to prepare AcNeu-glycosides. Although the 2,3-dehydroAcNeu methyl ester is a substrate for the hydration reaction, neither the AcNeu-α-methyl nor -β-methyl glycoside methyl esters are substrates for neuraminidase. The reaction mixture can be saponified, and the de-esterified product then tested as a potential substrate for the enzyme. If methanol is released, as a result of enzyme action, then the product must be alpha, since the anomeric specificity of neuraminidase is absolute.

ONDETTI: You do have tryptophans in the enzyme, don't you?

FLASHNER: Yes, the amino acid composition is known for the *Arthrobacter* neuraminidase and there are 10 tryptophans.

ONDETTI: Have you looked at the UV changes on the enzyme, when it is inactivated by N-bromosuccinimide? Is there any indication that a tryptophan is attacked?

FLASHNER: No, we have not done that and let me emphasize that with any of these "group specific" reagents, one has to clearly identify the amino acid residue which has been modified. We have not as yet done that and we will, of course, do it.

ONDETTI: I wonder what the tryptophans would be doing at the active site? Do you have any idea?

FLASHNER: By analogy with lysozyme, tryptophan residues may be involved in the distortion of the substrate.

CHOWDHRY: I am curious if you looked at the double bonded exocyclic C-1, because that would put only a formal sp^2 hybridization at C-2 without presumably upsetting too much C-3, though it will change the ring conformation, of course.

FLASHNER: No, we have not and that is a very interesting idea.

SILVERMAN: Can you tell me, why did you exclude an elimination mechanism possibility in favor of a double S_N2 displacement? This mechanism would also lead to an sp^2 carbon, which would be similar to your inhibitor.

FLASHNER: Essentially on the basis of literature information. We do not really have any evidence to talk about mechanism - it is a kind of working hypothesis. We drew heavily on Dr. Wolfenden's work, with β-galactosidase and its inhibition by galactal[1].

WOLFENDEN: I think that one reason for preferring an S_N2 displacement to elimination is that one does see accumulation of an intermediate. The only reason for not particularly liking that possibility, as I recall, had to do with some observations on isotope effects. I think that elimination still remains a possibility, since sp^2 hybridization would be expected either for a carbonium ion or for a compound containing a double bond between C-1 and C-2.

REFERENCE

1. Wentworth, D.F. and Wolfenden, R. (1974) Biochemistry 13, 4715-4720.

II
Suicide Inactivators

NATURAL AND SYNTHETIC K_{CAT}-INHIBITORS OF TRANSAMINASES AND DECARBOXYLASES

ROBERT R. RANDO

Department of Pharmacology, Harvard Medical School, Boston, MA   02115   USA

The problem of the identification and modulation of drug receptors is central to pharmacology. The specific chemical tagging of these receptors can be used as an approach to this problem. In the case of a membrane bound receptor which only has small molecule binding properties, the affinity labeling approach is usually used[1]. In this technique, a chemically reactive or photo-reactivatable group is attached to receptor ligand and upon binding a chemical reaction ensues between an active-site amino acid and the chemically reactive ligand (Fig. 1).

$$D + R \rightleftharpoons D{\cdot}R \qquad\qquad K_D = \frac{(D)\ (R)}{(DR)}$$

$$D + R - X \rightleftharpoons D{\cdot}X - R \longrightarrow D - X - R$$

X = chemically reactive moiety

D = drug

R = receptor

Figure 1

The specificity of labeling agents of this type are almost solely dependent on their dissociation constant (K_D). Because they contain chemically reactive groups, frequently even a very low dissociation constant is not enough to insure specificity of action. When enzymes are considered as receptors, however, a new dimension unfolds for their specific active-site labeling. Since enzymes catalyze chemical reactions, the possibility exists that the enzymes can be used to catalyze their own inactivation (Fig. 2). The advantage

$$E + S \rightleftharpoons ES \xrightarrow{k_{cat}} E \cdot I \xrightarrow{k_{inh}} E - I$$

Figure 2

of this mode of inactivation over affinity labeling is considerable since the actual chemically reactive inhibitor is generated and sequestered at the active site of the enzyme, thus preventing unwanted side reactions which ultimately lead to lack of specificity. In fact, inhibitors of this type are relatively common in pharmacology and biochemistry today as a consequence of a great deal of work done on their development in the past several years[2]. This work had its impetus in an important and serendipitous discovery made by Konrad Bloch and coworkers[3]. They demonstrated, in a particularly clear way, that β,γ acetylenic thioesters inactivated β-hydroxy decanoyl thioester dehydrase by a mechanism that required enzymatic participation. Namely, the enzyme catalyzed the formation of the highly reactive conjugated allenic thioester from the acetylene which led to alkylation of an active site histidine residue (Fig. 3).

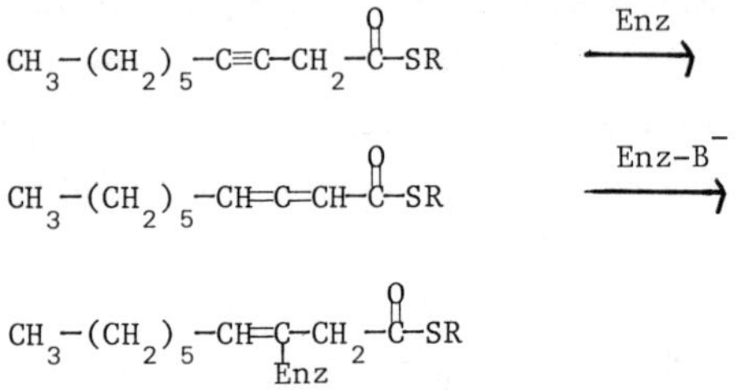

$$CH_3-(CH_2)_5-C{\equiv}C-CH_2-\overset{O}{\overset{\|}{C}}-SR \qquad \xrightarrow{\quad Enz \quad}$$

$$CH_3-(CH_2)_5-CH{=}C{=}CH-\overset{O}{\overset{\|}{C}}-SR \qquad \xrightarrow{\quad Enz-B^- \quad}$$

$$CH_3-(CH_2)_5-CH{=}\underset{Enz}{\overset{}{C}}-CH_2-\overset{O}{\overset{\|}{C}}-SR$$

Figure 3

The most important line of research on these inhibitors, which are termed either k_{cat} or suicide inhibitors, in the past several years has been to develop latent functional groups which could be exploited in the design of these inhibitors. Basically, there are three functional groups utilized in k_{cat} inhibitor design. The acetylenic functional group first introduced by Bloch, the olefinic group introduced by us and the fluorinated analogs introduced by Abeles and coworkers[2,3]. All of these functional groups are enzymatically activated to produce Michael acceptors at the enzyme's active-site. Since enzymes would be expected to possess nucleophilic groups at their active sites, it could be anticipated that the generation of Michael acceptors should result in the inactivation of the enzyme (Fig. 4). Furthermore, since

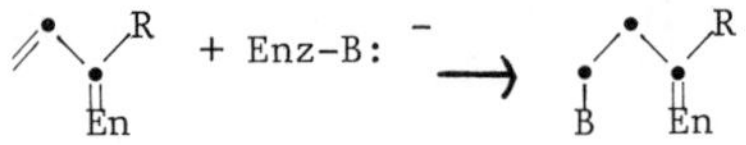

$$\text{En} = O, N, S$$

Figure 4

Michael acceptors of the kind shown here are readily enzymatically generated by the formal oxidation of β,γ olefenic substrate analogs it might be anticipated that allylic amines and alcohols would serve as potent k_{cat} inactivators of certain enzymes (Fig. 5). Since it is the purpose of this article to

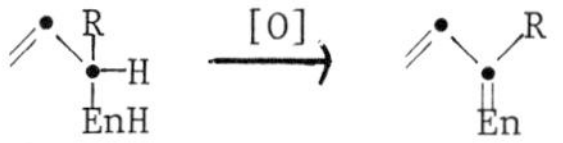

Figure 5

explore the inactivation of pyridoxal phosphate linked transaminases and to a lesser extent decarboxylases, I will concern myself with the interaction of unsaturated amino acids with these enzymes.

The simplest β,γ unsaturated amino acid is vinyl glycine 1, a molecule first synthesized by us in 1974. This simple molecule serves as a prototype for olefinic amino acid enzyme inactivators. We were able to show that vinyl glycine inactivates pyridoxal phosphate linked aspartate aminotransferase[4]. As expected, the enzyme was recalcitrant to inactivation in the pyridoxamine form or when it was resolved and was not protected from inactivation by nucleophilic trapping agents. Furthermore, the inhibitor is 90% efficient in that for every turnover there is a 90% chance that the enzyme will be inactivated[5]. This is shown by demonstrating that in the absence of α-ketoglutarate 90% of the enzyme is inactivated. Of course, the remaining 10% of the enzyme can be inactivated by adding α-ketoglutarate. This reagent drives the remaining 10% of the pyridoxamine form of the enzyme back to the pyridoxal form which is further inactivated. As to the stoichiometry of the inactivation process, it was determined that one molecule of inhibitor was incorporated per subunit of the dimeric enzyme. The vinyl glycine proved to be attached to Lys-258, the lysine residue presumed to be involved in Schiff base formation with the pyridoxal phosphate[5]. The overall mechanism of inhibition is shown below (Fig. 6):

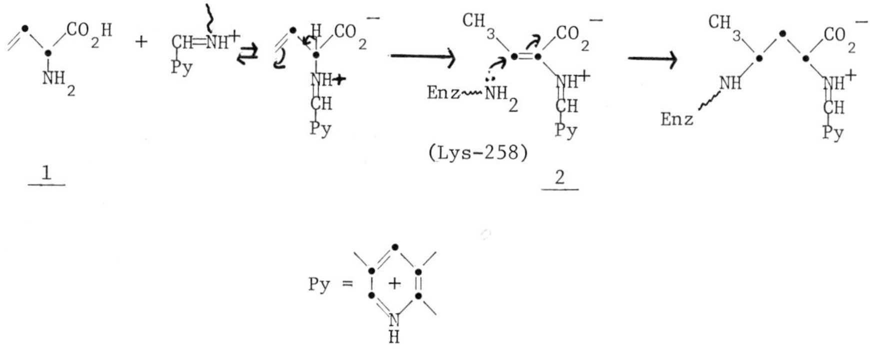

Figure 6

The isomerization route was demonstrated by showing the pyridoxal phosphate could be liberated from the inactivated enzyme. Direct transamination of the enzyme bound vinyl glycine to yield 3 doesn't seem to occur. It is interesting to note that simply heating vinyl glycine and pyridoxal phosphate in the presence of a transition metal ion affords intermediate 2 and not 3[6]. Thus

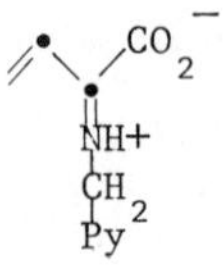

3

the formation of 2 is kinetically favored. Vinyl glycine will certainly not inactivate all pyridoxal phosphate linked enzyme that can utilize it as a substrate. For example, thieonine deaminase and methionine lyase both convert vinyl glycine to α-ketobutyrate without themselves being inactivated. Although one can rationalize why one enzyme and not another should be inactivated, there is no a priori way of knowing which enzyme will be susceptable to inactivation. It is of interest to note that vinyl glycine has been shown to be a natural product. The biological role of this material, if one exists, is not currently known. In fact, as we have pointed out before, many natural products function as k_{cat} inactivators, many of which are highly potent and specific.

Another β,γ unsaturated amino acid, L-2-amino-4-methoxy-trans-2-butenoic acid (AMB) 4 is a bacterial toxin which also inactivates aspartate aminotransferase[6,7]. The introduction of the OCH_3 group slightly increases the structural complexity of this inhibitor over that of vinyl glycine. This increased complexity manifests itself in the mechanism of action of the inactivator. The mechanism of this inactivation process involves the following:

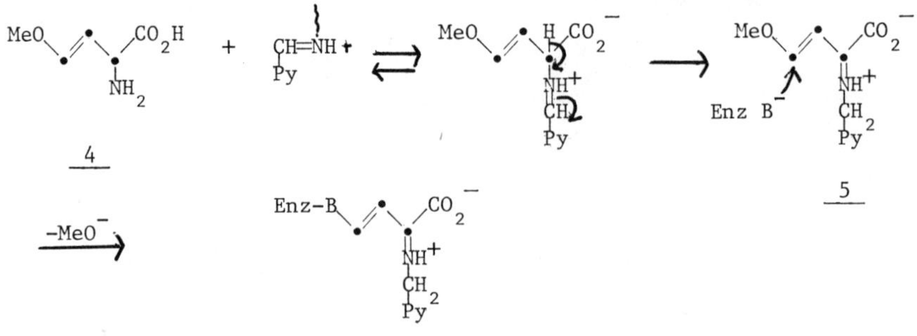

In this case, transamination does occur to yield 5, which engages in a Michael reaction followed by MeO⁻ elimination with the enzyme to afford inactivated enzyme 6. The fact that there is a leaving group here adds a note of complexity to the mode of inactivation over that of vinyl glycine. Again model studies are consistent with the enzymological results. Heating AMB with pyridoxal phosphate and transition metal ions affords virtually a quantitative yield of transaminated product[6]. Presumably the conjugative interactions between the methoxy group and the double bond resists isomerization. In addition to in-activating aspartate aminotransferase, AMB also inactivates tryptophan synthe-tase and inhibits methionine γ-lyase by a yet unknown mechanism[8]. The K_I for the competitive term is the inhibition of the latter enzyme by AMB is 5 μM, some 10^3 times lower than the K_I for methionine[9]. There seems to be a general tendency for trans-β,γ-unsaturated amino acids to bind more tightly to the target enzyme than does the saturated substrate. For example, trans-dehydro-ornithine binds some three orders of magnitude more tightly to ornithine decarboxylase than does ornithine[10]. In addition to inhibiting the foremen-tioned enzymes, AMB also interrupts ethylene production in plants, suggesting that it inactivates another pyridoxal phosphate linked enzyme, γ(β)-cystathion-ase[11]. It should be noted that rhizobitoxine (2-amino-4-(2-amino-3-hydroxy-propoxy-trans-3-butenoic acid) 7, another naturally occurring β,γ-unsaturated

HOCH₂—CH—CH₂—O ... CO₂H (7) with NH₂ groups

HO₂C—CH—CH₂—S—CH₂—CH₂—CH—CO₂H (8) with NH₂ groups

                7   8

amino acid, is also reported to inactivate β-cystathionase from plants and hence also prevents ethylene production[12]. The structural similarity of this compound to cystathionine 8 is obvious. One can speculate that the mechanism of the inactivation of cystathionine by rhizobitoxine is similar to the mechanism of the AMB induced inactivation of aspartate aminotransferase.

Other β,γ-unsaturated amino acids have also been shown to inactivate pyri-doxal phosphate linked enzymes. For example, vinyl GABA (4-amino-5-hexenoic acid) 9 has been shown to be a k_{cat} inactivator of GABA transaminase (GABA-T)[13].

CH₂=... CO₂H (9) with NH₂ group

NH₂CH₂ ...=... CO₂H (10)

                9   10

Presumably, the mechanism of inactivation is similar to that for the vinyl
glycine induced inactivation of aspartate aminotransferase. It is interesting

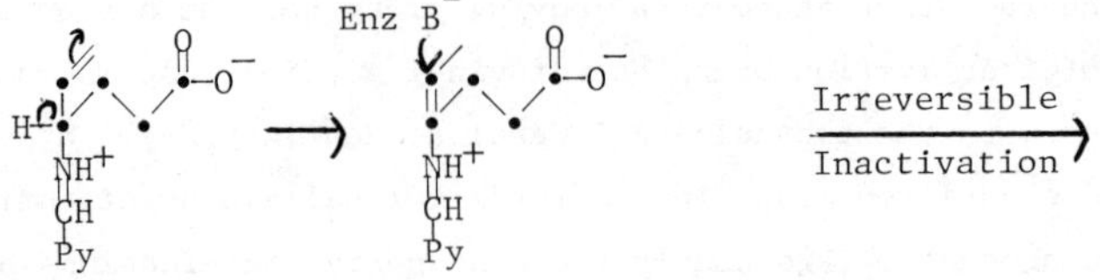

to note that when the double bond is placed in the GABA backbone, as in 10, no
inactivation of the enzyme is observed. In fact, 10 is a superb substrate for
GABA-T. GABA-T is the enzyme that terminates the action of the inhibitory
neurotransmitter GABA.

We have so far discussed some of the enzymological ramifications of placing
a double bond β,γ to a cleavable C–H bond. It is interesting to consider what
would happen if an additional double bond were added in conjugation with the
first 11 to increase the chemical complexity of the molecule. If compound 11

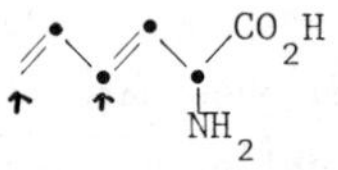

11

were enzymatically transaminated or decarboxylated, two sites, indicated by
the arrows, instead of one would be activated and made susceptable to a
Michael reaction. Of greater interest, however, is the case where the two
double bonds are tied back in ring 12. If compound 12 were decarboxylated, an
interesting thing happens, because the product 13 in addition to allowing for

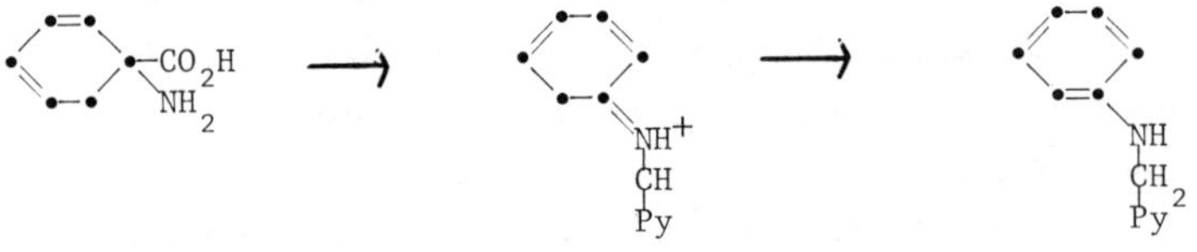

12   13   14

a Michael reaction at the indicated sites also can aromatize to yield 14,
which has covalently tied the cofactor to the substrate. Since this product
should bind very tightly to the enzyme, the enzyme would be rendered inactive.
Isomers of 12 should also be transaminase inactivators 15, 16 and 17. In
these cases, the transaminated products can aromatize to covalently tie the

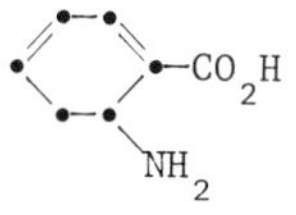

15 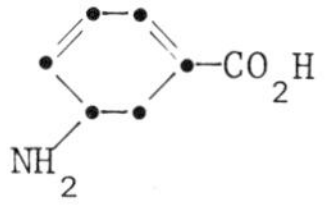   16 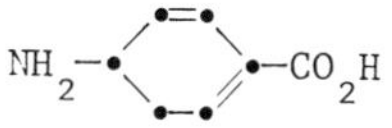   17

substrate to the cofactor. It turns out the compound 16, gabaculine, is a natural product[14]. It is an exceedingly potent inactivator of bacterial and mammalian GABA-T[15]. This enzyme is involved in the degradation of the inhibitory neurotransmitter γ-aminobutyric acid (GABA) in animals. The partial reaction for the enzyme is shown in Fig. 7.

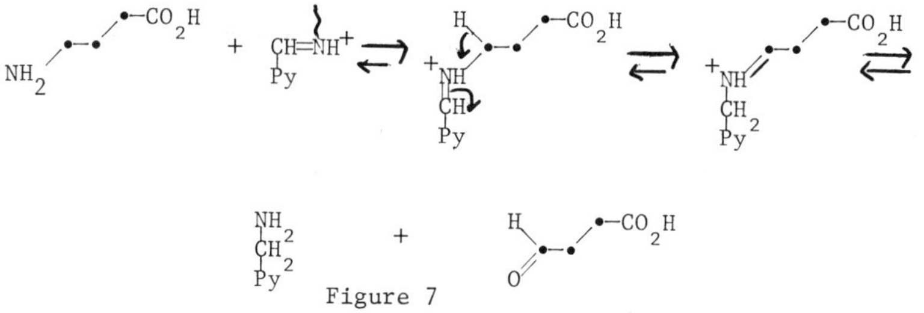

Figure 7

The pyridoxal form of the enzyme is again regenerated when α-ketoglutarate reverses the whole process to produce L-glutamate. When this enzyme is treated with gabaculine, it suffers rapid irreversible inactivation with first order kinetics. The inhibitor is completely efficient in that only one turnover is required to completely inactivate the enzyme. The inactivation process is stereospecific in inactivator (L form) and does not occur when the enzyme is in the pyridoxamine form. In addition to irreversibly inhibiting GABA-T, gabaculine binds to this enzyme some three orders of magnitude more tightly than does GABA[15]. The mechanism of the inactivation involves the following (Fig. 8):

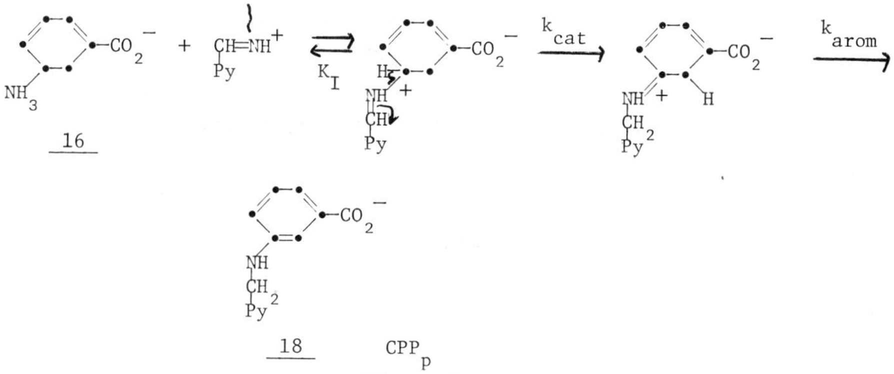

16

18   CPP$_p$

Figure 8

Meta-carboxyphenylpyridoxamine phosphate (CPP$_p$) <u>18</u> is generated at the active
site and binds so tightly to the enzyme that it can only be liberated under
denaturing conditions. The measured K_I (gabaculine) for the mouse brain
enzyme is 5.87×10^{-7}M and the $k_{cat} = 1.3 \times 10^{-3}$ sec^{-1} at $15°$[15]. It is of
interest to consider this latter term since it is of exceedingly small for an
enzyme catalyzed reaction. This means that gabaculine is a very weak substrate
for GABA-T. In general, this is what one finds for k_{cat} inactivators; they
are very poor substrates for their target enzymes. Since they are not often
isosteric with the natural substrates, this is not surprising. However,
operationally it doesn't matter if the k_{cat} inactivators are poor substrates.
This is because on a pharmacological time scale it is irrelevant if the <u>in</u>
<u>vivo</u> $T_{1/2}$ of an enzyme is 1 msec or 1 min. A further practical aspect of this
is that most published structure-activity relationships for enzyme substrates
are almost totally irrelevant as a starting point for k_{cat} inactivator design.
If a compound were found to be less than 1% as active as the natural substrate,
it would probably be reported as not being a substrate at all. However,
potent k_{cat} inactivators could be designed on the basis of much less than 1%
the rate of turnover of the natural substrate(s).

The rate-limiting step in the formation of CPP$_p$ is the k_{cat} step. This was
shown by demonstrating of deuterium isotope effect on the inactivation rate
with 5-deuterogabaculine. 6-deuterogabaculine inactivates GABA-T at the same
rate as does gabaculine[16]. That this proton is lost during the inactivation
process was shown by double labeling studies with 6-^{3}H-1-^{14}C-gabaculine. The
^{3}H/^{14}C ratio of the gabaculine inactivated enzyme proved to be approximately
1/2 that of gabaculine[16]. Proof that CPP$_p$ actually was generated during the
inactivation process was shown by isolating radiolabeled enzyme and showing
that the compound liberated under denaturing conditions was chemically identical to an authentic sample of CPP$_p$. Again model studies with gabaculine and
pyridoxal phosphate mirrored the enzymological results. Simply heating gabaculine with pyridoxal phosphate led to the formation of CPP$_p$ as the sole
product[17]. This reaction does not occur at room temperature and has an E_A of
24.8 kcal/mole. Thus, gabaculine is not a general pyridoxal phosphate antagonist but requires enzymatic conversion. The mechanism of action of gabaculine

gabaculine   α-gabaculine   β-gabaculine

predicts that isomers of this molecule should also inactivate GABA-T.   There
are three stable isomeric gabaculines.   Upon transamination all three compounds
should afford CPP_p. α-gabaculine has recently been synthesized and it indeed
inactivates GABA-T as expected[18].   In addition to being of theoretical interest,
gabaculine is also a potent inactivator of GABA-T in vivo[19].   It is able to
cross the blood-brain barrier in animals and achieve inactivation of the brain
GABA-transaminase. When given to mice i.p. a rapid and irreversible inactivation
of the brain enzyme ensues with a concomitant increase in brain GABA levels.
The behavioral pattern that develops is quite similar to that reported for the
human molecular disease hypergabanuria, where seizures occur followed by long
periods of somnolence[20].   The fact that gabaculine raises whole brain GABA
levels means that it may prove to be of clinical importance in the treatment
of certain convulsive disorders and Huntingtons disease.   In fact, it has
recently been shown that gabaculine exhibits anti-convulsive activities in
animals.   It should be emphasized that although gabaculine is an exceptionally
potent inactivator of GABA-T, it has little affinity for either the presynaptic
GABA uptake system or the GABA receptor.   Interactions with these latter
elements occur in the millimolar range which is approximately 10^3-fold higher
than the K_I for GABA-T inactivation.

  The highly novel mechanism for the gabaculine induced inactivation of GABA-
T is of great interest for a variety of reasons.   Foremost, is that it points
to a new mode of enzyme inactivation.   Since the gabaculine transformation
product need not react with the enzyme, propinquous active-site residues of
the correct chemical type are not required in order for inactivation to proceed.   Since information about the active-site of an enzyme is generally not
available prior to inactivating it, the rational design of inhibitors is not
easily imagined.   Thus the aromatization mechanism of inactivation should be
easily generalized to other pyridoxal phosphate linked enzymes.   For example,
compounds 19 should inactivate the appropriate decarboxylase depending on R,

    19   20   21

20 should inactivate aromatic amino acid transaminases, and 21 should inactivate
the appropriate α-amino acid transaminase.   Furthermore, it should be possible
to extend the aromatization mechanism of inactivation to enzymes other than
pyridoxal phosphate dependent ones.   For example, the flavin cocatalyzed

enzymes should be amenable to inactivation by these inhibitors.

As mentioned earlier, GABA-T is the enzyme responsible for the degradation of the major inhibitory neurotransmitter GABA. The enzyme involved in the biosynthesis of GABA is L-glutamate decarboxylase, also a pyridoxal phosphate linked enzyme. In the standard mechanism of action of this enzyme a carbanion is generated on C-2 as a result of the decarboxylation event (Fig. 9).

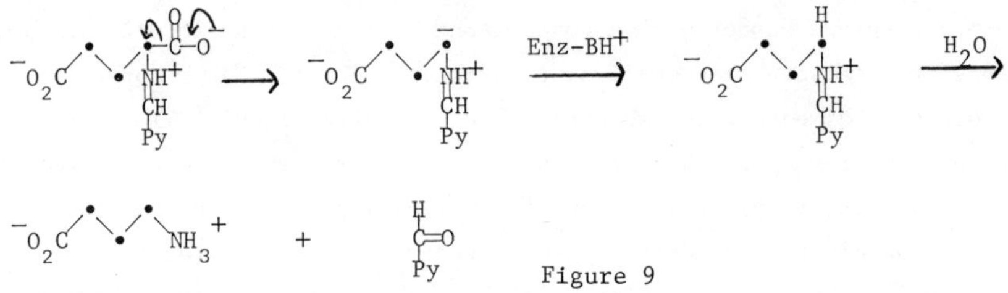

Figure 9

It would be highly useful to have an inactivator of glutamate decarboxylase as such a compound would allow for the net depletion of brain GABA and thus allow for an understanding of its in vivo roles. Furthermore, for the first time an inhibitor of this type coupled with the GABA-t inactivators would allow for the specific modulation of a neurotransmitter levels in vivo. To these ends α-methyl dehydroglutamate was synthesized 22. The methyl was added

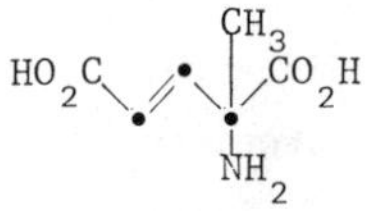

22

to the molecule to prevent it from inhibiting the many glutamate dependent transaminases that exist in cells. Since α-methyl glutamate is a substrate for glutamate decarboxylase, albeit a weak one, it was reasoned that α-methyl dehydroglutamate 22 should also be a substrate for the enzyme. This compound proved to be an inactivator of chick embryo brain glutamate decarboxylase[21]. The inhibition cannot be overcome by pyridoxal phosphate so that interaction with the cofactor cannot be at the heart of the observed inhibition which is irreversible. The typical Kitz-Wilson plot for the inactivation scheme shows that saturation occurs and that the K_I = 6.6 x 10^{-4}M and the k_{cat} for turnover is 1.01 x 10^{-3} sec^{-1}[21]. Furthermore, the substrate L-glutamate slows down the rate of inactivation which is expected if the molecule is active site directed. Preliminary studies suggest that catalytic turnover by the enzyme must occur prior to inactivation. For example, neither the apoenzyme nor hydrazine treated

holoenzyme are effected by the inhibitor . In addition, several glutamate
dependent enzymes such as ornithine decarboxylase, aspartate aminotransferase
and alanine aminotransferase have been tested and shown not to be effected by
the inhibitor. Plausable mechanisms of action for this inhibitor are indicated
in Fig. 10. Further studies will determine which, if either, of these two

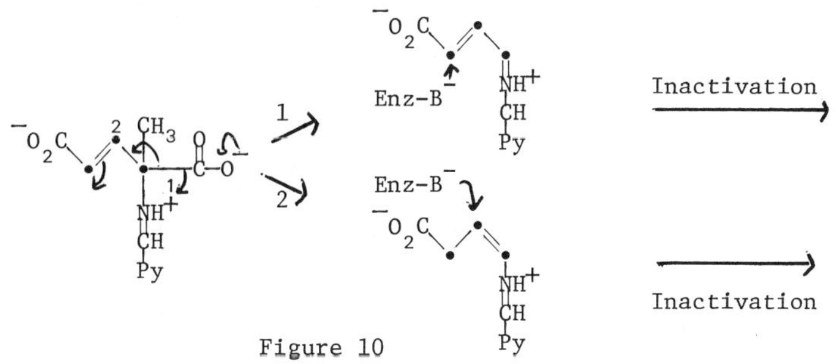

Figure 10

mechanisms describe the inhibitory process. Although preliminary tissue
culture studies suggest that the inhibitor will be a useful tool, further
studies will be required to determine the specificity of action of this
inhibitor.

SUMMARY

Vinyl glycine serves as a prototypical β,γ-unsaturated enzyme inactivator.
The introduction of double bonds β,γ to an atom suffering a formal oxidation
serves as a useful starting point in the design of k_{cat} enzyme inactivators.
For example, potent inactivators of GABA-transaminase and glutamate decarboxylase have been designed using this principle. The introduction of multiple
double bonds into a substrate leads to a new kind of irreversible enzyme
inactivator as described in the example of gabaculine where enzymatic turnover
results in the chemical linking of the substrate to the cofactor.

Acknowledgements

The work reported here was funded by U.S. Public Health Service Research
Grant NS 11550 and Research Career Development Award GM 00014, from the
National Institutes of Health.

REFERENCES

1. Baker, B.R. (1967) Design of Active-Site Directed Irreversible Enzyme
   Inhibitors. Wiley, New York.

2. Rando, R.R. (1974) Science, 185, 320–324; Abeles, R.H. and Maycock, A.L. (1976) Acct. Chem. Res., 9, 313–319.
3. Bloch, R. (1969) Acct. Chem. Res., 2, 193–202.
4. Rando, R.R. (1974) Biochem., 13, 3859–3863.
5. Ghring, H., Rando, R.R. and Christen, P. (1977) Biochem., 16, 4832–4836.
6. Rando, R.R., Relyea, N. and Cheng, L. (1976) J. Biol. Chem., 251, 3306–3312.
7. Rando, R.R. (1974) Nature, 250, 586–587.
8. Miles, E.W. (1975) Biochem. Biophys. Res. Commun., 66, 94.
9. Soda, K. and Rando, R.R. (unpublished experiments).
10. Relyea, N. and Rando, R.R. (1975) Biochem. Biophys. Res. Commun., 67, 392–402.
11. Personal Communication from Professor N. Anmrhein.
12. Giovanelli, I., Owens, L.D., and Mudd, S.H. (1971) Biochim. Biophys. Acta, 227, 671–682.
13. Lippert, B., Metcalf, B.W., Jung, M.J. and Casara, P. (1977) Eur. J. Biochem., 74, 441–446.
14. Mishima, H., Kurihara, H., Kobayashi, K., Miyazawa, S. and Terahara, A. (1976) Tett. Lett., 7, 537.
15. Rando, R.R. (1977) Biochem., 16, 4606–4610; Rando, R.R. and Bangerter, F.W. (1976) J. Amer. Chem. Soc., 98, 6762–6764.
16. Rando, R.R., unpublished experiments.
17. Rando, R.R. and Bangerter, F.W. (1977) J. Amer. Chem. Soc., 99, 5141–5145.
18. Metcalf, B., unpublished experiments.
19. Rando, R.R. and Bangerter, F.W. (1977) Biochem. Biophys. Res. Commun., 76, 1276–1281.
20. Scriver, C.R. and Perry, T.L. (1972) in The Metabolic Basis of Inherited Disease, 3rd Edition, Stanbury, J.B., Wyngaarden, D.B. and Frederickson, D.S., eds., Chapter 25, McGraw Hill, New York.
21. Chrystal, E.J.T., Bey, P. and Rando, R.R. (1979) J. Neurochem., in press.

DISCUSSION

KORYTNYK: We have synthesized the 4-vinyl analog of pyridoxal phosphate and

found it to be a potent inhibitor of pyridoxine phosphate oxidase[1] (K_i=5.3x10^{-7} M). It is also active for certain apoenzymes, e.g., it binds to apo-arginine decarboxylase very tightly (K_i=2.5x10^{-8}M), but in contrast, it has no effect with apo-D-serine dehydratase, even at a concentration of 500-fold over that of pyridoxal phosphate. We do not profess to understand the selectivity of this action, but it certainly shows that vitamin B_6 cofactor binding sites can be highly selective for very close structural analogs for the natural coenzyme.

COWARD: Have you looked at the reversible inhibition of the m-carboxyphenyl-pyridoxamine phosphate or the anthranylate analog and compared it with the measured K_i-values?

RANDO: No, the problem with the bacterial enzyme that we have used is that we cannot dissociate that material from the enzyme without denaturing the enzyme. Now, I think there are other transaminases, where in fact you can resolve the complex - maybe Dr. Walsh would like to comment on that.

WALSH: We have looked at homogeneous bacterial transaminase from *Pseudomonas* which has some advantages, you can get 100 mg of it pure, so you can easily determine the stoichiometry and reversible inhibition by m-carboxyphenyl-pyridoxamine-P - and all the kinetic and equilibrium constants bear out this mode of inhibition.

CHWANG: In one of your previous publications, you proposed that penicillin works not as a transition state analog, but rather acts as a k_{cat} inhibitor. Do you have any data to substantiate this?

RANDO: The point of that was that many of naturally occuring products in fact are substrates for their target enzymes, *e.g.*, the inhibition of acetylcholine esterase by physostigmine, which goes through an acyl-enzyme intermediate, that are hydrolyzed exceedingly slowly compared to the true substrates. There are several notions of penicillin action. One of the possibilities that penicillin is simply a substrate analog for D-alanyl-D-alanine dipeptide and in fact goes through the same acyl enzyme intermediate, but penicillin having that large bulky group does not allow the lysine to come in. So, the whole notion was simply that it could be a substrate which one might consider as one of the plausible mechanisms (still true today!). However, the absence of data with the isolated enzymes, there could be any number of mechanisms operative*.

CHU: Is it possible that the dihydro compound is not a suicide inhibitor of the transaminase, but just an inhibitor of pyridoxal phosphate? It seems to me that it inhibits pyridoxal phosphate, instead of the enzyme.

RANDO: No, it does not interact with pyridoxal phosphate, *per se*. It should be very similar to vinyl-GABA, which also, as far as I know does not react with pyridoxal phosphate. Dihydrogabaculine is not at all an inactivator of the bacterial GABA-transaminase and an exceedingly weak one of the mammalian enzyme. Earlier, we were wondering whether the aromatization mechanism does occur, so we were interested in looking at the dihydro derivative, which of course could not aromatize and indeed the mechanisms are totally different.

---

*See also Dr. Holden's paper[2] and Dr. Boyd's comments following that paper.

60

REFERENCES

1. Korytnyk, W., Hakala, M.T., Potti, P.G.G., Angelino, N. and Cheng, S.C. (1976) Biochemistry, 15, 5458.
2. Holden, K.G., Gleason, J.G., Huffman, W.F. and Perchonock, C.D. (1979) this volume.

THE MICROSCOPIC REVERSIBILITY PRINCIPLE IN ENZYME INHIBITION

BRIAN METCALF AND ALBERT SJOERDSMA
Merrell Research Center, Merrell-National Laboratories
Division of Richardson-Merrell Inc.,
2110 East Galbraith Road, Cincinnati, Ohio

INTRODUCTION

An enzyme inhibitor which requires transformation by the target enzyme prior to that enzyme's irreversible inhibition should be extremely specific, because it will inactivate only those enzymes which can accept it as a substrate. Such known inhibitors are usually analogues of the natural substrate, however, less obviously, in view of the microscopic reversibility principle, they may conceptually be analogues of the product. An example of inhibition induced by a substrate analogue is the irreversible inhibition of γ-aminobutyric acid-(GABA)-α-ketoglutarate transaminase (GABA-T) by the synthetic GABA analogue, 4-aminohex-5-ynoic acid (γ-acetylenic GABA, 1).[1,2] It was expected that the inhibition of this enzyme, the major metabolizing enzyme for the inhibitory neurotransmitter, GABA, should result in elevated brain levels of this substance. Furthermore, such an elevation could have a beneficial effect in human diseases such as Huntingtons chorea,[3] epilepsy and schizophrenia[4] where a deficiency in GABA function has been demonstrated or implicated. The proposed mechanism of inhibition of GABA-T, a pyridoxal phosphate (Py CHO) dependent enzyme by 4-aminohex-5-ynoic acid (1) is shown in Figure 1. Thus, if 4-aminohex-5-ynoic acid (1) could enter the catalytic cycle in the same manner as GABA itself, Schiff's base formation with PyCHO would occur. The usual transamination reaction, induced by abstraction of the proton α to the Schiff's base could then lead to the tautomeric imine (path a). As a result, the acetylenic function would enter into conjugation with the imine and hence be transformed into an alkylating reagent. Irreversible inhibition would then result from the covalent linkage of a nucleophilic residue (Nu) in the active site to the transformed inhibitor. Alternatively (path b) the proton abstraction described above could initiate the formation of an allene. Such an allene, being conjugated to the pyridine ring of the co-enzyme, would also be an active alkylating agent.

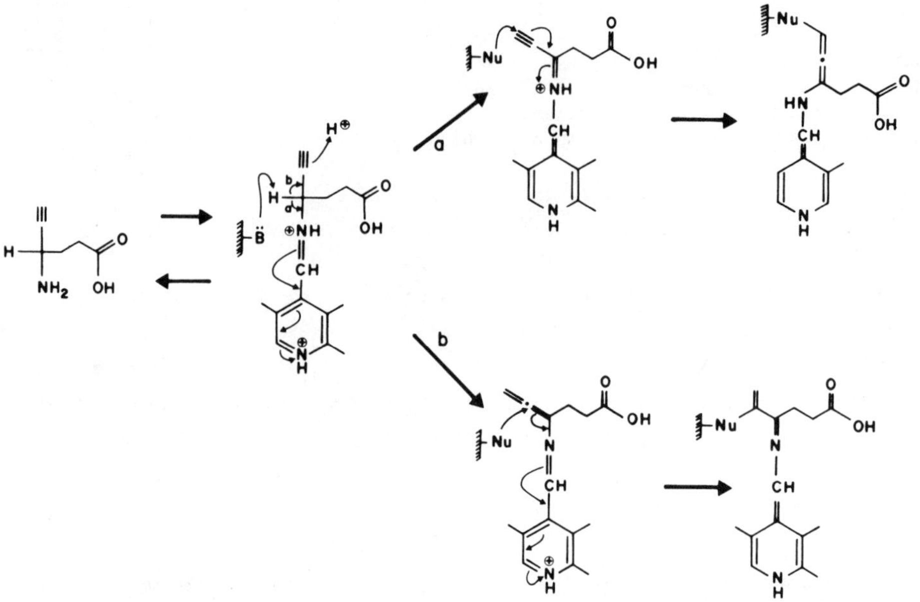

Fig. 1. Proposed mechanism of inhibition of GABA-T by (±)-4-aminohex-5-ynoic acid (1).

In practice, 1 does irreversibly inhibit GABA-T in vitro. That the inactivation process is active-site directed and involves a catalytic turnover is demonstrated by the protective effect of GABA in the absence of α-ketoglutarate. In the presence of α-ketoglutarate this protective effect is lost.[2] 1 also is active in vivo, the blockade in GABA metabolism inducing a long-lasting elevation in brain GABA levels.[5] Surprisingly, further in vivo studies revealed that the GABA synthesizing enzyme, glutamic acid decarboxylase (GAD), another PyCHO-dependent enzyme, is also inhibited by 1, although to a lesser extent than is GABA-T.

As GAD normally catalyses the loss of CO_2 from the α-amino acid glutamate, its inhibition by a propargylic amine, 4-aminohex-5-ynoic acid (1) was unexpected because, according to our initial premise, for inhibition to occur 1 must be a substrate for the target enzyme so that it can be activated as a consequence of the enzyme's usual mechanism of action. It was at this point, with the microscopic reversibility principle in mind, that we decided to probe further the mechanism of the inhibition of GAD by 1.

63

BACTERIAL GLUTAMIC ACID DECARBOXYLASE

Commercially-available bacterial GAD was chosen for further in vitro study.
A major consideration guiding the choice of the bacterial and not the mammalian
enzyme in the initial studies was that the stereochemistry of the replacement
of carboxyl by hydrogen in the decarboxylation reaction had been determined with
the bacterial enzyme and had been found to proceed with retention of configuration.[6]

Incubation of GAD from E. coli with 1 results in a time-dependent loss of
enzyme activity which follows pseudo first order kinetics until the inhibition
is essentially complete[7] (Figure 2). Protection against inactivation is
afforded by 2-methylglutamate and by L-glutamate itself, suggesting that the
inactivation process is active-site directed. A kinetic isotopic effect of 2.5
at 0.33 mM inhibitor is found when the rate of inhibition induced by 4-deuterio-
4-aminohex-5-ynoic acid is compared with that observed with 1, demonstrating
that inhibition involves a catalytically-functioning enzyme and requires
abstraction of the propargylic hydrogen. The inhibition is also stereospecific
as (±) 1 was resolved and the inhibitory activity found to reside with the

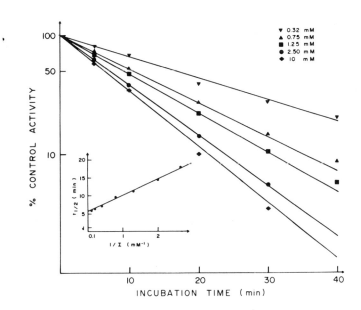

Fig. 2. Inhibition of bacterial GAD by (±)-4-aminohex-5-ynoic acid (1).

(-) isomer. This was assigned the R absolute configuration as oxidation with RuO₄ afforded R(-)glutamate, while the (+) isomer yielded S(+)glutamic acid.[7]

As illustrated below, these results are compatible with a mechanism of inactivation which relies on the microscopic reversibility principle. Figure 3 shows the normal mechanism for the enzymatic replacement of CO_2 with H. As this reaction occurs with retention of configuration at the α-carbon,[6] it is the pro-4 R hydrogen of GABA which is potentially labile in the reverse direction. If 4(R)-4-aminohex-5-ynoic acid, which bears a proton stereochemically corresponding to that which replaces CO_2 in 2(S)glutamic acid, can replace GABA in the active site, then the proton abstraction implicit in the reverse reaction should lead to the formation of a propargylic anionic intermediate which could induce irreversible inactivation of the enzyme by either of paths a or b (Figure 4). Although proton exchange of the 4-pro R hydrogen of GABA catalyzed by GAD has not been detectable,[6] it is feasible that with 4(R)-4-aminohex-5-ynoic acid, this proton abstraction is facilitated by the adjacent acetylenic group.

Exploitation of the microscopic reversibility principle presages a new concept for the irreversible inhibition of amino acid decarboxylases. The next section describes its successful application to the inhibition of mammalian ornithine decarboxylase.

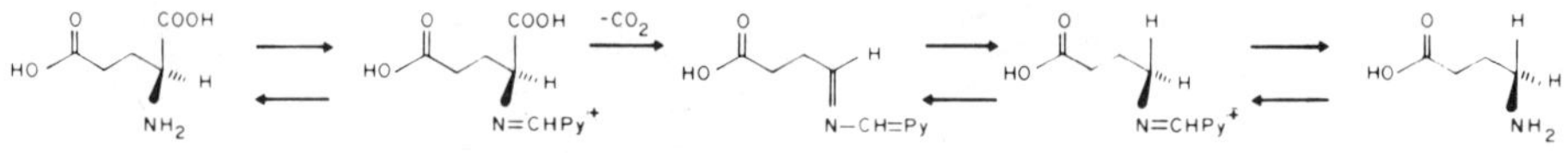

Fig. 3. Decarboxylation of 2(S)-Glutamic Acid by GAD.

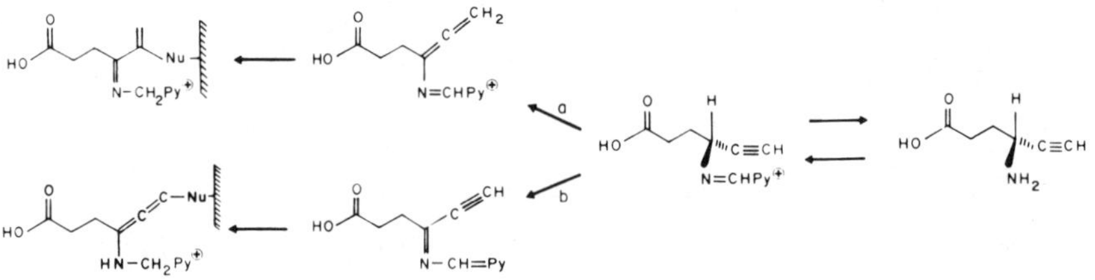

Fig. 4. Proposed mechanism of inhibition of bacterial GAD by 4(R)-4-aminohex-5-ynoic acid.

ORNITHINE DECARBOXYLASE

Ornithine decarboxylase (ODC) is another PyCHO-dependent enzyme which catalyzes the conversion of ornithine to putrescine. Putrescine is in turn converted to the higher polyamines spermidine and spermine[8] (Figure 5). These
polyamines have been implicated in the regulation of growth processes and an
induction of ODC, with the resultant elevation of polyamine levels, has been
correlated with conditions of rapid cell proliferation.[9]

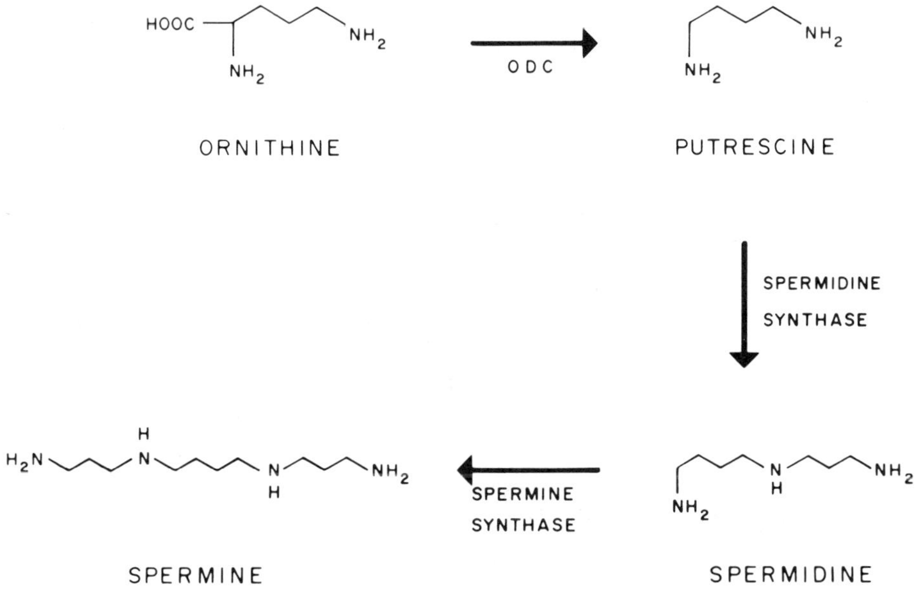

Fig. 5. Polyamine biosynthetic pathway.

With the intention of exploiting the microscopic reversibility principle, the
putrescine analogues 5-hexyne-1,4-diamine (2) and trans-5-hexyne-1,4-diamine-
but-2-ene (3) were synthesized and their inhibitory activity towards ODC
assessed.[10] The unsaturated analogue 3 was included in the study because
Relyea and Rando[11] had shown that trans-1,4-diaminobut-2-ene (dehydroputrescine)
has an affinity for ODC more than 10,000 times that of putrescine itself and
had suggested that this is due, in part, to a preferential binding of the
extended conformer.

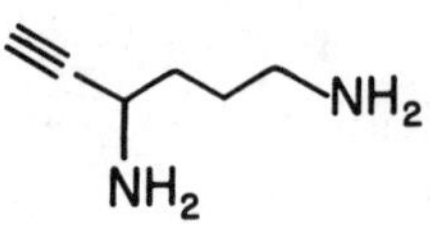

2 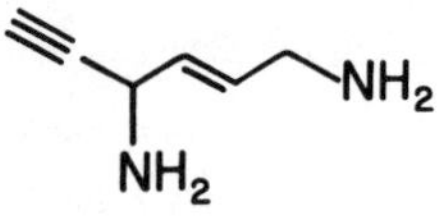   3

Incubation of the enzyme preparation obtained from livers of thioacetamide-
treated rats at pH 7 with 2 resulted in a time-dependent loss of enzyme activity
which followed pseudo-first-order kinetics for at least two half lives (Figure
6). Over longer time periods, the semilogarithmic plots deviated from linearity.
However, incubation with 2 at 0.1 mM concentration resulted in 95% inactivation
of ODC after 10 min. Prolonged (24 h) dialysis of enzyme previously inactivated
by 2 against a buffer solution containing phosphate (30 mM), pyridoxal phosphate
(0.1 mM), and dithiothreitol (5 mM) (conditions where the native enzyme is
stable) did not lead to regeneration of enzyme activity, thus demonstrating the
irreversibility of the process. That the inhibition of ODC is active site
directed is shown by the protective effects of the natural substrate L-ornithine,
of a competitive inhibitor 2-methylornithine[12] and of putrescine, the product of
decarboxylation, against induced inactivation (Figure 6). The presence of
dithiothreitol (5 mM) in the preincubation medium and the absence of lag time
before the onset of inhibition rule out the possibility of inhibition via an
affinity labeling mode by a diffusible alkylating species. The unsaturated
analogue 3 gave similar results, although was found to be more active (Table 1).

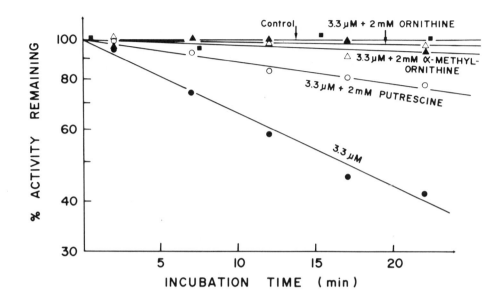

Fig. 6. Irreversible inhibition of rat liver ODC by (±) 5-hexyne-1,4-diamine
(2).

Further evidence for the involvement of the enzyme's active site in the
inhibitory process comes from the observed saturation effect (Table 1) on the
rate of inactivation (demonstrated by plotting t 1/2 as a function of 1/I
according to Kitz and Wilson).[13]   Moreover, with 2, the inhibitory activity
resides with only one optical isomer ((-)-2), the other isomer being essentially
inactive.

TABLE 1

KINETIC CONSTANTS FOR THE IRREVERSIBLE INHIBITION OF RAT LIVER ODC

Compound	K_I, μM	τ_{50}, min	k inact, S^{-1}
2	2.3	9.7	1.2×10^{-3}
[^{2}H]-2	4.3	9.6	1.2×10^{-3}
3	1	5	2.3×10^{-3}

K_I = apparent dissociation constant
τ_{50} = half life at infinite inhibitor concentration
k inact = inactivation rate constant

When the rate of inhibition induced by 4-deuterio-hex-5-yne-1,4-diamine
($[^2H]\underline{2}$) was compared with that observed with $\underline{2}$, no kinetic isotope effect on
the inactivation rate constant was observed, but rather a primary kinetic
isotope effect on the apparent Michaelis constant is measured (Figure 7).
Proton abstraction hence must occur, but is not rate limiting. We have observed
a comparable isotopic effect on the apparent binding constants for GAD with the
isotopes of $\underline{1}$, while Belleau and Moran[14] have attributed a similar effect
observed with monoamine oxidase to some degree of bond elongation taking place
during the binding step.

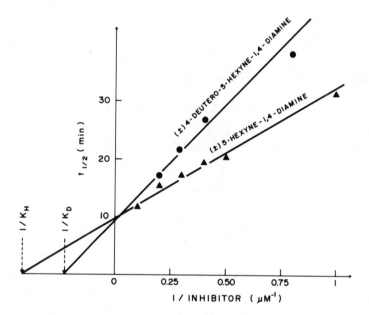

Fig. 7. Isotope effects.

$\underline{2}$ and $\underline{3}$ inhibit ODC in vivo,[15] with a single dose of 100 mg/kg of either
compound in rats producing a near-total decrease of ornithine decarboxylase
activity in prostate and to a lesser extent in thymus and testis (Figure 8).
Three doses of 100 mg/kg of $\underline{2}$ during a 24 hour period markedly decreased
putrescine concentrations in the three organs studied, while spermidine levels
were also lowered in the prostate.

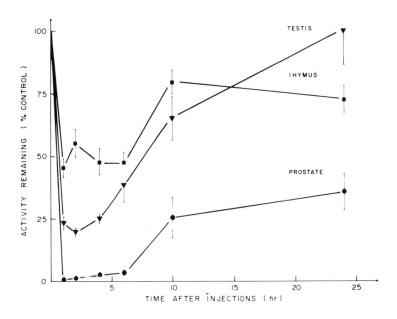

Fig. 8. Effects of a single dose of 5-hexyne-1,4-diamine (2) 100 mg/kg ip on rat prostate, thymus and testis ODC activities (Mean ± Sem, n = 5)[15]

Prolonged treatment of rats with 2 induces behavior reminiscent of that of animals which had received the GABA-T inhibitor 4-aminohex-5-ynoic acid (1). It has now been confirmed that 2 is converted to 1 via a mitochondrial pathway involving monoamine oxidase.[16] It was hoped that the allylamine analogue 3 would not be subject to an analogous transformation because allylamine itself had previously been shown to be a pseudo-irreversible inhibitor of monoamine oxidase.[17] This, however, is not the case, as administration of 3 also leads to an inhibition of brain GABA-T, as well as of prostatic ODC. This unwanted transformation has been overcome using the analogue 4, which, being an α-disubstituted amine, is no longer a substrate for monoamine oxidase. ODC inhibitory activity, however, is retained.[18]

4

PERSPECTIVE

That the microscopic reversibility principle can be used to advantage in the design of enzyme-activated irreversible inhibitors has been hitherto unexploited. Thus, inhibition by product analogues offers to be a powerful complement to the more common use of substrate analogues. In the context of α-amino acid decarboxylases, loss of carbon dioxide from an enzyme-bound substrate analogue should also lead to carbanion formation in the active site. α-acetylenic-α-aminoacids hence could be expected to be irreversible inhibitors of the corresponding amino acid decarboxylases. We have recently synthesized α-acetylenic glutamate[19] and α-acetylenic ornithine[20] which have been found to be irreversible inhibitors of GAD and ODC respectively.[21] On the other hand, α-acetylenic DOPA[22,23] inhibits aromatic amino acid decarboxylase in a competitive manner (K_I = 0.3 μm), the irreversible component, although present, is rather weak.[24] It has also been reported that α-difluoromethylornithine is an irreversible inhibitor of ODC,[10] while several monofluoromethyl amino acids and amines irreversibly inhibit the corresponding amino acid decarboxylases.[25,26] At the moment, it is difficult to predict for a given decarboxylase whether the substrate or product analogue will prove to be a more effective inhibitor.

The situation is further complicated by our finding that in contrast to the inhibition of bacterial GAD by 4(R)-4-aminohex-5-ynoic acid, mammalian GAD is inhibited by the 4(S) isomer.[7] As mammalian GAD has recently been shown to decarboxylate glutamate with retention of configuration[27] it appears that a mechanism other than microscopic reversibility can be operative for inhibition by product analogues in some cases. This is further borne out by the report[25] that (R)-fluoromethyldopamine irreversibly inhibits aromatic amino acid decarboxylase, while (S)-fluoromethyl histamine inhibits histidine decarboxylase.

ACKNOWLEDGEMENTS

The work described above has been carried out in the Centre de Recherche Merrell International, Strasbourg, France in collaboration with Michel Jung, Patrick Casara, Charles Danzin, Bruce Lippert, Karin Jund, Edith Bonilavri, and Benoit Reger.

Figure 1 is reproduced from B. W. Metcalf et al, "γ-Acetylenic GABA and γ-vinyl GABA-two enzyme-activated irreversible inhibitors of GABA aminotransferase" in "GABA Neurotransmitters," Alfred Benzon Symposium 12, Munksgaard, 1978. Figures 2, 3, and 4 are reprinted from M. J. Jung et al, Biochemistry, 17, 2628-2632 (1978). Figure 8 is reproduced from C. Danzin et al, Biochem. Pharmacol., 28, 627-631 (1979).

REFERENCES

1. Metcalf, B.W. and Casara, P. (1975) Tetrahedron Lett., 3337-3340.
2. Jung, M.J. and Metcalf, B.W. (1975) Biochem. Biophys. Res. Commun., 67, 301-306.
3. Bird, E.D., Mackay, A.V.P., Raynor, C.N. and Iverson, L.L. (1973) Lancet, 1, 1090-1092.
4. Roberts, E. (1974) Biochem. Pharmacol., 23, 2637-2649.
5. Jung, M.J., Lippert, B., Metcalf, B.W., Schechter, P.S., Böhlen, P., and Sjoerdsma, A. (1977) J. Neurochem., 28, 717-723.
6. Yamada, Y. and O'Leary, M.H. (1978) Biochemistry, 17, 669-672.
7. Jung, M.J., Metcalf, B.W., Lippert, B. and Casara, P. (1978) Biochemistry, 17, 2628-2632.
8. Russell, D.H. (1973) "Polyamines in Normal and Neoplastic Growth," Raven Press, New York, N.Y.
9. Mamont, P.S., Böhlen, P., McCann, P.P., Bey, P., Schuber, F. and Tardif, C. (1976) Proc. Nat. Acad. Sci., U.S.A., 73, 1626-1630.
10. Metcalf, B.W., Bey, P., Danzin, C., Jung, M.J., Casara, P., and Vèvert, J.P., (1978) J. Amer. Chem. Soc., 100, 2551-2553.
11. Relyea, N. and Rando, R.R. (1975) Biochem. Biophys. Res. Commun., 67, 392-397.
12. Abdel-Monem, M.M., Newton, N.W., and Weeks, C.E. (1974) J. Med. Chem., 17, 447-451.
13. Kitz, R., Wilson, I.B. (1964) J. Biol. Chem., 237, 3245-3249.
14. Belleau, B. and Moran, J. (1963) Ann. N.Y. Acad. Sci., 107, 822-839.
15. Danzin, C., Jung, M.J., Metcalf, B.W., Grove, J., and Casara, P. (1979) Biochem. Pharmacol., 28, 627-631.
16. Danzin, C., Jung, M.J., Seiler, N., and Metcalf, B.W. (1979) Biochem. Pharmacol., 26, 633-639.
17. Rando, R.R., and Eigner, A. (1977) Molecular Pharmacology, 13, 1005-1013.
18. Metcalf, B.W., Bonilavri, E., Danzin, C., and Jung, M.J., unpublished work.
19. Casara, P. and Metcalf, B.W. (1978) Tetrahedron Lett., 1581-1584.
20. Casara, P., Jund, K. and Metcalf, B.W., unpublished work.
21. Casara, P., Danzin, C., Jung, M.J., and Metcalf, B.W., unpublished work.
22. Metcalf, B.W. and Jund, K. (1977) Tetrahedron Lett., 3689-3692.
23. Taub, D. and Patchett, A.A. (1977) Tetrahedron Lett., 2745-2747.
24. Ribereau-Gayon, G., Danzin, C., Palfreyman, M.G., Aubry, M., Wagner, J., Metcalf, B.W., and Jung, M.J., Biochem. Pharmacol., in press.
25. Kollonitsch, J., Patchett, A.A., Marburg, S., Maycock, A.L., Perkins, L.M., Doldouras, G.A., Duggan, D.E., and Aster, S.D. (1978) Nature, 274, 906-908.
26. Jung, M.J., this symposium.
27. Bouclier, M., Jung, M.J., and Lippert, B. (1979) Eur. J. Biochem., in press.

DISCUSSION

WALSH: Can you distinguish between the two alternative mechanisms of the addition of the enzymic nucleophile, whether it attacks the allene after the postulated propargylic rearrangement, or if it attacks the acetylenic terminus, in the case of the acetylenic Michael?

METCALF: We would like to do this. We see no other way to find out whether it is an allenic rearrangement, except to degrade the inactivated enzyme, but we have not done this yet.

WALSH: We have similar problems, I just wondered, if you had resolved it.

METCALF: No, we have not.

P. BARTLETT: Speaking to the point which Prof. Walsh raised, perhaps you could distinguish between the two mechanisms of inactivation by considering the following. It is reasonable to assume that the rate limiting step of inactivation in each case would involve nucleophilic attack by the enzyme-bound group. You could distinguish presumably the mechanism of the substitution of the allene vs. the conjugate addition to the acetylene by deuterium isotope effect of the acetylenic proton. If you replace the acetylenic hydrogen with deuterium, you would expect to see an isotope effect if there were direct attack on that carbon, converting it from sp to sp^2 hybridized. Whereas, if you do a direct attack on allenic carbon that should not effect the terminus, in which the deuterium resides.

METCALF: That is a nice idea. Thank you.

FEDOR: Picking up on that last point, on the acetylenic spermine derivative (2) I recall that you used the deuterium substituted compound and found no isotope effect on inactivation, but found one on binding. If allene formation is necessary for inactivation, I wonder if one could consider the possibility that the proton transfer step out is not in fact rate determining, as the lack of isotope effect suggests, but possibly proton transfer back into the acetylenic carbon to give the allene might be rate determining, which point might be addressed by running the reaction in D_2O. In base catalyzed isomerization of β,γ-unsaturated ketones to α,β-unsaturated ketones, deprotonation at α-C is fast and protonation at γ-C is rate determining.[1]

METCALF: We have not tried to run the reaction in D_2O. We should do it.

CHOWDHRY: I think you said in the acetylenic GABA case one of enantiomers inactivated, the other one protected by way of binding, but no inactivation occurred.

METCALF: Yes. In the case of glutamic acid decarboxylase the (+) isomer protected against the inactivation by the (-) isomer.

CHOWDHRY: I am curious to know whether or not you get racemization accompanying the inactivation by one enantiomer? Essentially, what is the partitioning of the proton going back, as opposed to inactivation event?

METCALF: We have not followed it long enough. For the time periods in which we followed this, each isomer seems to retain its integrity, but we have not followed this for very long times.

CHOWDHRY: If that ratio is large, you have to follow it for quite sometime, before you would be able to detect it.

METCALF: Probably. Yes.

CHOWDHRY: These compounds apparently are active *in vivo* and I am curious, if you know anything about the transport mechanism across the blood brain barrier for these compounds?

METCALF: We measured the concentrations of each inhibitor in the brain after administration and there is a very small amount, which enters. Probably does not enter any better than GABA itself, or maybe slightly better. Of course the amount which enters must simply be enough to inhibit the enzyme.

CHOWDHRY: Over long term administration, I am curious, whether you might get inactivation of the transport system itself and whether that may be one of the side effects?

METCALF: We followed inactivation over long periods of time and enzyme levels remained low, suggesting that the compounds still get in over a long period of time.

REFERENCE

1. Whalen, D.L.; Weimaster, J.F.; Ross, A.M.; Radhe, R. (1976) J. Am. Chem. Soc. 98, 7319.

Published 1979 by Elsevier North Holland, Inc.
Kalman, ed. Drug Action and Design: Mechanism-Based Enzyme Inhibitors

SURVIVAL AND RECOVERY: THE REVERSIBILITY OF COVALENT DRUG-ENZYME INTERACTIONS

THOMAS I. KALMAN AND JACK C. YALOWICH
State University of New York at Buffalo, Departments of Medicinal Chemistry and
Biochemical Pharmacology, School of Pharmacy, Amherst, New York 14260

INTRODUCTION AND REVIEW

Brian Metcalf demonstrated in his presentation[1] that in agreement with the
principle of microscopic reversibility some enzymes may commit suicide by
allowing the proper inhibitory analogs to enter the inactivation pathway
from either the substrate or the product side of the catalytic reaction
sequence and thus become trapped in the covalent E-I complex (see Figure 1,
solid arrows). The same principle predicts that there must be a finite

Figure 1.

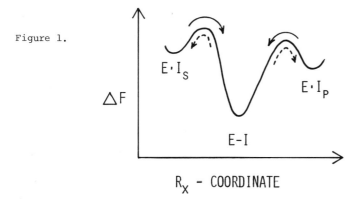

probability of escaping from the trap by the exact reversal of the inactivation
reaction (see Figure 1, *broken arrows*). The efficiency of such a reactivation
process is inversely related to the relative heights of the energy barriers
confronting the E-I complex. Unless the reversal reaction coincides with the
lowest energy pathway (which the escape route must follow), the microscopic
reversibility principle will not apply. Thus, if the relative stability of
the E-I complex permits significant decomposition to occur with concomitant
recovery of catalytic activity, one may encounter different types of enzyme
reactivation mechanisms.

Mechanisms of Spontaneous Regeneration of Catalytic Activity from Covalent
Enzyme-Inhibitor Complexes

In the context of the topics of this Symposium it is of interest to review briefly the main types of spontaneous enzyme reactivation mechanisms which may also occur *in vivo*, since the dynamics of drug action at the target site is one of the critical factors determining pharmacological activity.

The following 3 representative mechanisms were chosen for this discussion:

(1) slow turnover;

(2) reversal of the inactivation reaction;

(3) degradation of enzyme-bound inhibitor.

It should be emphasized that we are concerned with *spontaneous* reactivation processes which require the structural and functional integrity of the active site and therefore can be considered 'enzyme-catalyzed'. The release of a radioactive inhibitor from the covalent complex usually takes place under native conditions. Unless the linkage is thermodynamically unstable, denaturation leads to the permanent attachment of the label to the protein and separation cannot be affected without resorting to appropriate chemical treatment.

(1) Slow turnover. Physostigmine (eserine), a drug which has been used for a century in the treatment of glaucoma and a large number of other parasympathomimetic carbamates inhibit acetylcholinesterase, because they are "substrates with exceptionally low turnover rates"[2] (see scheme below, $k_3 \ll k_2$; $k_{-2}=0$). The rate of enzymatic hydrolysis of physostigmine is some 7 orders

$$ E + I \xrightleftharpoons[k_{-1}]{k_1} E\cdot I \xrightleftharpoons[k_{-2}]{k_2} E\text{-}I \xrightarrow{k_3} I' \qquad (1) $$

of magnitude slower than that of acetylcholine, indicating the relative stability of the carbamylated enzyme (E-I) toward hydrolysis ($k_3=0.018\text{min}^{-1}$).[3] Organic phosphate inhibitors of cholinesterases act in an analogous way.[4-6] The turnover rate of dimethyl-4-nitrophenylphosphate is $3.5\text{x}10^7$ times slower than that of acetylcholine.

(2) Reversal of the inactivation reaction. Enzyme reactivation following this mechanism, in accordance with the microscopic reversibility principle, leads to the reformation of the original structure of the inhibitor and the enzyme (including the coenzyme), irrespective of whether the inhibitor is an analog of the substrate, the product, an activated intermediate (or transition state). Thus, according to the scheme $k_{-2}>0$; $k_3 \geqq 0$.

The reversibility of the inactivation process depends on the nature of the chemical reaction leading to the formation of the covalent complex. For instance, if a leaving group other than hydrogen ion (or water) is involved, its diffusion away from the reaction site will preclude an effective back-reaction, even when an intrinsic reversibility persists. Often, in the presence of a very large concentration of the free leaving group, reversibility in this type of reaction can still be demonstrated. Acetylcholinesterase from electric eel is inactivated by diethyl phosphorofluoridate through phosphorylation of the active site serine residue. The enzyme can be reactivated[7] by fluoride *via* reversal of the phosphorylation reaction (see scheme below). The actual values for k_{inact} and k_{react} are 2.3×10^5 $M^{-1} min^{-1}$ and 10 $M^{-1} min^{-1}$, respectively.

$$HO-ENZ \; + \; (ETO)_2\overset{\overset{\displaystyle O}{\|}}{P}-F \; \underset{k_{REACT}}{\overset{k_{INACT}}{\rightleftharpoons}} \; (ETO)_2\overset{\overset{\displaystyle O}{\|}}{P}-OENZ \cdot H^+ \; + \; F^- \qquad (2)$$

If the leaving group remains attached to the inhibitor after covalent complex formation, like in the case of *cyclic* esters (such as lactones, sultones, and cyclic phosphodiesters) the spontaneous reversal of the reaction is possible even when the reformation of the cyclic structure is thermodynamically unfavorable (the reversal is then under kinetic control). This was clearly demonstrated by Kaiser *et al.*[8] in the case of the phosphorylation of chymotrypsin by catechol cyclic phosphate. The kinetic constants characterizing the system outlined in Figure 2 are:

$k_2 k_1 / k_{-1} = 3 \times 10^2$ $M^{-1} sec^{-1}$; $k_{-2} = 3.8 \times 10^{-4} sec^{-1}$ and $k_3 = 3.4 \times 10^{-7} sec^{-1}$.

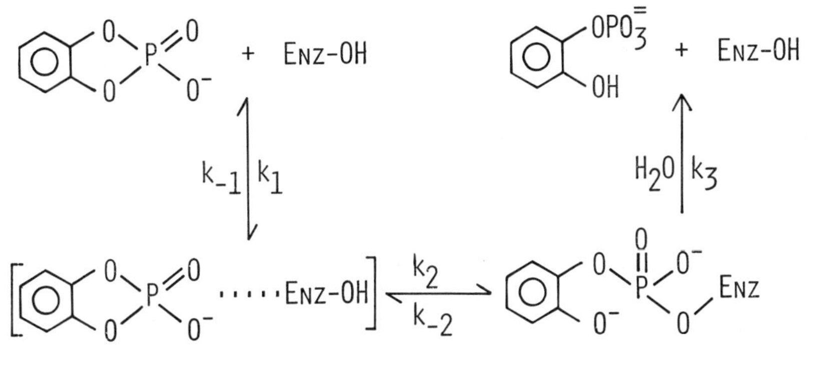

Figure 2. Reversible phosphorylation of chymotrypsin by catechol cyclic phosphate.[8]

A large number of potentially reversible reactions fall into the category of *addition to unsaturation*. Aldehyde inhibitors[9-14] of serine and cysteine proteases form covalently linked hemiacetals and thiohemiacetals, respectively, which mimic the structure of the tetrahedral transition states involved in the enzyme catalyzed reaction (see following scheme, x = 0 or S).

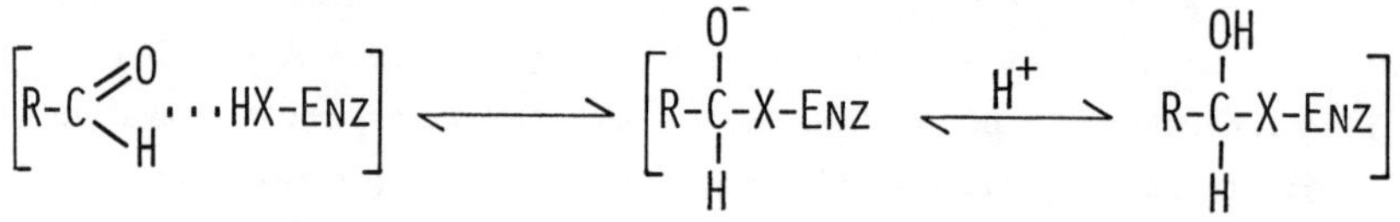

$$\left[R-C\overset{O}{\underset{H}{\diagdown}}\cdots HX-Enz\right] \longrightarrow \left[R-\overset{O^-}{\underset{H}{\underset{|}{\overset{|}{C}}}}-X-Enz \overset{H^+}{\longleftarrow} R-\overset{OH}{\underset{H}{\underset{|}{\overset{|}{C}}}}-X-Enz\right]$$

In the case of the inhibition of α-chymotrypsin by N-benzoyl-L-phenyl-alaninal, the rate constant for the breakdown of the tetrahedral hemiacetal is only about 10^3-fold lower than that for its formation.[13] Reversible tetrahedral adduct formation with boronic acid derivatives of substrates also occurs with the active site serine-OH of proteolytic enzymes[15-17] and acetylcholine esterase.[18]

The interaction of cyclopropanone hydrate with sulfhydryl enzymes, as exemplified by the reversible inactivation of aldehyde dehydrogenase[19,20] involves the reversible formation of the corresponding tetrahedral thio-hemiketal:

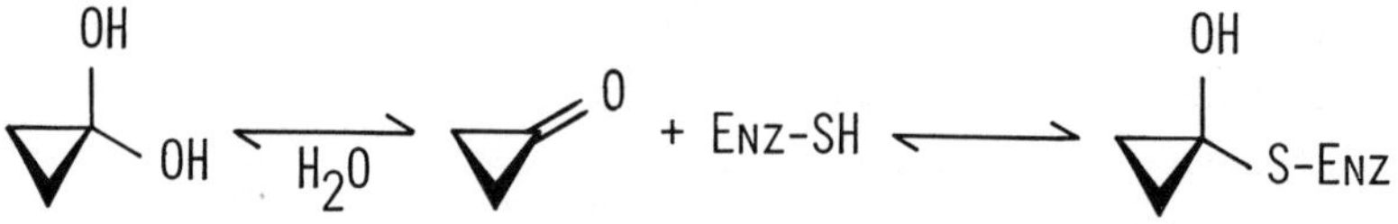

Addition of enzymic SH-groups to activated carbon-carbon double bonds can also occur in a reversible fashion as part of the catalytic mechanism.[21] Thymidylate (dTMP) synthetase is inactivated by certain 5-substituted deoxy-uridylate (dUMP) analogs, through the reversible formation of 5,6-dihydro-pyrimidine adducts[22] with an active site SH-group[22-25]. Thus, in the presence[26] or absence[27,28] of the cofactor, the 5'-monophosphate of the antiviral[29,30] 5-nitro-2'-deoxyuridine[26,29,31] inactivates L. casei dTMP synthetase by forming an "enzyme generated transition state analog (or reactive intermediate)"[32] via reversible covalent interaction with an active site cysteine residue[26] as outlined below (see also Dr. Santi's paper).[33]

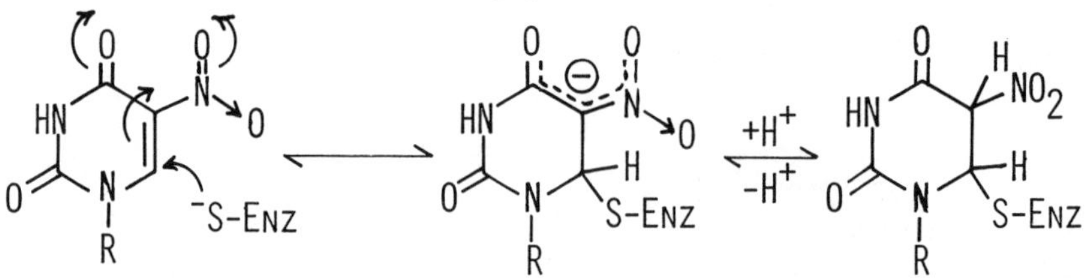

Studies with mammalian cellular systems[30,33-35] established the inhibition of dTMP synthetase in vivo, when cells are exposed to 5-nitro-2'-deoxyuridine.

Suicide inactivators bearing a vinyl or ethynyl group[36-38] with prior catalytic activation[39] can accept nucleophiles of the enzyme or coenzyme and the resulting adducts may, in principle, decompose by reversal of the conjugate addition leading to their formation. Additional chemical transformations, however, often divert the product from the truly reversible pathway.

Enzyme catalyzed reversal of covalent bond formation between a coenzyme and an inhibitor was elegantly demonstrated in the case of pyruvate dehydrogenase.[40,41] Methyl acetylphosphonate is an analog of pyruvate and inhibits the enzyme with a K_i-value of 5×10^{-8} M; a mechanism outlined below was postulated to account for the high affinity.[40] The proposed intermediate analog methyl

1-ethane-(2'-thiamine diphosphate)phosphonate was prepared and incubated with apo-pyruvate dehydrogenase, lacking thiamine diphosphate. The enzyme converted one enantiomer to thiamine diphosphate (and methyl acetylphosphonate) on the basis of the principle of microscopic reversibility and reconstituted the active holoenzyme.[41]

It is tempting to speculate that the extremely tight but reversible binding of methotrexate to dihydrofolate reductase may reflect covalent interaction between the inhibitor and the active site aspartate[42] residue (see Figure 3), forming a carboxylate adduct at C-8a of the diamino pteridine. This hypothesis is not inconsistent with the x-ray structure[43] of the drug-enzyme-NADPH ternary complex and a recent analysis of available nmr data.[44]

(3) Degradation of enzyme-bound inhibitor. The covalently bound inhibitor may undergo enzyme mediated transformation(s) and become released as one or more structures which are distinct from the product(s) of a normal catalytic turnover. As expected, this process also leads to spontaneous enzyme reactivation. The fragmentation of penicillins and cephalosporins by various penicillin binding target enzymes is an interesting example of this process, which depends on the structure of the β-lactam antibiotic and the type and source of the binding protein.[46-48] For instance, the stability of the covalent benzylpencillin-DD-carboxypeptidase complex from different bacterial species varies widely: the characteristic half-life values range for < 5 min to > 4 hrs.[46]

There are many more examples for reactivation mechanisms involving the

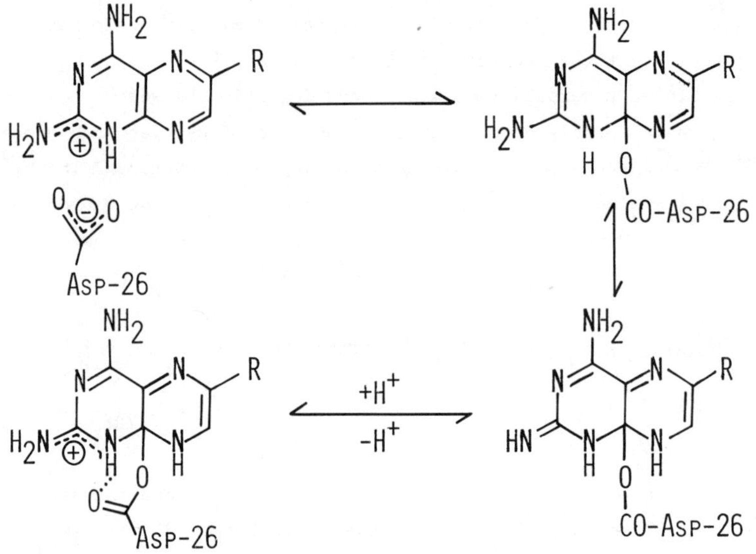

Figure 3.   Postulated reversible covalent binding of methotrexate to
            L. casei dihydrofolate reductase. *

release of the inhibitor from the covalent complex with a permanent loss of
the drug's ability to inactivate the enzyme, due to a structural change taking
place within the complex.   Many of these examples were subject of discussion
during this Symposium.

Alanine racemase is reversibly inactivated by D- and L-fluoroalanine.[49]
D-Cycloserine inactivates serine transhydroxymethylase involving transamination.[49]   The same enzyme can regain its catalytic activity under the
proper circumstances after inactivation by D-fluoroalanine, with the concomitant conversion of the latter to pyruvate.[49]

The mechanism of inactivation of dopa decarboxylase by α-vinyldopa and
α-ethynyldopa[50,51] is complex, but the inhibition is largely reversible and
the analogs are decarboxylated during their interaction with the enzyme.[50]

Mitochondrial monoamine oxidase inactivated by N-cyclopropylbenzylamine
can be reactivated by dialysis at pH 9.0 or gel filtration, but the released
inhibitor is no longer N-cyclopropylbenzylamine.[52]

---

* A detailed description of the model will be presented elsewhere.[45]

Significance of Spontaneous Regeneration of Catalytic Activity from Covalent
Enzyme-Inhibitor Complexes

The pharmacological activity and ultimately the therapeutic effectiveness
of drugs which act as tight binding inhibitors of enzymes, is greatly influenced and often determined by the dynamics of drug-target interactions, representing 'bioavailability at the molecular level'. After the elimination of
99%+ of a single dose of a drug, the target site occupancy of a stiochiome-
trically binding inhibitor is still 100%. Once the free drug concentration
drops below that of the target enzyme, the reappearance of catalytic activity
will depend only on 2 factors: the 'residence time' of the drug in the inactive
enzyme complex and the rate of new enzyme synthesis. If the rate of enzyme
reactivation is effectively zero or slower than that of new enzyme synthesis,
the speed of the recovery process and the duration of drug action will become
a drug-independent variable. It is clear that in many situations this would
be highly undesirable. Silverman[52] alluded to the idea of using potentially
reversible monoamine oxidase inhibitors to safeguard against dietary hypertensive crises.

If the rate of enzyme reactivation is faster than that of new enzyme
synthesis then the relative speed of the recovery process will depend on the
molecular mechanism of the drug-target interaction, which is influenced by
the structure of the drug, as discussed above. Thus, if it is of therapeutic
advantage to control *both* the inactivation and the reactivation of a target
enzyme, then there is an additional dimension in the design of mechanism-based
enzyme inhibitors, which medicinal chemists could take into consideration.

In the following section, we will discuss some of our studies relating to
the reversibility of the inactivation of thymidylate synthetase by 5-substituted
pyrimidine nucleotide analogs using a purified bacterial enzyme and a mammalian
intact cell system.

RESULTS AND DISCUSSION

The most potent inhibitor of thymidylate (dTMP) synthetase[53] *in vitro* and
in vivo is 5-fluoro-2'-deoxyuridylate (FdUMP) the active form[54] of the anti-
neoplastic 5-fluoropyrimidines.[55] Our current knowledge about the catalytic
mechanism of dTMP synthetase[33,56] and its interaction with FdUMP[33,56,57] has
mostly been gained through the study of the purified enzyme[58] from a methotrexate resistant mutant strain of *Lactobacillus casei*.[59] Recently, the
complete amino acid sequence of this enzyme was reported.[60]

The postulated structure of the enzyme-bound drug in the inactive ternary complex is shown in Figure 3 of Dr. Santi's paper.[33] Denaturation leads to permanent attachment of the tetrahydrofolate cofactor-linked FdUMP to the polypeptide, through the sulfur of Cys-198 of the *L. casei* enzyme[25,60] (see Figure 4).

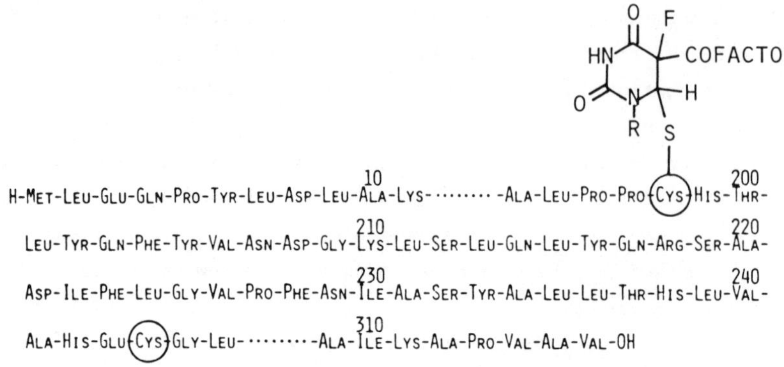

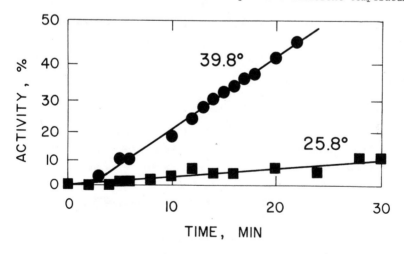

Figure 4.   Partial sequence of *L. casei* dTMP synthetase (after Maley *et al.*[60]) and the point of covalent attachment of FdUMP to the active site cysteine residue.

Studies of the Reactivation of *L. casei* Thymidylate Synthetase

The FdUMP-treated enzyme can be reactivated according to the principle of microscopic reversibility, yielding fully active enzyme and unchanged FdUMP, if reassociation of the drug is prevented by high excess of the substrate, dUMP.[61] Figure 5 shows typical results of the reappearance of catalytic activity upon incubation of the inactive enzyme at 2 different temperatures.

Figure 5.   Reactivation of thymidylate synthetase.

The reversal of the formation of the covalent complex necessitates braking of 2 covalent bonds: a C-S bond at position 6 and a C-C bond at position 5. Thus, the stability of the drug-enzyme complex is very much dependent on the temperature; the activation energy required for this porcess was found to be 26.5 kcal/mole.[61] Table 1 lists the half-times of the regeneration of enzymic activity at different temperatures.

TABLE 1

TEMPERATURE DEPENDENCE OF THE REACTIVATION OF FdUMP-INACTIVATED THYMIDYLATE SYNTHETASE

Temperature °C	$t_{\frac{1}{2}}$ of reactivation min
25.8	183
35.2	39.6
37.0	32.5
39.8	22.4
44.4	11.9
53.9	3.8

Evidence for the reformation of the 5,6-double bond of FdUMP during enzyme reactivation was obtained by demonstrating that a significant secondary deuterium isotope effect at position 6 of FdUMP is associated with the process,[62] due to the accompanying $sp^3 \to sp^2$ rehybridization of C-6:

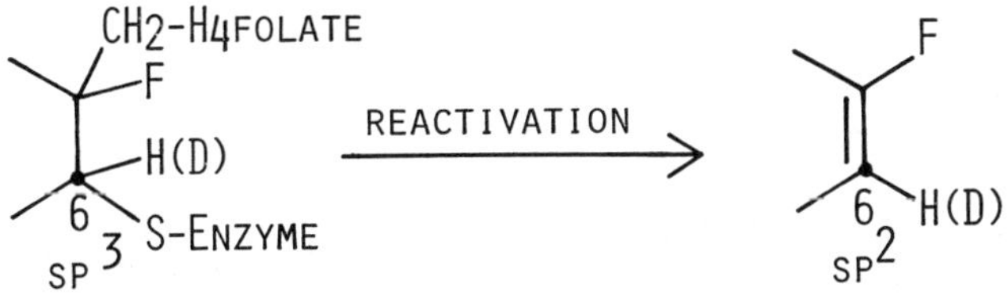

The results are shown in Figure 6, which illustrates the first order rates of reactivation of dTMP synthetase inactivated by FdUMP and FdUMP-6-d, respectively. The rate difference corresponds to an isotope effect of $k_H/k_D = 1.24$, which is considerably higher than the measured secondary tritium isotope effect associated with the decomposition of the covalent complex.[63] An explanation for this apparent discrepency has been offered.[64] No isotope effect could be detected, when the reactivation was performed with a covalent complex prepared using CD_2-H_4folate in comparison with CH_2-H_4folate,[63] which indicates that C-C bond cleavage at position 5 does not contribute to the rate of

84

reactivation.

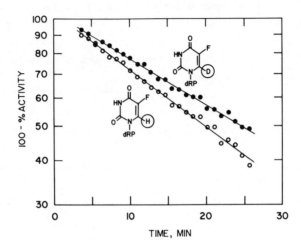

Figure 6. Secondary deuterium isotope effect on the rate of enzyme reactivation.
Thymidylate synthetase of *L. casei* was inactivated at 30° by FdUMP
or FdUMP-6-*d*. The rate of regeneration of enzyme activity was
followed spectrophotometrically[65] at 40° in the presence of 20 mM
dUMP (10^6-fold excess over FdUMP concentration). Experimental
points are averages of 6 independent determinations.[62]

Studies of the Reactivation of Thymidylate Synthetase in Intact Leukemia L-1210 Cells

We have recently developed an assay method suitable for the determination
of the catalytic turnover of intracellular dTMP synthetase.[66-68] The cells
are incubated with labelled metabolic precursors of 5-^{3}H-dUMP and the tritium
released during the enzyme catalyzed reaction is measured.[68]

$$5\text{-}^3\text{H-dUrd} \xrightarrow{\text{cell}\atop\text{membrane}} 5\text{-}^3\text{H-dUrd} \xrightarrow{\text{thymidine}\atop\text{kinase}} 5\text{-}^3\text{H-dUMP} \xrightarrow{\text{dTMP synthetase}\atop\text{CH}_2\text{H}_4\text{folate}} \text{dTMP} + {}^3\text{H-H}_2\text{O}$$

Leukemia L1210 cells preincubated with 5-fluoro-2'-deoxyuridine (FdUrd)
rapidly lose their thymidylate synthetase activity.[66,67] Following subsequent
washing and resuspension, the cells show a pseudo first order rate of recovery
of enzyme activity (see Figure 7).

The acetylenic thymine analog, 5-ethynyluracil, the free base of 5-ethynyl-
2'-deoxyuridine,[69,70] was postulated by Rando[71] to be a potential suicide
inhibitor of dTMP synthetase. Although 5-ethynyluracil lacks significant
activity, 5-ethynyl-dUrd showed potent cytotoxic effect (50% growth inhibitory
concentration against L1210 in culture: $I_{50} = 2\times10^{-8}$ M).[70] Inhibition

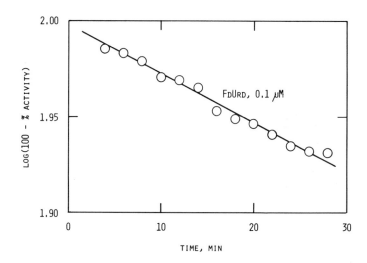

Figure 7.   Recovery of dTMP synthetase activity in L1210 cells. Enzyme was
            inactivated by 40 min preincubation with 10^{-7} M FdUrd at 37° followed
            by measurement of enzyme activity[68] in drug-free medium.

analysis[70] together with some preliminary studies in cell free systems pointed

to the possibility of dTMP synthetase as a site of action of this new anti-

metabolite. In our intact cell enzyme assay, dTMP synthetase was inhibited[72]

with an I_{50}-value of 2.7×10^{-7} M by 5-ethynyl-dUrd.

Cellular enzyme activity was recoverable upon incubation after the removal

of the inhibitor (see Figure 8). The rate of reactivation was dependent on the

extracellular concentration of the analog during the preincubation period.

The reactivation rates followed pseudo first order kinetics. This is illus-

trated in Figure 9. It is also shown, that the recovery of enzyme activity

after 10^{-6} M 5-nitro-dUrd treatment is about 5-fold slower than that in the

case of 5-ethynyl-dUrd, in spite of the fact that both analogs show the same

I_{50}-value in this system [72] (see also Table 2).

It is apparent that by lowering the concentration of 5-ethynyl-dUrd during

preincubation the rate of reactivation increases and then levels off and

reaches a maximum at ca.10^{-6} M concentration. By increasing the concentration

of inhibitors during preincubation, the reactivation rate usually decreases

and reaches a lower limit.

The maximum rate may correspond to the intrinsic dissociation of the

drug-enzyme complex. The low external concentration during the inactivation

period does not permit significant build up of an intracellular free drug

level and the resulting reassociation of the released inhibitor with the enzyme.

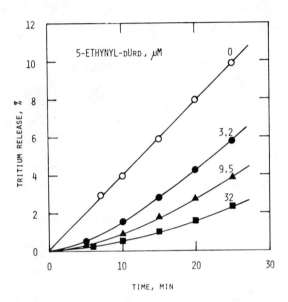

Figure 8. Reactivation of intracellular dTMP synthetase after treatment
of L1210 cells with 0-32 μM 5-ethynyl-dUrd at 37° for 40 min.
Tritium release was measured[68] after resuspension of the cells
in drug-free medium.

The minimum rate may be the consequence of the saturation of the uptake-
phosphorylation step at high extracellular drug concentrations leading to a
maximum intracellular pool of the drug which is no longer affected by further
increase in the external drug concentration.

Some of the relevant data obtained in the L1210 intact cell enzyme system
with the three 5-substituted dUrd analogs are summarized in Table 2.

TABLE 2

ACTIVITY OF THYMIDYLATE SYNTHETASE INHIBITORS IN L1210 CELLS

5-X-dUrd X	I_{50}* μM	Concentration** μM	$t_{\frac{1}{2}}$ of reactivation hr
F	0.006	0.1	2.0
NO$_2$	0.3	1.0	2.1
C≡CH	0.3	1.0	0.4

* I_{50} - values determined using 1.0 μM 5-^{3}H-dUrd, as described.[68]
** Concentrations used in reactivation experiments.

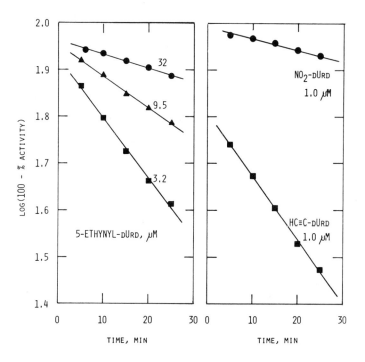

Figure 9. Kinetics of regeneration of dTMP synthetase activity after
incubation by 5-ethynyl- and 5-nitro-2'-deoxyuridine.

The I_{50}-value of 5-ethynyl-dUrd for growth inhibition of L1210 cells in
culture is only 10-fold higher than that of FdUrd,[70] yet the intracellular
inhibition of dTMP synthetase is much less effective and the recovery of enzyme
activity is much faster with the acetylenic inhibitor, using the intact cell
dTMP synthetase assay system.[66-68]

The molecular mechanism of interaction of 5-ethynyl-dUMP is currently under
study using the purified L. casei enzyme. Several structures can be considered
for the covalently linked inhibitor generated via the initial nucleophilic
attack of the active site cysteine-S⁻ at C-6 of the pyrimidine ring (see
Figure 10), forming the Michael-adduct 2. Protonation can lead to the reactive enzyme-bound allenic intermediate (4), in agreement with Rando's
predictions.[71] Nucleophilic attack on the central C-atom of the allene may
result in the formation of either 5 followed by 6 or 7. The formation of all

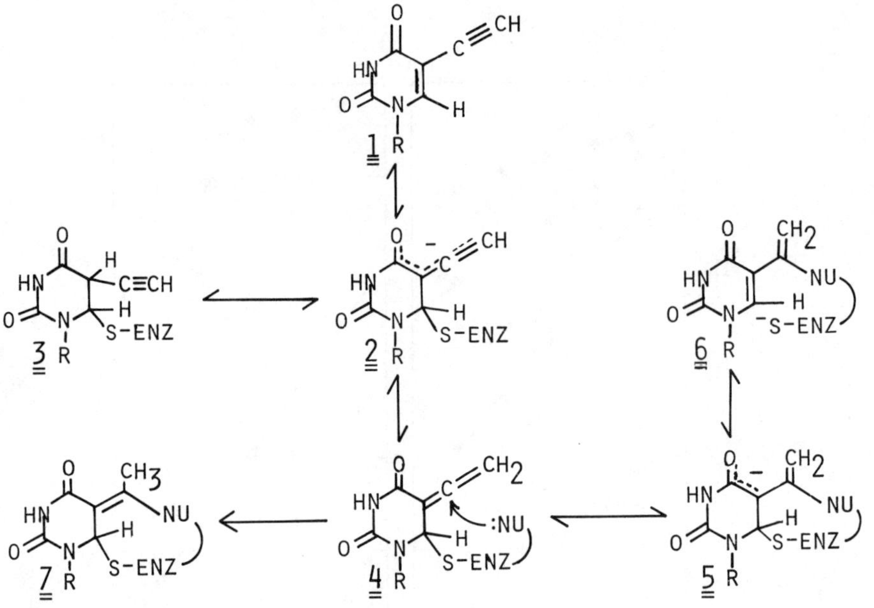

Figure 10. Possible structures involved in the covalent interaction of
5-ethynyl-dUMP (1) with dTMP synthatase.

the structures is reversible, with the apparent exception of structure 7.
If one considers the possibility that the nucleophile attacking the allene
(4) is an amine, one can also write a mechanism for the liberation of 5-acetyl-
dUMP (9) as outlined in Figure 11, and active enzyme. It was reported that

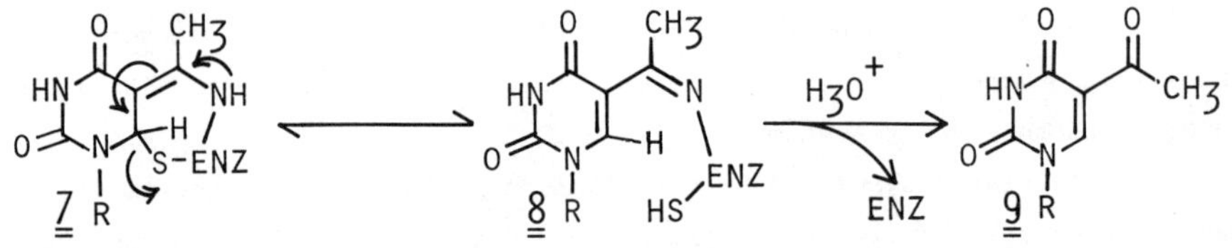

Figure 11.

5-acetyl-dUMP does not inhibit dTMP synthetase to any significant extent.[73]

CONCLUSIONS

A brief review of the reversibility of covalent drug-enzyme interactions reveals that there are a number of different molecular mechanisms responsible for the spontaneous regeneration of the catalytic activity of covalently inactivated enzymes. The characteristic involvement of catalytic functional groups in most mechanism-based inactivation reactions may also be responsible for the lowering of the activation energy required for the decomposition of the covalent drug-enzyme complex. The extent and rate of the reversibility of drug induced enzyme inactivation reactions may have important pharmacological consequences. It is conceivable that by rational design the dynamics of these covalent molecular interactions may be successfully influenced to achieve enhanced therapeutic effectiveness of many drugs acting *via* mechanism-based enzyme inhibition.

ACKNOWLEDGMENTS

This work was supported in part by research grant CA13604 and Research Career Development Award GM34138 (T.I.K.) and training grant GM07145 (J.C.Y.) from the National Institutes of Health, USPHS. We thank Dr. M. Bobek for an authentic sample of 5-ethynyl-2'-deoxyuridine.

REFERENCES

1. Metcalf, B., and Sjoerdsma, A. (1979), this volume.
2. Goldstein, A. (1951) Arch. Biochem. Biophys. 34, 169.
3. Wilson, I.B., Harrison, M.A. and Ginsburg, S. (1961) J. Biol. Chem. 236, 1498.
4. Wilson, I.B. (1951) J. Biol. Chem. 190, 111.
5. Aldridge, W.N. (1953) Biochem. J. 53, 110; 117.
6. Aldridge, W.N. (1953) Biochem. J. 54, 442.
7. Wilson, I.B. and Rio, R.A. (1965) Mol. Pharmacol. 1, 60.
8. Kaiser, E.T., Lee, T.W.S. and Boer, F.P. (1971) J. Amer. Chem. Soc. 93, 2351.
9. Westerik, J.O. and Wolfenden, R. (1972) J. Biol. Chem. 247, 8195.
10. Thompson, R.C. (1973) Biochemistry, 12, 47.
11. Rawn, J.D. and Lienhard, G.E. (1974) Biochemistry, 13, 3124.
12. Lewis, C.A., Jr. and Wolfenden, R. (1977) Biochemistry, 16, 4890.
13. Kennedy, W.P. and Schultz, R.M. (1979) Biochemistry, 18, 349.
14. Chen, R., Gorenstein, D.G., Kennedy, W.P., Lowe, G., Nurse, D. and Schultz, R.M. (1979) Biochemistry, 18, 921.
15. Koehler, K.A. and Lienhard, G.E. (1971) Biochemistry, 10, 2477.
16. Rawn, J.D. and Lienhard, G.E. (1974) Biochemistry 13, 3124.
17. Lindquist, R.N. and Terry, C. (1974) Arch. Biochem. Biophys. 160, 135.
18. Koehler, K.A. and Terry, C. (1974) Biochemistry, 13, 5345.
19. Wiseman, J.S. and Abeles, R.H. (1979) Biochemistry, 18, 427.
20. Abeles, R.H. (1978) Enzyme-Activated Irreversible Inhibitors, Seiler, N., Jung, M.J. and Koch-Weser, J., eds., Elsevier/North Holland, Amsterdam, p.1.

21. Kalman, T.I. (1972) Intra-Science Chem. Rept. 6(4), 35.
22. Kalman, T.I. (1971) Biochemistry, 10, 2567.
23. Kalman, T.I. (1971) Ann. N.Y. Acad. Sci. 186, 166.
24. Kalman, T.I. (1972) Biochem. Biophys. Res. Commun. 49, 1007.
25. Bellisario, R.L., Maley, G.F., Galivan, J.H. and Maley, F. (1976)
    Proc. Natl. Acad. Sci. USA, 73, 1848.
26. Kalman, T.I., Goldman, D. and Hsiao, M.C., to be published.
27. Matsuda, A., Wataya, Y. and Santi, D.V. (1978) Biochem. Biophys. Res.
    Commun. 84, 654.
28. Mertes, M.P., Chang, C.T.-C., De Clercq, E., Huang, G.-F. and Torrence, P.
    F. (1978) Biochem. Biophys. Res. Commun. 84, 1054.
29. Kluepfel, D., Murthy, Y.K.S. and Sartori, G. (1965) Il Farmaco (Ed. Sci.)
    20, 757.
30. De Clercq, E., Descamps, J., Huang, G.-F. and Torrence, P.F. (1978)
    Mol. Pharmacol. 14, 422.
31. Huang, G.-F. and Torrence, P.F. (1977) J. Org. Chem. 42, 3821.
32. Westerik, J.O. and Wolfenden, R. (1974) J. Biol. Chem. 249, 6351.
33. Washtien, W.L. and Santi, D.V. (1979) this volume.
34. Washtien, W., Matsuda, A., Wataya, Y. and Santi, D.V. (1978) Biochem.
    Pharmacol. 27, 2663.
35. Kalman, T.I., Thomas, L.K. and Yalowich, J.C., to be published.
36. Rando, R.R. (1974) Science, 185, 320.
37. Abeles, R.H. and Maycock, A.L. (1976) Accounts Chem. Res. 9, 313.
38. Walsh, C. (1977) Horizons Biochem. Biophys. 3, 36.
39. Seiler, N., Jung, M.J. and Koch-Weser, J. eds., (1978) "Enzyme-
    Activated Irreversible Inhibitors", Elsevier/North Holland, Amsterdam.
40. Kluger, R. and Pike, D.C. (1977) J. Amer. Chem. Soc. 99, 4504.
41. Kluger, R. and Pike, D.C. (1979) J. Amer. Chem. Soc. 101, in press.
42. Freisheim, J.H., Kumar, A.A. and Blankenship, D.T. (1979) in Chemistry
    and Biology of Pteridines, Kisliuk, R.L. and Brown, G.M. eds., Elsevier
    North-Holland, N.Y., p. 419.
43. Matthews, D.A., Alden, R.A., Bolin, J.T., Filman, D.J., Freer, S.T.,
    Hamlin, R., Hol, W.G.J., Kisliuk, R.L., Pastore, E.J., Plante, L.T.,
    Xuong, N., and Kraut, J. (1978) J. Biol. Chem. 253, 6946.
44. Matthews, D.A. (1979) Biochemistry, 18, 1602.
45. Kalman, T.I., in preparation.
46. Frere, J.-M. (1977) Biochem. Pharmacol. 26, 2203.
47. Ghuysen, J.-M. (1977) J. Gen. Microbiol. 101, 13.
48. Spratt, B.G. (1978) Sci. Prog. (Oxford) 65, 101.
49. Walsh, C., Shannon, P. and Wang, E. (1979) this volume.
50. Maycock, A.L., Aster, S.D. and Patchett, A.A. (1979) this volume.
51. Jung, M.J., Palfreyman, M.G., Ribereau-Gayon, G., Bey, P., Metcalf, B.W.,
    Koch-Weser, J. and Sjoerdsma, A. (1979) this volume.
52. Silverman, R.B. and Hoffman, S.J. (1979) this volume.
53. Friedkin, M. (1973) Adv. Enzymol. 38, 235.
54. Cohen, S.S., Flaks, J.G., Barner, H.D., Loeb, M.R. and Lichtenstein, J.
    (1958) Proc. Natl. Acad. Sci. USA 44, 1004.
55. Heidelberger, C. (1965) Progr. Nucleic Acid Res. Mol. Biol. 4, 1.
56. Pogolotti, A.L., Jr. and Santi, D.V. (1977) in Bioorganic Chemistry,
    van Tamelen, E.E., ed., Vol. 1 Academic Press, New York, p. 277.
57. Danenberg, P.V. (1977) Biochem. Biophys. Acta, 473, 73.
58. Leary, R.P. and Kisliuk, R.L. (1971) Prep. Biochem. 1, 47.
59. Crusberg, T.C., Leary, R. and Kisliuk (1970) J. Biol. Chem. 245, 5292.
60. Maley, G.F., Bellisario, R.L., Guarino, D.U. and Maley, F. (1979) J. Biol.
    Chem. 254, 1301.
61. Kalman, T.I. (1974) Intra-Science Chem. Rept. 8, 139.
62. Kalman, T.I. (1975) Ann. N.Y. Acad. Sci. 255, 326.

63. Kalman, T.I., unpublished results.
64. Kalman, T.I. (1977) in Isotope Effects on Enzyme-Catalyzed Reactions, Cleland, W.W., O'Leary, M.H. and Northrop, D.B. eds., University Park Press, Baltimore, pp. 118-119.
65. Wahba, A.J. and Friedkin, M. (1961) J. Biol. Chem. 236, PC 11.
66. Kalman, T.I. and Yalowich, J.C. (1977) Amer. Chem. Soc. 174th Meeting, Abstracts, BIOL 127.
67. Kalman, T.I. and Yalowich, J. (1978) Proc. Amer. Assoc. Cancer Res. 19, 153.
68. Kalman, T.I. and Yalowich, J.C. (1979) in Chemistry and Biology of Pteridines, Kisliuk, R.L. and Brown, G.M. eds., Elsevier North-Holland, N.Y. p. 671.
69. Perman, J., Sharma, R.A. and Bobek, M. (1976) Tetrahedron Lett. 2427.
70. Bobek, M. and Bloch, A. (1978) in Chemistry and Biology of Nucleosides and Nucleotides, Harmon, R.E., Robins, R.K. and Townsend, L.B. eds., Academic Press, New York, p. 135.
71. Rando, R.R. (1977) Methods Enzymol. 46, p. 164.
72. Kalman, T.I. and Yalowich, J.C., in preparation.
73. Kampf, A., Barfknecht, R.L., Shaffer, P.J., Osaki, S. and Mertes, M.P. (1976) J. Med. Chem. 19, 903.

Published 1979 by Elsevier North Holland, Inc.
Kalman, ed. Drug Action and Design: Mechanism-Based Enzyme Inhibitors

NEW SUICIDE SUBSTRATES FOR PYRIDOXAL PHOSPHATE DEPENDENT ENZYMES

C. WALSH, P. SHANNON AND E. WANG
Departments of Chemistry and Biology, Massachusetts Institute of
Technology, Cambridge, Massachusetts 02139

SUMMARY

The mechanism of action of some suicide substrates[1-5] on two pyridoxal
phosphate (PLP) linked enzymes, alanine racemase (EC 5.1.1.1) from
Escherichia coli B and serine transhydroxymethymethylase (EC 2.1.2.1) from
rabbit and lamb liver are studied. With alanine racemase,[3,4] both the D and L
isomers of β-fluoroalanine and β-chloroalanine partition between (a) α,β-
elimination to pyruvate, ammonia, and halide ion or (b) inactivation. No racemization is detectable. The V_{max} for pyruvate formation from L-chloroalanine
is about 50-fold lower than from the D-isomer of chloroalanine or either
fluoroalanine. However both enantiomeric pairs partition identically - about
830 turnovers per inactivating event. This invariant partition ratio suggests
that a common intermediate, the eneamino-PLP complex, is the species responsible
for inactivation, probably by Michael attack from a nucleophilic residue at
the enzyme active site. O-Carbamoyl-D-serine, O-acetyl-D-serine, O-propionyl-
D-serine, and O-butyryl-D-serine also undergo enzyme-catalyzed elimination for
830 turnovers before causing irreversible inactivation, presumably from the
same intermediate. In contrast, the L isomers of these β-substituted serines
do not eliminate or induce inactivation, but serve merely as reversible,
competitive inhibitors of the enzyme. This indicates asymmetric binding
regions for bulky substituents at the active site and suggests that D isomers
of substituted β-alanine would be more effective enzyme inactivators. D-Cycloserine also inactivates alanine racemase in a time-dependent fashion.

Active site-directed inactivation of alanine racemase by D- and L- difluoroalanine and D,L-trifluoroalanine has been examined and is compared to monofluoroalanine inactivation. A β-elimination of fluoride from these compounds
generates a fluoro-substituted eneamine intermediate, which induces inactivation. The new properties conferred upon the aminoacrylate by fluorine
substitution are reflected in a significant change in the partition ratio,
difluoroalanine > monofluoroalanine >> trifluoroalanine, the rate of elimination
of fluoride, and the stability of the enzyme-inactivator adduct. The D- and
L-difluoroalanine-inactivated racemase is reactivated to about 50% of its
original activity after dialysis while the mono- and trifluoroalanine induced

inactivations are stable. A mechanism consistent with these observations is proposed.

Serine transhydroxymethylase (STHM) also catalyzes a β-elimination of fluoride from D-fluoroalanine to form pyruvate, ammonium ion, and fluoride, and homogeneous enzyme from rabbit or lamb liver is inactivated concomitantly with catalytic turnover.[5] Both turnover and inactivation are accelerated greatly by tetrahydrofolate. Consistent with observations about enzyme inter-action with D-alanine[6,7] D-fluoroalanine also transaminates rabbit and lamb STHM, forming pyridoxamine, fluoropyruvate and apoenzyme. D-Chloroalanine and D-serine also partition between β-elimination and inactivation. This fact suggests that a common inactivating intermediate - the eneamino-PLP complex - is formed.

Isolation of radioactive S-carboxyhydroxyethyl cysteine and lanthionine among the products of hydrolysis of borohydride reduced, [^{14}C]-D-fluoro-alanine-inactivated rabbit and lamb STHM implicates cysteine as the active site nucleophile. One mole of [^{14}C]-D-fluoroalanine is incorporated per mole subunit in both lamb and rabbit STHM. Dialysis of D-fluoroalanine-inactivated STHM with 30% ammonium sulfate followed by phosphate buffer containing PLP and dithiothreitol will release most of the label and restore most of the activity. Both D-fluoroalanine-inactivated enzymes retain much of the original PLP, and the observed reactivation is caused by a β-elimination of sulfur to yield pyruvate, PLP, and native enzyme.

D-Cycloserine also induces a time-dependent, pseudo first order inactivation of STHM,[5] and the inactivation rate is also accelerated by tetrahydrofolate. However, this inactivation is completely reversible, and inactivation is caused by transamination. The transamination of STHM by D-cycloserine in the absence of tetrahydrofolate is similar to that by D-alanine: the rates of trans-amination are the same, although the K_i for D-cycloserine is much smaller.

The nature of tetrahydrofolate stimulation of β-elimination was also studied by using other D- and L-β-substituted amino acids as substrates and pterin analogues as effectors in D-fluoroalanine elimination.

Lysine ε-aminotransaminase is reversibly inactivated[8] by three unsaturated lysine analogues, 2,6-diamino-4-hexynoate, cis-2,6-diamino-4-hexenoate, and trans-2,6-diamino-4-hexenoate to produce three spectroscopically distinct forms of modified enzyme. The acetylenic analogue partitions in a 40 to 1 ratio between production of a 4-substituted picolinate and enzymic alkylation with a first order rate constant for alkylation of 0.07 s^{-1}. The cis and trans analogue partition ratios were found to be 1700 and 160, respectively, with inactivation rate constants of 0.20 s^{-1} *(cis)* and 0.13 s^{-1} *(trans)*. Both olefinic analogues produced varying amounts of picolinate during catalysis.

REFERENCES

1. Walsh, C. (1977) "Recent Developments in Suicide Substrates and Other Active Site-Directed Inactivating Agents of Specific Target Enzymes", Horizons Biochem. Biophys. 3, 36-81.
2. Walsh, C. (1978) "Chemical Approaches to the Study of Enzymes Catalyzing Redox Transformations", Ann. Rev. Biochem. 47, 881-931.
3. Wang, E. and Walsh, C. (1978) "Suicide Substrates for the Alanine Racemase of *Escherichia coli* B", Biochemistry, 17, 1313-1321.
4. Walsh, C., Johnston, M., Marcotte, P. and Wang, E. (1978) "Studies on Suicide Substrates for Pyridoxal-P and Flavin-Linked Enzymes" in Enzyme-Activated Irreversible Inhibitors, Seiler, N., Jung, M.J. and Koch-Weser, J., eds., Elsevier/North Holland, Amsterdam, pp. 177-185.
5. Wang, E., Kallen, R. and Walsh, C. (1979) "D-Fluoroalanine: A Suicide Substrate for Serine Hydroxymethylase" in Chemistry and Biology of Pteridines, Kisliuk, R.L. and Brown, G.M. eds., Elsevier North-Holland, New York, pp. 507-512.
6. Schirch, L. and Jenkins, W.T. (1964) J. Biol. Chem. 239, 3797-3800.
7. Schirch, L. and Jenkins, W.T. (1964) J. Biol. Chem. 239, 3801-3807.
8. Shannon, P., Marcotte, P., Donovan, J. and Walsh, C. (1979) "Studies with Mechanism-Based Inactivators of Lysine ε-Transaminase from *Achromobacter liquidum*", Biochemistry, 18, in press.

DISCUSSION

COWARD: Have you looked at O-phosphoserine in your system?

WALSH: Yes, we studied the effects of various β-substituents. We looked at the pK$_a$ of the conjugate acid of the prospective leaving groups and it looks like we need general acid catalysis when the leaving group gets above pK 5 or 6. Halide ions will depart, of course and with such nonbasic anions we have no problem. Acetate will depart, nothing much with a pK above that. We have not checked all the alternatives on this.

COWARD: Do I understand it correctly that the lysine acetylene analog inactivates ornithine transaminase? In other words, there is no apparent specificity between ornithine and lysine in this enzyme system?

WALSH: Let me clarify that. Only the *trans*-olefin inactivates purified rat liver ornithine-δ-transaminase in the hands of David Vallee and in our hands, as well. The acetylene does not, nor does the *cis*-olefin. That of course, raises a problem of why the specificity? Maybe it needs a transoid configuration. And why doesn't the acetylene work, I do not know. But it has also been reported that lysine is not a substrate for ornithine-δ-transaminase, but of course "not a substrate" is an absolute term. One of the things useful about suicide substrates is that if they are highly efficient, all you need is one turnover. Let us make the following argument. Pure ornithine-δ-trans-

aminase has a specific activity of about 15 units/mg (μmoles/mg). Subunit
molecular weight, let us assume is 50,000 - Michel (Jung) may say it is
different. If it is 50,000 - then that is a turnover number of about 1,000/min
for ornithine. Let us say lysine or the *trans*-lysine analog reacted only 0.1
moles/min. Four orders of magnitude below. You would not pick that up in a
catalytic assay, but if one molecule inactivates efficiently, then you will
see 0.1 inactivations per minute, the enzyme will be dead in less than 10
minutes. So you see, if an enzyme processes with low partitioning ratio, it
can take a suicide substrate, which has really a very low k_{cat} and kill itself
in quite a short observational time scale.

COWARD: And those rate differences are seen, when you compare ornithine
and lysine?

WALSH: In the literature it is reported that lysine is not a substrate.
We have not gone to limits of catalytic detection to see.

COWARD: I do not mean as regular substrate, but comparing the Merrell
compound with your lysine derivative.

WALSH: Maybe Dr. Jung would like to comment on that.

JUNG: We did not see inhibition by the vinyl GABA-analog in the absence of
α-ketoglutarate, since it has been looked at by Fowler[1] in presence of α-ketoglutarate, and he sees a very slow time-dependent inhibition of ornithine
transaminase.

WALSH: The GABA analogs have of course only one amino group; the distal one,
they do not have the proximal one, which the lysine analogs do.

JUNG: You looked at the polyhaloalanine analogs, difluoro- aand trifluoro-
methyl, on the alanine racemase. Did you find different partition ratios?

WALSH: Yes. For monofluoro D- or L-alanine the *E. coli* racemase is killed
with a partition ratio of 830:1. The trifluoroalanine shows less than 10 turnovers. We cannot detect any turnover - our limit would be if we would pick up
10. So, the trifluoro is much more efficient, it may be completely efficient
and that is consistent with what Silverman and Abeles found for a variety of
pyridoxal enzymes[2]. The difluoro is anomalous. The difluoro turns over
100,000 times; that is wrong! It is not wrong in the experimental sense,
because in fact the enzyme can be killed to 98% with the difluoroalanine, but
it stays at 2% level, as long as you want, until it has chewed through all of
the difluoroalanine. The reason for that, we hypothesize, is that the difluoroalanine adduct is kinetically labile, and I tell you my molecular interpretation.
I think the enzyme nucleophile, which adds is a lysine. In the case of monofluoroalanine, you get an amine, it is at the alcohol oxidation state, if you

will. In the case of trifluoroalanine Abeles and Silverman showed very
elegantly[2], you can kick out all 3 fluorines and get to the acyl oxidation
state. In the case where nitrogen has added, that's an amide and it is
kinetically stable in water. In the difluoro case we get to the aldehyde
oxidation state and if it is an imine - and you either have an enamine or an
imine tautomer and those I think are sufficiently hydrolytically labile - it
just comes off and so the enzyme keeps turning over and it sits in the steady
state - 98 out of 100 molecules are alkylated in the steady state, and so the
partition ratio there was anomalous; it tipped us off to worry about the
chemistry and I think that that is a reasonable interpretation, not completely
iron clad yet.

JUNG: If you are really interested in inhibition of ornithine γ-aminotrans-
aminase, I think you should look at something more efficient with a lower ratio
than your *trans*-dehydro analog has. You generate a lot of unsaturated aldehyde.

WALSH: I am certainly hoisted by my own petard there. We do not know how
many, in the sense that if indeed there are a large number of turnovers, we
are going to have a problem of specificity, no question, but the partition
ratios I have in the lecture were for the bacterial lysine-ε-transaminase. We
do not know what they are yet for the rat liver ornithine-γ-transaminase.
There are a couple ways of doing it. One is this C-14 assay, which was started
- the other is, what is the minimal molar excess that you need, to titrate away
an activity? It looks pretty low - I do not know the numbers yet, but I do
not think it will generate a dramatic number of olefinic aldehyde molecules.

CHU: You explained the difference between the D- and the L-O-acetylserine
and O-carbamylserine on steric grounds. Would it be possible to explain the
difference by a reversed Michael addition, which would be stereoselective?

WALSH: Let us assume for the moment that in the D- and L- isomers, the
R-group points in two different directions and one goes through the elimination
process and one gets X$^-$ sitting at the active site. Then you want it kinetically to be able to get out if it came out as the D-amino acid, but not to get
out in the case of the L-amino acid for physical reasons, let us say. It sits
there sufficiently long for a nucleophile to read 100% of the time. It is
conceivable, but then you also have to suggest to me that the α-H is held
totally sequestered from bulk solvent, because we have looked and there is
absolutely no α-H exchange, although there is with some other L-amino acids.
I think that makes too many restrictions, for me to believe that it is likely.

CHU: If the reaction goes both ways from L to D, then why is the D more
specific than the L?

WALSH: Given that the enzyme is providing a chiral, asymmetric microenvironment; only L-amino acid side chains are there - that is asymmetric.
When it interacts with D-amino acid to form an E·S complex and then for this
transition state it has a certain activation energy to get over those barriers.
When it forms a complex with an L-amino acid, it will have a different activation barrier, because in fact, these are diastereomeric complexes and
transition states. That is an energetic argument. The structural argument
is that in the active site, the R-groups point in different directions. We
started out as a premise in that, when it points in one direction there is
simply more room than in the other. Why does alanyl racemase let that happen?
The answer is that it could be, anthropomorphically, that is, when the group
is small enough, e.g., a methyl, it does not matter, does not cause a problem,
but as soon as you start putting bigger groups on, which are not physiologically encountered, so there is no evolutionary pressure on E. coli alanine
racemase to evolve to avoid that, you begin to pick it up.

CHU: What is the situation with the β-bromoalanine?

WALSH: We have not looked at that in this case. We have made β-bromoalanine for other purposes. What we know is that L-fluoro is as good as
D-fluoro, but L-chloro is 50 times worse; so I think L-bromo would be crummy,
but we have not done it, specifically.

ONDETTI: Is it known which amino acid residue is playing the role of
abstracting the proton from the α-position in any of the enzymes you have been
dealing with?

WALSH: There is no evidence. That is a very difficult question to answer,
because I think anytime you use a modifying reagent, whether it is an affinity
label or mechanism based one, what you are doing is trapping the kinetically
competent nucleophile. Now, it is true that things, which can react as nucleophiles can also react as general bases, but that does not mean that what you
have trapped out as nucleophile functions catalytically as a general base.
That ambiguity always persists no matter what modifying reagent you use. That
is why I say there is no evidence. Now, if I had seen some proton seques-
trations and internal transfers, I could begin to make arguments about how many
protons the base has in its conjugate acid form. For the moment, I do not have
any. One knows that lysine is there and in the aspartate aminotransferase
story, which Rando and Christen have done[3] - there they have trapped lysine-258
in that enzyme. Is that acting as the general base? I do not know. In serine
transhydroxymethylase, is that cysteine SH-group acting as the α-H base? I do
not know. It is there, it is certainly competent to do so. But, I cannot

answer with any certainty. Can you? Do you have some better way of resolving it?

ONDETTI: No, I was more or less thinking in terms of whether you have displaceable group at the α-position, that you can actually build a covalent intermediate with the nucleophile on the enzyme.

WALSH: Do S_N2 chemistry on the α-carbon? It is conceivable. This enzyme seems to have sufficiently facile elimination chemistry. If you have a displaceable group on α-carbon, you are going to have problems with stability of that amino acid, aren't you?

ONDETTI: Yes. You have a problem actually to make the compound.

WALSH: If it is good enough to be displaced, it is going to be hard to keep. I think, if you let the enzyme do it, that is fine, but it is going to be hard to get started, if the α-carbon is blocked.

KALMAN: The serine transhydroxymethylase inhibitors you used were not very effective. Indeed, there is no potent and specific inhibitor known for this enzyme. The mutants Jim Coward mentioned, the Chinese hamster ovary cells defective in folylpolyglutamate synthetase, require glycine, adenosine and thymidine for growth[4]. In addition to an apparent requirement for the polyglutamate form of the tetrahydrofolate coenzyme in the serine transhydroxymethylase reaction in these cells, auxotrophy for glycine indicates that the enzyme has an essential function. In the metabolic cycle you outlined earlier, the other 2 enzymes, thymidylate synthetase and dihydrofolate reductase are susceptible to inhibition by a wide variety of extremely potent inhibitors. So are, for that matter, most of the pyridoxal phosphate dependent enzymes.

Would you like to speculate about the possible reasons for why so far no inhibitors were found, which can effectively block this enzyme in the cell?

WALSH: For the isolated enzyme, there are some reported, which are pretty awful, e.g., glycidaldehyde phosphate has been reported and you can use haloketones, like bromopyruvate, but I do not imagine anyone would think those endoalkylating reagents have any utility. If you say to me, why we have not found something - that is a difficult question. O-Carbamylserine, e.g., kills alanine racemase. Why did we find that? I think, in many cases it depends on how you do the inhibition assay, as to whether you find an irreversible component to the inactivation.

Certainly, there are hundreds of folate analogs, which may have been tried and screened against serine hydroxymethylase. As far as I know, nothing, which is folate based, has turned up that is useful. There are, I guess some compounds of B.R. Baker, some sulfonyl fluorides, which people have said have some promise. The fact one has not found a potent inhibitor yet means that one has not been a clever enough chemist to design one. Let me take that as a prejudice.

As to the question of the physiological role of serine transhydroxymethylase; is it an essential 1-carbon donor? Can you knock it out and still keep the cells healthy? Well, Puck reported some years ago[5,6] that he had some auxotrophic mutants, which did not have much serine transhydroxymethylase activity and he raised the question, is the enzyme essential? But those mutants were never mapped in any effective genetic way.* The point is, there may be other enzymes to provide flux. Certainly you know you can come through 5,10-methylenetetrahydrofolate dehydrogenase from the methenyltetrahydrofolate. But I cannot really say just how much of the thymidylate methyl group biosynthetic flux does serine transhydroxymethylase provide.

REFERENCES

1. John, R.A., Charteris, A.T. and Fowler, L.J. (1978) in Enzyme-Activated Irreversible Inhibitors, Seiler, N., Jung, M.J. and Koch-Weser, J. eds. Elsevier/North-Holland, Amsterdam, p. 109.
2. Silverman, R.B. and Abeles, R.H. (1976) Biochemistry, 15, 4718.
3. Gehring, H., Rando, R.R. and Christen, P. (1977) Biochemistry, 16, 4832.
4. McBurney, M.W. and Whitmore, G.F. (1974) Cell, 2, 173.
5. Kao, F.T., and Puck, T.T. (1968) Proc. Nat. Acad. Sci. USA, 60, 1275.
6. Kao, F.T., and Puck, T.T. (1969) J. Cell. Physiol. 74, 245.
7. Zelikson, R. and Luzzati, M. (1976) Eur. J. Biochem. 64, 7.

---

*Editor's note: There is an interesting thymidylate requiring mutant of yeast, tmp^3, which has lost its mitochondrial serine transhydroxymethylase isozyme[7] and also has requirements for methionine, adenine and histidine in spite of the presence of the cytoplasmic enzyme.

IN VITRO AND *IN VIVO* STUDIES OF MECHANISM-BASED INHIBITION OF
THYMIDYLATE SYNTHETASE

WENDY L. WASHTIEN AND DANIEL V. SANTI
Department of Pharmaceutical Chemistry and Department of Biochemistry and
Biophysics, University of California, San Francisco, California 94143, USA

INTRODUCTION

Thymidylate (dTMP) synthetase catalyzes the reductive methylation of 2'-
deoxyuridylate (dUMP) to dTMP with concomitant conversion of 5,10-methylene-
tetrahydrofolic acid (CH_2-H_4folate) to 7,8-dihydrofolate. Studies leading to
the currently accepted minimal mechanism for this enzyme (Fig. 1) have recently

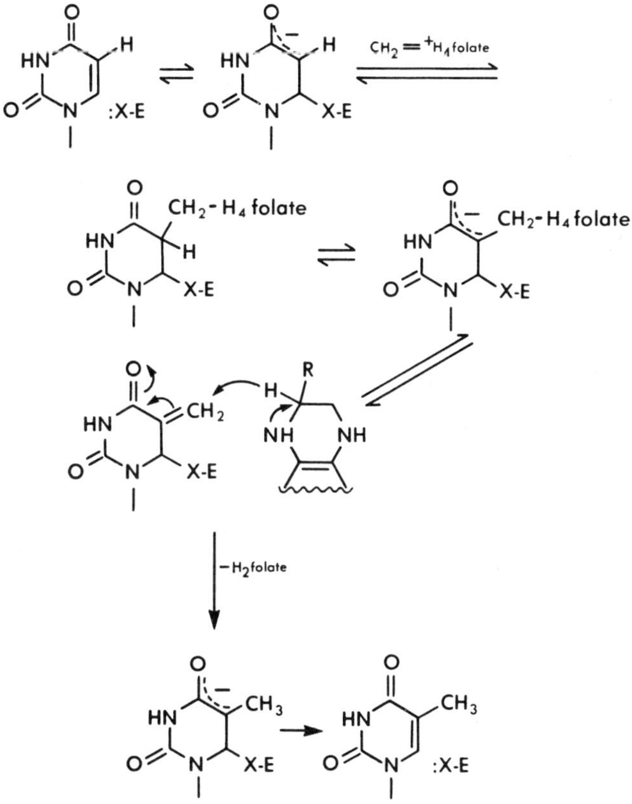

Fig. 1. Mechanism of Thymidylate Synthetase

been reviewed.[1] Because this enzyme represents the sole *de novo* pathway for
dTMP synthesis, it has received much attention as a target for inhibitors of
DNA synthesis with potential chemotherapeutic utility. A number of these
inhibitors (Fig. 2) are analogs of the substrate dUMP which have been substituted at the 5-position.

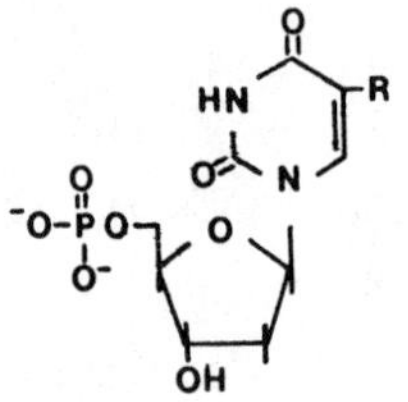

F (FdUMP)

NO_2 (NO_2dUMP)

CF_3 (CF_3dUMP)

CH=CHCF$_3$ (CF$_3$CH=CHdUMP)

Fig. 2. dUMP analogs.

An initial event in the normal catalytic reaction (Fig. 1) involves formation of a covalent bond between a nucleophilic group of the enzyme and the
6-position of dUMP. The most important aspect of *mechanism-based* inhibitors
of dTMP synthetase which are 5-substituted dUMP's is that they first interact
with the enzyme to form a reversible E--I complex and then form a covalent bond
with a nucleophilic catalyst of the enzyme. Depending on the inhibitor, the
covalent bond formed is either sufficiently stable to permit isolation (*e.g.*,
FdUMP, NO$_2$dUMP) or it activates a latent reactive chemical group at the 5-
position of the analog (*e.g.*, CF$_3$dUMP, CF$_3$CH=CHdUMP).

In this paper we briefly describe two inhibitors which form a stable covalent bond with the 6-position of dTMP synthetase. These include 5-fluoro-2'-
deoxyuridylate (FdUMP), which was a known inhibitor of thymidylate synthetase
before it was determined to be effective *via* mechanism-based inhibition, and
5-nitro-2'-deoxyuridylate (NO$_2$dUMP), which was designed after the mechanism of
the enzyme was established. We also describe studies which demonstrate the
utility of these mechanism-based inhibitors in studies of the *in vivo* action
of inhibitors of thymidylate synthetase.

In Vitro Studies. The prototype mechanism-based inhibitor of dTMP synthetase is FdUMP; this interaction is more fully described elsewhere.[1,2] In the
presence of CH$_2$-H$_4$folate this analog rapidly reacts with the enzyme in a manner
analogous to the first two steps depicted in Fig. 1. At this stage--where a
proton from C-5 of the covalently bound dUMP is removed in the normal enzymic
reaction--the stability of the C-F bond results in accumulation of a covalently

bound complex which may be considered analogous to a steady-state intermediate
of the normal enzyme reaction (Fig. 3). In this tight, ternary complex, the
6-position of FdUMP is covalently bound to the enzyme and CH_2-H_4folate is bound
at the 5-position of FdUMP. This complex can readily be isolated by nitrocellulose filtration, gel filtration or acid precipitation. The properties of
the covalent ternary complex are summarized in Table 1.

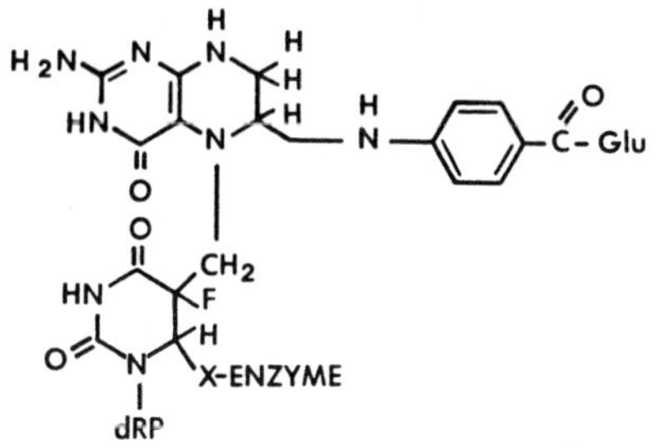

Fig. 3. Structure of the FdUMP-CH_2-
H_4folate-dTMP synthetase complex.

TABLE 1

PROPERTIES OF COVALENT COMPLEX BETWEEN TS[a] AND 5-SUBSTITUTED dUMP COMPOUNDS

Property	FdUMP	NO_2dUMP
Complex formation requires CH_2-H_4folate	yes	no
Stable to:		
Sephadex gel filtration	yes	yes
nitrocellulose filtration	yes	yes
TCA	yes	no
SDS	yes	no
Dissociated by heating (65°, 15 min)	yes	yes

[a]TS = dTMP synthetase

We have observed[3] that NO_2dUMP forms a reversible complex with dTMP synthetase with an apparent K_i = 2 x 10^{-8} M. As NO_2dUMP is highly ionized at the pH
utilized in this assay, the actual K_i is calculated to be approximately 100-
fold lower. After formation of a reversible complex, this compound rapidly
inactivates the enzyme; unlike FdUMP, CH_2-H_4folate is not required for inactivation by NO_2dUMP. At 25° at least 80% of enzyme activity is lost within 1 min

and at 0° the half-life of the first-order inactivation at saturating NO_2dUMP is *ca.* 13 min. It was not experimentally feasible to obtain complete inactivation kinetics even at 0°, and we resorted to the use of including dUMP in the reaction mixture in an attempt to slow the reaction. Two relevant points emerged from this experiment. First, it is clear that dUMP protects the enzyme against inactivation by NO_2dUMP, which suggests that the inhibitor binds at the same site as the substrate. Second, the inactivation of dTMP synthetase by NO_2dUMP clearly follows first-order kinetics indicative of reversible binding of the inhibitor followed by irreversible (or pseudo-irreversible) inhibition. Further evidence that structural changes occur in the heterocycle of NO_2dUMP was obtained by uv difference spectra. The uv difference spectra of enzyme plus NO_2dUMP *vs* NO_2dUMP shows a peak at 345 nm with an isosbestic point at 321 nm. Difference spectra-titration (at 345 nm) of dTMP synthetase with $5-NO_2dUMP$ demonstrates that 2 mol of inhibitor are bound per mol enzyme. More recently, utilizing $[6-^3H,^{14}C]NO_2dUMP$, we have demonstrated that the complex can be isolated by gel filtration or nitrocellulose filtration in the absence of CH_2-H_4folate. With the enzyme from *L. casei*, it has been shown that the complex is reversible with $k_d = 0.53$ hr^{-1}, when excess NO_2dUMP is added to the preformed complex to prevent reassociation of the radioactive ligand. The radioactive ligand dissociated either as described above or by treatment with SDS was shown to be NO_2dUMP by HPLC. Further, utilizing NO_2dUMP labeled with tritium at the 6-position, a secondary hydrogen isotope effect of $k_H/k_T = 1.19$ was observed upon dissociation, suggesting that the 6-position of the enzyme-bound inhibitor is sp^3 hybridized. From the aforementioned results, the mechanism shown in Fig. 4 has been proposed for the interaction of NO_2dUMP with dTMP synthetase. The properties of this complex are summarized in Table 1.

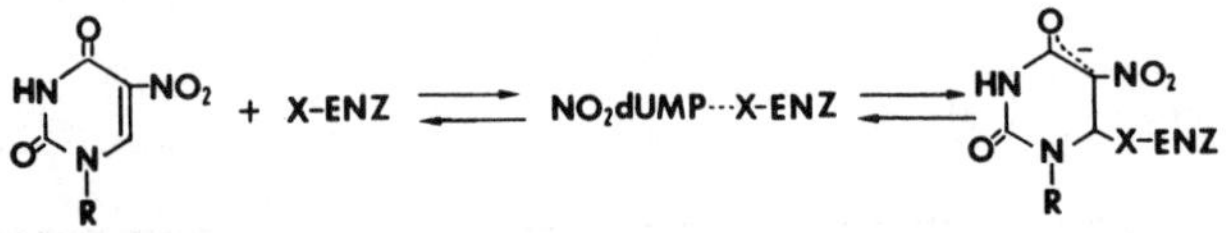

Fig. 4. Proposed mechanism of interaction of NO_2dUMP with dTMP synthetase; R = 5-phospho-2-deoxyribosyl.

In Vivo Studies. The remainder of this paper deals with preliminary studies of the utilization of these mechanism-based inhibitors of dTMP synthetase for studies in tissue culture. As shown in Table 2, both NO_2dUrd and FdUrd are cytotoxic to a variety of tissue culture cells.[4] Cells exposed to NO2dUrd show

TABLE 2

CYTOTOXICITY OF NO_2dUrd AND FdUrd $(EC_{50}, \mu M)$ [a]

Compound	Cell line [b]		
	S-49	L1210	HTC
NO_2dUrd	0.030	0.033	0.25
FdUrd	0.001	0.0005	0.005

[a]Dose response curves were constructed from a minimum of 12 points in which concentrations of inhibitor spanned 3-log units.
[b]HTC is a subclone of buffalo rat hepatoma tissue culture cells. S-49 are mouse lymphoma cells. L1210 are mouse leukemia cells.

a decrease in the incorporation of dUrd into DNA, but no effect on the incorporation of dThd into DNA or Urd into RNA. A number of biochemical parameters of cells treated with $[6-^3H]NO_2dUrd$ were ascertained. When cytosol from such cells was passed through Sephadex G-25, macromolecular radioactivity was isolated in the void volume of the column. In accord with the aforementioned properties of the NO_2dUMP-dTMP synthetase complex, when this fraction was heated at 65° for 15 minutes macromolecular bound radioactivity was no longer present and the released radioactivity was identified as NO_2dUMP by HPLC. These results indicated that there was negligible incorporation of the inhibitor into nucleic acid ($< 3 \times 10^{-8}$ pg NO_2dUMP/pg DNA) and it was concluded that the sole intracellular target for NO_2dUrd, after its conversion to the nucleotide was indeed thymidylate synthetase. Analysis of the metabolites formed after treatment of cells with $[6-^3H]NO_2dUrd$ indicated that no di- or tri-nucleotides were produced. Details of these studies will be published elsewhere.

A more extensive study of the utility of the mechanism-based inhibitor FdUMP for *in vivo* studies was performed.[5] Here, the objective was to develop methodology which would permit determination of several important aspects of FUra and FdUrd metabolism using a single small sample of cells. It was anticipated that if a number of parameters could be assessed easily, one or more might correlate with the observed drug cytotoxicity and provide insight into the possible differential effects of FUra on various cells. The procedures developed are summarized in Figure 5 and utilize the aforementioned properties of the ternary $FdUMP-CH_2-H_4folate$-dTMP synthetase complex. Cells are exposed to the radioactive drug, harvested and washed with cold phosphate-buffered saline. The combined media and washings can be analyzed by HPLC to identify

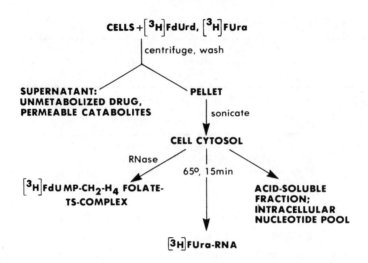

Fig. 5. Summary of methods for analysis of FdUrd, FUra metabolism.

and quantitate unreacted drug and cell permeable metabolites. After disruption of cells, gel filtration or TCA precipitation is used to separate macromolecules from low molecular weight compounds. The latter fraction may be directly applied to HPLC for assessment of the metabolism of the radioactive drug. In addition, the acid soluble fraction can be analyzed by HPLC to determine the effect of the drug on nucleotide pool sizes. Analysis of the radioactivity in the macromolecular fraction provides an assessment of the amount of drug both incorporated into RNA and bound to thymidylate synthetase. When incorporation of the drug into both components is possible, techniques are employed which selectively destroy each *prior* to analysis of macromolecular radioactivity. RNA can be hydrolyzed by RNase under conditions where the $FdUMP-CH_2-H_4$folate-TS complex is stable. Likewise, the ternary $FdUMP-CH_2-H_4$folate-TS complex can be disrupted by heating at 65° without destruction of RNA. Thus, using 10^6-10^8 cells, it is feasible to analyze FUra incorporation into RNA, FdUMP bound to thymidylate synthetase, drug metabolites and nucleotide pool sizes.

When HTC cells are exposed to $[6-^3H]FdUrd$ for 2 hours, all intracellular macromolecular-bound radioactivity is present as an $FdUMP-CH_2-H_4$folate-TS complex (Fig. 6). This is demonstrated by comparison of the properties of this macromolecular-bound radioactivity with those of the complex formed using $[6-^3H]FdUMP$, CH_2-H_4folate and cytosol from untreated cells, as well as with

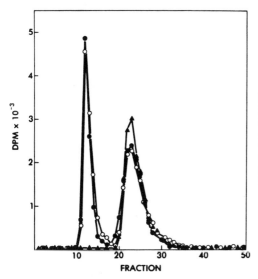

Fig. 6. Sephadex G-25 Chromatography of cytosol from HTC cells incubated with [6-^{3}H]FdUrd. Aliquots of cytosol were subjected to chromatography untreated (●—●—●); after treatment with 1% SDS, 100° for 2 min (o—o—o); or after heating at 65° for 15 min (▲—▲—▲).

the well-characterized ternary complex formed with *L. casei* thymidylate synthetase.[6,7] As with complexes formed *in vitro* (Table 1), macromolecular-bound radioactivity isolated from cells treated wtih [6-^{3}H]FdUrd was resistant to RNase, precipitated with TCA, stable to SDS and could be dissociated to provide free [^{3}H]FdUMP by heating at 65°. In addition, the only low molecular weight intracellular drug metabolite found by HPLC analysis was FdUMP. The radioactive macromolecular fraction migrated in SDS gel electrophoresis with a subunit molecular weight of 35,000 daltons, which is similar to the molecular weight reported for FdUMP-CH$_2$-H$_4$folate-TS complex by others.[8,9]

Treatment of cells with excess [6-^{3}H]FdUrd permits titration of intracellular levels of thymidylate synthetase. Formation of the intracellular FdUMP-CH$_2$-H$_4$folate-TS complex is complete within 40-60 min. As the intracellular level of thymidylate synthetase is likely to be one of the factors involved in the susceptibility of cells to FUra and FdUrd,[10] this simple procedure may be useful in predicting the responsiveness of cells towards these drugs. Indeed, with the cell lines used here, there is a good correlation between the intracellular levels of thymidylate synthetase and the cytotoxicity of FdUrd; that is, cells which possess more enzyme are more resistant to the cytotoxic effects of FdUrd (Table 3).

We have also measured certain kinetic parameters of the intracellular FdUMP-CH$_2$-H$_4$folate-TS complex. When cells treated with [6-^{3}H]FdUrd to allow

TABLE 3

CYTOTOXICITY OF FdUrd AND MEASUREMENT OF FdUMP-CH$_2$-H$_4$FOLATE-TS COMPLEX

Cell Type	EC$_{50}$FdUrd (nM)[a]	FdUMP-CH$_2$-H$_4$folate-TS Complex (pmol/10^6 cells)	
		Intracellular[b]	In Vitro
S-49	0.84	0.18	0.3
S-49/TK$^-$	< 2000	< 0.04	0.4
HTC	5	0.87	1.2

[a]Determined as described in Table 2.
[b]Cells in exponential growth were spun down and resuspended at a density of 5 x 10^6 cells/ml in fresh media. [6-^{3}H]FdUrd and folinic acid were added and the suspensions incubated at 37° for 1 hr. At the end of this time, cell cytosol was prepared and the amount of [^{3}H]FdUMP-CH$_2$-H$_4$folate-TS complex determined by Sephadex G-25 chromatography.
[c]Determined by direct titration of cell cytosol with [6-^{3}H]FdUMP and CH$_2$-H$_4$folate, followed by Sephadex G-25 chromatography.

formation of the ternary complex are subsequently exposed to excess unlabeled FdUrd, [^{3}H]FdUMP which has dissociated from the complex is replaced by unlabeled FdUMP; the loss of macromolecular bound radioactivity reflects the intrinsic rate of dissociation of the intracellular complex. This is a first-order process with $t_{\frac{1}{2}} \simeq 6.2$ hrs. Interestingly, the rate of dissociation of the intracellular complex is slower than that of the complex in cytosol ($t_{\frac{1}{2}} \simeq$ 2 hrs), indicating that an apparent stability is provided by the intracellular environment. When cells possessing the [^{3}H]FdUMP-CH$_2$-H$_4$folate-TS complex are washed and resuspended in media possessing no unlabeled FdUrd, there is no decrease apparent in the amount of intracellular complex over a period of 7 hrs. Given the measured half-time for dissociation, the observed stability of the intracellular complex can best be explained by the persistance of an intracellular pool of [^{3}H]FdUMP sufficient to saturate the enzyme. That is, even though [^{3}H]FdUMP dissociates from the enzyme with a finite rate, association to reform the complex is more rapid than degradation and subsequent efflux of radioactivity from the cell.

While most of the studies described here utilize FdUrd, the methodology has been developed to be equally adaptable to similar studies employing FUra and such studies are ongoing in this laboratory. The utility of these procedures is illustrated in a preliminary experiment designed to examine FUra metabolism in L1210 cells exposed to [6-^{3}H]FUra (Fig. 7). When radioactivity in the acid soluble fraction from these cells was analyzed by HPLC, [^{3}H]FdUMP

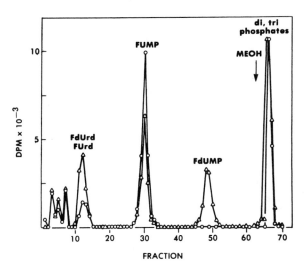

Fig. 7. Analysis of radioactivity present in the intracellular nucleotide pool following incubation of L1210 cells with [6-^{3}H]FUra. Intracellular metabolites were extracted from the cytosol either before (O-O-O) or after (Δ-Δ-Δ) the cytosol was heated at 65° for 15 min.

could not be detected. Similar findings have recently been reported.[11] However, when the cytosol was heated at 65° prior to acid precipitation, [^{3}H]FdUMP was shown to be present at levels of *ca.* 50 fmol/10^6 cells. This demonstrated that all of the intracellular FdUMP present at the time of analysis was bound to thymidylate synthetase and illustrates how direct analysis of acid soluble fractions could be misleading in interpreting studies of the metabolism of this drug. Furthermore, although these studies have employed radioactive drug, the methods for FdUMP-CH$_2$-H$_4$folate-TS complex isolation and FdUMP ligand dissociation described here could easily be adapted to procedures which have been previously employed for measuring free non-radioactive FdUMP levels.[12] In this manner, determinations of both free and enzyme-bound FdUMP can be made in situations which are not amenable to the use of radioactive drugs. Therefore, without major modification, the methods described here should be applicable for a variety of *in vivo* studies of FUra and FdUrd action.

In summary, the properties of two mechanism-based inhibitors of dTMP synthetase have been described. FdUMP is the prototype inhibitor which was important in elucidating the mechanism of this enzyme. With such knowledge, a new mechanism-based inhibitor, NO$_2$dUMP, was designed and its interaction with dTMP synthetase described. Using appropriate nucleoside precursors of these inhibitors, aspects of the effects of mechanism-based inhibition of dTMP synthetase on tissue culture cells have been examined.

ACKNOWLEDGEMENTS

This study was supported by Grant CA 14394, awarded by the National Cancer Institute, DHEW. DVS is the recipient of an NIH Career Development Award. WLW was a Leukemia Society of America Fellow, 1976-1978.

REFERENCES

1. Pogolotti, A.L. Jr. and Santi, D.V. (1977) in Bioorganic Chemistry, Vol. 1, Academic Press, N. Y., pp. 277-311.
2. Danenberg, P.V. (1977) Biochim. Biophys. Acta, 473, 73-92.
3. Matsuda, A., Wataya, Y. and Santi, D.V. (1978) Biochem. Biophys. Res. Comm., 84, 654-659.
4. Washtien, W., Matsuda, A., Wataya, Y. and Santi, D.V. (1978) Biochem. Pharm., 27, 2663-2666.
5. Washtien, W. and Santi, D.V. (1979) Cancer Res., in press.
6. Santi, D.V., McHenry, C.S. and Sommer, H. (1974) Biochemistry, 13, 471-481.
7. Danenberg, P.V., Langenbach, R.J. and Heidelberger, C. (1974) Biochemistry, 13, 926-933.
8. Dunlap, R.B., Harding, N.G.L. and Huennekens, F.M. (1971) Biochemistry, 10, 88-97.
9. Ullman, B., Lee, M., Martin, D.W. Jr. and Santi, D.V. (1978) Proc. Natl. Acad. Sci. USA, 75, 980-983.
10. Wilkinson, D.S., Solomonson, L.P. and Cory, J.G. (1977) Proc. Soc. Exp. Biol. and Med., 154, 368-371.
11. Laskin, J.D., Evans, R.M., Slocum, H.K., Burke, D. and Hakala, M.J. (1979) Cancer Res., 39, 383-390.
12. Myers, C.E., Young, R.C., Johns, D.G. and Chabner, B.A. (1974) Cancer Res., 34, 2683-2688.

DISCUSSION

KALMAN: I would like to emphasize in connection with the last part of your presentation that it is indeed of great importance to evaluate the differential sensitivities of various tissues and cells to drugs. In other words, these approaches permit the determination of inherent drug sensitivities of cells, which have not yet been exposed to drugs, as well as the resistance of cell populations developed by selection in the presence of the drug, e.g., resistant cells, which are incapable of activating an antimetabolite.

SANTI: Like the TK⁻ cells, in the case of 5-fluorodeoxyuridine.

KALMAN: That's right. We have been studying a different intact cell system of L1210 leukemia, as an experimental therapeutic model and developed a means of measuring intracellular thymidylate synthetase activity in an attempt to use this as an indicator for the evaluation of drug action and effectiveness among the antimetabolites of the pyrimidine nucleoside analog and antifolate variety[1,2]. It is interesting that when we looked at the recovery of enzyme activity after 5-NO_2-dUrd and FdUrd treatment, both occurred and with a shorter half-life[3] than what you indicated for the decomposition of the [6-^{3}H]-FdUrd-labelled complex. This may be due to differences in the respective methodologies, at least in the case of the fluoro-analog. With respect to 5-NO_2-dUMP - you mentioned that the cofactor is not required for tight complex formation with thymidylate synthetase, in contrast to the case with FdUMP. Did you observe any stabilizing effect of 5,10-methylenetetrahydrofolate on the 5-NO_2-dUMP-enzyme complex, once it is formed?

SANTI: We have looked at that with a large excess of cofactor after prolonged incubation and analyzed the complexes to find out what fraction is bound to cofactor plus inhibitor *vs.* inhibitor alone. We found a small amount, about 5%, which corresponded to the ternary complex. That is probably because the bound carbanion is so well stabilized.

MALOCHE: Is there any information about the nature of the group of the enzyme that attacks C-6 of the pyrimidine ring?

SANTI: Yes, the information is based not on direct studies of the complex, but on sequence studies of the peptide that is in the complex, by Frank Maley[4] who has determined the complete sequence of the enzyme recently. From his studies he would suggest and I think most people would that a cysteine is involved in that complex. We are in the process of sequencing the peptide directly with 5-fluoro-dUMP attached. We have not chewed into it far enough yet. It is still being done.

MALOCHE: Can the enzyme be crystalized?

SANTI: Yes, it crystalizes very easily.

MALOCHE: Is anyone doing X-ray work on it?

SANTI: There is a lot of people trying, but to my knowledge no one has obtained crystals suitable for X-ray work.

SCHINAZI: Is the 5'-phosphate necessary for binding to thymidylate synthetase?

SANTI: Yes, as far as I know, all analogs that bind, require the phosphate.

KISLIUK: When you presented the dissociation of the FdUMP methylenetetrahydrofolate ternary complex, the comparable data for the NO_2-compound were without the cofactor. I would like to know, what it is with the cofactor?

SANTI: With the cofactor we do not see very much ternary complex formed; we notice something like a 5% difference, in the rate of dissociation in the presence or absence of cofactor, but I think this may be within experimental error. I would say in the presence of the cofactor it is essentially the same.

KISLIUK: When you react the 5-NO$_2$-dUMP with enzyme you get a stoichiometry of two. Is that in the presence of mercaptoethanol? Because this is different, when you react the enzyme with the substrate, then you get just one, at least under our conditions.

SANTI: That is right, but this forms a covalent bond. It is in the presence of mercaptoethanol.

KISLIUK: You would get a stoichiometry of 2 even if you did not have mercaptoethanol present?

SANTI: As long as the enzyme is pretreated with thiols.

KISLIUK: Even if it has never seen mercaptoethanol?

SANTI: You do see the difference spectra in the absence of mercaptoethanol, but I do not recall if we titrated the enzyme under these conditions. I do not know if I can really answer your question.

CHWANG: Do you know, whether 5-nitro-2'-deoxyuridine is incorporated into DNA?

SANTI: If so it is less than 3×10^{-8} pgm/pgm DNA.

CHWANG: What is the dose for 50% kill in a cell line? For FdUrd, *e.g.*, it is in the nanomolar range. How about 5-NO$_2$-dUrd?

SANTI: It depends upon the tissue culture line. It is about 20-fold poorer than dFUrd in most tissue culture systems - about $1-5 \times 10^{-8}$ M.

CHWANG: Does trifluoromethyl-dUMP require the cofactor for inactivation of thymidylate synthetase?

SANTI: The reaction of CF$_3$dUMP with dTMP synthetase is very interesting. We do not really know what is going on. It definitely causes time-dependent inactivation of the enzyme. It will do it in the presence or absence of the cofactor, apparently by different mechanisms. The reason I say I do not understand it is that it is probably the only example I know of, when one of these suicide inhibitors that kills the enzyme is not ultimately covalently bound to the enzyme, for some unknown reason.

COWARD: Is the C-nucleoside, corresponding to FdUrd - with the N-1 missing - known?

SANTI: I do not know. Does anyone know? Has it been made?

VOICE from the audience: No, it has not been made.

COWARD: That would be interesting to try and separate out the DNA- from the RNA-effect.

MARQUEZ: Have you thought of using other heterocyclics, which would allow the enzyme to attack the 6-positon? I am thinking of something like 5-azadeoxyuridine. Something, which will enhance the activity, in terms of building a different heterocyclic nucleus.

SANTI: I know workers doing such things. We are not doing that.

KALMAN: Let me comment on this. 5-Aza-2'-deoxyuridine has a very short half life in aqueous solutions and falls apart to the ring-opened N-formyl-biuret derivative[5]. The more stable 5-aza-2'-deoxycytidine also made in Prague[6,7] is more cytotoxic and is presumably deaminated to the corresponding 5-azauracil derivatives *in situ* , since there is evidence for the involvement of thymidylate synthetase inhibition in its mode of action. We have made the stable 1-deaza-5-aza-dUMP *i.e.*, 2'-deoxypseudouridylate[8], which inhibits *L. casei* thymidylate synthetase competitively with a K_i-value of 4.6×10^{-7} M.

A variety of modifications in the heterocyclic moiety of pyrimidine nucleosides as a part of a general strategy of drug design, and the resulting biological activities have been reviewed by Bloch[9].

REFERENCES

1. Kalman, T.I., and Yalowich, J.C. (1977) Amer. Chem. Soc. 174th Meeting, Abstracts, BIOL 127.
2. Kalman, T.I., and Yalowich, J.C. (1979) in The Chemistry and Biology of Pteridines, Kisliuk, R.L. and Brown, G.M., Eds., Elsevier North-Holland N.Y., p. 671.
3. Kalman, T.I., and Yalowich, J.C. (1979) this volume.
4. Maley, G.F., Bellisario, R.L., Guarino, D.U., and Maley, F. (1979) J. Biol. Chem. 254, 1301.
5. Čihák and Šorm, (1972) Biochem. Biophys. Res. Commun. 46, 1194.
6. Pliml, J. and Šorm, F. (1964) Collect. Czech. Chem. Commun. 29, 2060.
7. Šorm and Veselý (1968) Neoplasma 15, 339.
8. Kalman, T.I. (1972) Biochem. Biophys. Res. Commun. 46, 1194.
9. Bloch, A. (1973) in Drug Design, Vol. IV, Ariëns, E.J. Ed., Academic, New York, p. 306.

SUICIDE INACTIVATION OF DECARBOXYLASES

A. L. MAYCOCK, S. D. ASTER AND A. A. PATCHETT
Merck Sharp & Dohme Research Laboratories, Division of Merck & Co., Inc.
P.O. Box 2000, Rahway, New Jersey 07065, USA

INTRODUCTION

The importance of amino acid decarboxylases in mammalian systems is well known and a great deal of effort has been directed toward the design and synthesis of highly specific inhibitors of them. We have studied a number of α-substituted amino acids as potential suicide inactivators[1-6] (also called k_{cat} inhibitors and enzyme activated irreversible inhibitors) of the respective decarboxylases. Suicide inactivators are chemically non-reactive compounds which are converted to reactive species by the action of the target enzyme and subsequently cause irreversible inhibition (inactivation) of the enzyme. The design of such compounds for decarboxylases has been discussed earlier by several workers[6] and is based on the known mechanism by which pyridoxal phosphate dependent enzymes catalyze their respective reactions.[7] Briefly, all such reactions involve formation of a delocalized carbanion (quinoid) intermediate ($\underline{1}$), usually by loss of CO_2 (decarboxylases) or a proton (racemases,

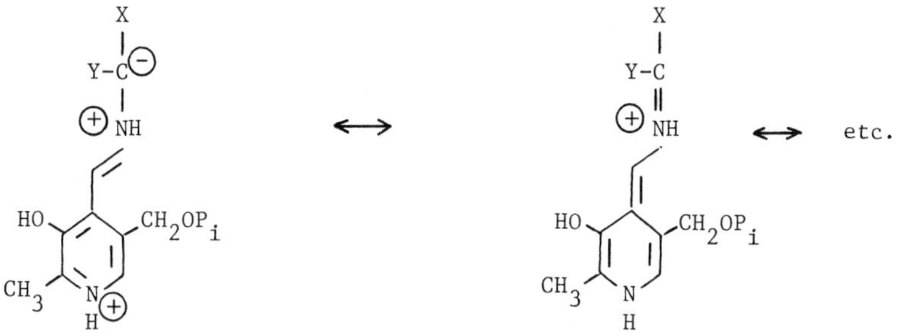

$\underline{1}$

β-replacement enzymes). Subsequently, these intermediates undergo either protonation or elimination which eventually leads to the normal reaction product. In designing suicide inactivators for pyridoxal phosphate dependent enzymes, one considers substrate analogs which are capable of forming quinoid intermediates that subsequently react to generate reactive (usually electrophilic) species at the enzyme active site. Before escaping the enzyme, this intermediate may in turn interact with fortuitously located nucleophilic groups at (or near) the active site, leading to formation of an enzyme-inhibitor covalent adduct which is catalytically inactive.

One of the earliest examples of suicide inactivation of a pyridoxal phosphate dependent enzyme was that of alanine racemase by 3-fluoro-D-alanine,[8] an effective antibacterial compound.[9,10] Although it was only recently verified that 3-fluoro-D-alanine is a suicide inactivator,[11] the possibility was recognized earlier by one of us (A. A. Patchett) and others,[12,13] and led at Merck to the design and synthesis[14-17] of the α-substituted amino acids which we have studied.

Two types of compounds have been evaluated: compounds such as 2 where X is a potential leaving group and unsaturated compounds such as 3 and 4. Neither

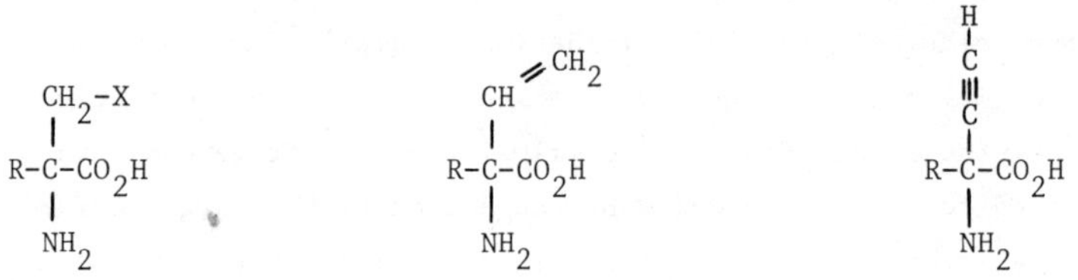

$$
\begin{array}{ccc}
\text{CH}_2\text{-X} & \text{CH}\!\!=\!\!\text{CH}_2 & \text{H-C}\!\!\equiv\!\!\text{C} \\
| & | & | \\
\text{R-C-CO}_2\text{H} & \text{R-C-CO}_2\text{H} & \text{R-C-CO}_2\text{H} \\
| & | & | \\
\text{NH}_2 & \text{NH}_2 & \text{NH}_2 \\
\underline{2} & \underline{3} & \underline{4}
\end{array}
$$

type of compound is inherently chemically reactive under physiological conditions. However, enzyme catalyzed decarboxylation of such compounds could lead to reactive species through either elimination or protonation of the respective intermediates:

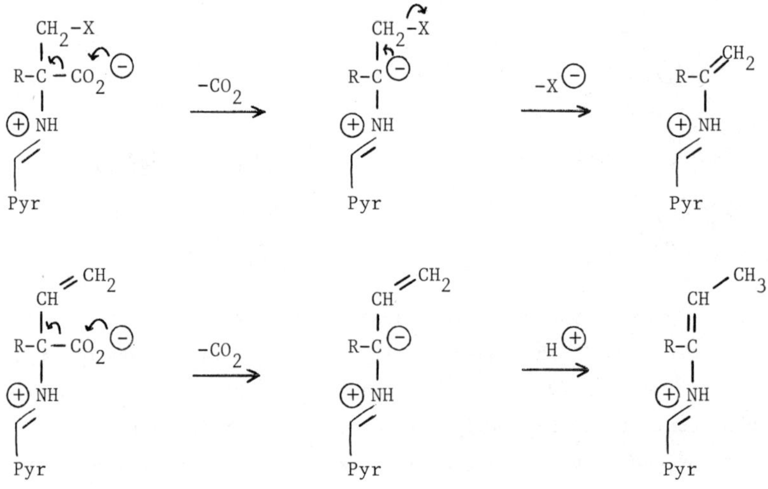

(PyrCHO is enzyme bound pyridoxal phosphate)

Subsequent Michael addition of an enzyme nucleophile would lead to a covalent enzyme-inhibitor adduct.

MATERIALS AND METHODS

Inhibitors. Synthesis of the inhibitors has been described[15-19]. Unless otherwise indicated, the racemic (R,S) mixtures were used.

Enzymes and assays. Enzymes were isolated and assayed as previously described.[15] Preincubation experiments were carried out by treating enzyme with inhibitor under normal assay conditions but in the absence of substrate. At appropriate time intervals, aliquots of the preincubation mixture were removed, diluted into assay mixtures containing substrate and assayed in the usual manner.

RESULTS AND DISCUSSION

Aromatic amino acid (dopa) decarboxylase. A number of compounds were studied as potential inactivators of dopa decarboxylase (Table 1). All of the

TABLE 1

EFFECTS OF POTENTIAL INACTIVATORS ON DOPA DECARBOXYLASE (HOG KIDNEY)

Inhibitor	Nature of Inhibition
α-Fluoromethyldopa	Time dependent, rapid[a], irreversible
α-Chloromethyldopa	Time dependent, rapid
α-Difluoromethyldopa	Time dependent, rapid
α-Hydroxymethyldopa	No inhibition
α-Fluoromethyldopamine	Time dependent, rapid, irreversible
α-Trifluoromethyldopamine	No time dependence
α-Vinyldopa	Time dependent, rapid, incomplete
α-Vinyldopamine	Time dependent, slow
α-Ethinyldopa	Time dependent, rapid, incomplete
α-Ethinyldopamine	Time dependent, slow
α-Vinyltyrosine	No inhibition
α-Vinyl-m-tyrosine	Time dependent, rapid, incomplete
α-Fluoromethyltyrosine	Time dependent, slow
α-Fluoromethyl-m-tyrosine	Time dependent, rapid

[a]Rapid signifies 50% inactivation in <20 min.

α-halomethyldopas were rapid, time-dependent inhibitors, α-fluoromethyldopa
(FMDopa) being the most rapid at low (micromolar) concentration. α-Vinyldopa
(VDopa) and α-ethinyldopa (EDopa) also caused rapid, time-dependent inhibition,
but it was not complete. According to the literature p-tyrosine itself is a
poor substrate for the enzyme, but m-tyrosine is an excellent one. In line
with this substrate specificity we found α-fluoromethyl-p-tyrosine to be a
very slow time-dependent inhibitor of dopa decarboxylase, whereas α-fluoro-
methyl-m-tyrosine produced extremely rapid time-dependent inhibition. A similar pattern was observed with the α-vinyltyrosines. No inhibition was observed with the para isomer, whereas the meta isomer behaved in a manner
analogous to VDopa. Of the dopamine analogs studied, all except α-trifluoro-
methyldopamine produced time-dependent inhibition of the enzyme. Again, the
α-monofluoromethyl compound caused the most rapid inactivation at low concentrations.

Based on the observed time-dependent inhibition which suggests the possibility of suicide inactivation, three compounds, FMDopa, VDopa, and EDopa were
selected for further study.

FMDopa.[15,19] When dopa decarboxylase was treated with FMDopa, a rapid time-
dependent loss of enzyme activity was observed (Fig. 1). Although most (85-
95%) of the activity was lost rapidly, there was always a slower second phase.
This behavior has also been observed by other workers.[20] The reason for this
biphasic inactivation has not been ascertained. The inactivation was further
characterized as being independent of the presence of exogenous pyridoxal
phosphate, stereospecific (only the S isomer inactivated), irreversible
(dialysis) and active site directed (α-methyldopa diminished the inactivation
rate). These data are all consistent with the postulated mode of inactivation, namely enzyme catalyzed decarboxylation leading to formation of a reactive electrophilic species at the active site which then causes irreversible
inhibition.

In order to further characterize the process we used isotopically labelled
samples of FMDopa. When pure enzyme was treated with [ring-^{3}H]FMDopa, one
mole of tritium became associated with protein per mole enzyme inactivated.
On the other hand, when enzyme was treated with [carboxyl-^{14}C]FMDopa, <0.02
equivalents of inactivator became associated with dead enzyme. Furthermore,
only 1.25 moles of $^{14}CO_2$ was evolved from [carboxyl-^{14}C]FMDopa per mole of
enzyme inactivated. Concomitantly, less than 0.05 moles of the "normal" decarboxylation product, R-α-fluoromethyldopamine (FMDopamine) was formed. In
another experiment 1.1 mole of fluoride was released from FMDopa per mole of

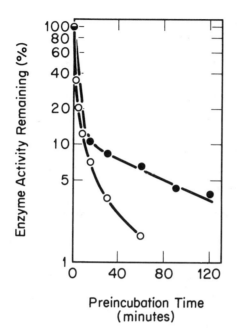

Fig. 1. Time-dependent inhibition of dopa decarboxylase caused by preincu-
bating it with R,S-α-FMDopa. Different enzyme samples treated with 5 μM
R,S-α-FMDopa: fully purified enzyme, specific activity 11200 units/mg (●);
enzyme from ammonium sulfate fractionation, specific activity 110 units/mg (O).

tritium incorporated into enzyme from [ring-^{3}H]FMDopa. These data show that
the inactivation of hog kidney dopa decarboxylase by FMDopa results in the
formulation of a 1:1 covalent inhibitor-enzyme adduct which lacks the fluorine
and the carboxyl group originally present in the inactivator. Furthermore, the
concomitant production of only 1.25 equivalents of CO_2 and essentially no
FMDopamine shows that the inactivation is highly efficient, i.e. virtually
every FMDopa molecule which is decarboxylated causes inactivation. This
efficiency can be expressed as a partitioning ratio[21] (moles of inactivator
processed/mole of enzyme killed) of approximately 1. The desirability of low
partitioning ratios for compounds which might be used in in vivo situations
has been discussed.[21] The inactivation data are summarized in Table 2.

Interestingly, although free FMDopamine itself is not produced during the
inactivation of dopa decarboxylase by FMDopa, the amine itself is a stereospecific (R), stoichiometric, and irreversible inactivator of the enzyme. We
suggest that this process may be an example of the microscopic reversibility
principle which allows, in principle at least, the suicide inactivation of

TABLE 2

CHARACTERISTICS OF INACTIVATION OF DOPA DECARBOXYLASE BY α-FLUOROMETHYLDOPA

Time dependent
Rapid at low concentration
Irreversible
Active-site directed
Stereospecific
[ring-^{3}H] Inhibitor labels enzyme stoichiometrically
[1-^{14}C] Inhibitor does not label enzyme, but 1.25 equivalents of CO_2 are liberated
An equivalent of $F^{\ominus}$ is lost per equivalent of ^{3}H incorporated
Less than 0.05 equivalents of α-fluoromethyldopamine are formed

enzymes by product analogs as well as by substrate analogs. (See Metcalf, this volume for other examples.)

A plausible mechanism for inactivation of dopa decarboxylase by S-FMDopa and by R-FMDopamine is shown in Scheme 1.

SCHEME 1

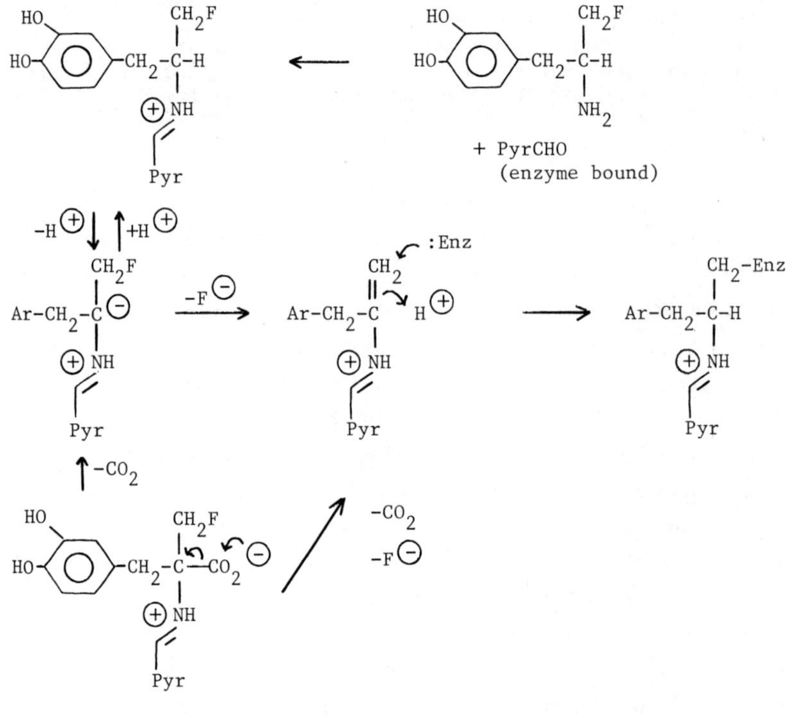

In summary, we believe our data are consistent with FMDopa being a highly effective suicide inactivator of dopa decarboxylase, and we have identified the chemical transformations (i.e. loss of CO_2 and $F^{\ominus}$) which are responsible for the compound's effects.

In vivo studies (rats) show that FMDopa causes inactivation of dopa decarboxylase with a resultant lowering of catechol amine levels.[22,23] Administration of FMDopa to spontaneously hypertensive (SH) rats also causes a lowering of the mean arterial blood pressure.[22] Given this fact alone, one might suppose that the mechanism by which FMDopa produces hypotension is similar to that postulated for ALDOMET (α-methyldopa), namely decarboxylation in the brain and subsequent β-hydroxylation to the active compound, α-methylnorepinephrine.[24,25] (Scheme 2). A similar sequence of reactions would result

SCHEME 2

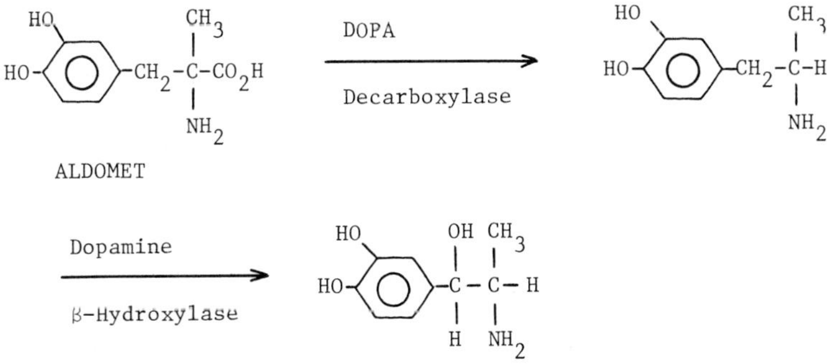

HO- (ring) -HO   CH$_3$ DOPA Decarboxylase   →   HO- (ring) -HO   CH$_3$

CH_2-C-CO_2H with NH_2 ALDOMET   → CH_2-C-H with NH_2

Dopamine β-Hydroxylase →

HO- (ring) -HO   OH CH$_3$ -C-C-H with H and NH_2

α-Methylnorepinephrine

in the production of α-fluoromethylnorepinephrine from FMDopa. However, if our in vitro results with hog kidney dopa decarboxylase can be extrapolated to in vivo situations, we would expect dopa decarboxylase to be inactivated by FMDopa and no free α-fluoromethyldopamine to be produced. Hence the pathway of Scheme 2 should not be possible with FMDopa. Taken together, these data suggest that α-methyldopa (ALDOMET) and α-fluoromethyldopa must produce antihypertensive effects by fundamentally different mechanisms.

α-Vinyldopa (VDopa) and α-ethinyldopa (EDopa). These two compounds were also studied extensively as inactivators and were found to behave very differently in some respects from FMDopa.

Treatment of dopa decarboxylase with α-ethyldopa, VDopa or EDopa gave the results shown in Fig. 2. The saturated compound produces no inactivation, whereas both unsaturated analogs cause rapid, time dependent, but incomplete

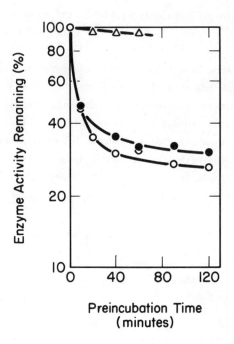

Fig. 2. Preincubation of dopa decarboxylase with 32 μM R,S-α-vinyldopa (O), 32 μM R,S-α-ethinyldopa (●), and 1000 μM R,S-α-ethyldopa (Δ) at room temperature.

loss of enzyme activity, a result very different from the situation observed with FMDopa. Some of the residual activity (<10%) is due to partial reactivation of enzyme during the assay. This incomplete inactivation could be due to multiple forms of enzyme, some susceptible to inactivation and others not, or to modification of all enzyme molecules in such a manner that the activity of each enzyme molecule has been altered. Presently we favor the former explanation, although as yet we have not rigorously excluded the latter.

The inactivation caused by VDopa and by EDopa differs from that caused by FMDopa in another important respect: it is largely (but never completely) reversible. Approximately 70-85% of the original activity is recovered after extensive dialysis or after a preincubation mixture is diluted and allowed to stand at room temperature.

Additional experiments, similar to those described for FMDopa were performed to further characterize the inactivation caused by VDopa and EDopa.

The results of those experiments are summarized in Table 3. Some of the data
have been presented earlier.[18] As with FMDopa, when [ring-^{3}H]VDopa or

TABLE 3

CHARACTERISTICS OF INHIBITION OF DOPA DECARBOXYLASE BY α-VINDYDOPA AND α-
ETHINYLDOPA

Time dependent, rapid
Pseudo-first order
Incomplete
Largely reversible
Retarded in the presence of substrate
Occurs in competition with CO_2 production
Accompanied by loss of absorption band near 420 nm
[ring-^{3}H] Inhibitors label enzyme
Most ^{3}H is lost upon reactivation
[carboxyl-^{14}C] Inhibitors do not label enzyme

[ring-^{3}H]EDopa was employed 0.8-1.2 equivalents of radioactivity became associated with inactivated enzyme, indicating the formation of an enzyme-inactivator adduct. During reactivation, most of the radioactivity was lost. After
extensive dialysis, the residual radioactivity associated with protein corresponded approximately to the amount of enzyme activity which was not
recoverable. When [carboxyl-^{14}C]VDopa or [carboxyl-^{14}C]EDopa was employed, no
radioactivity was associated with inactivated enzyme, indicating that the
enzyme-inhibitor adduct lacked the carboxyl group of the inhibitor. When CO_2
evolution from the ^{14}C inhibitors was monitored during inactivation, it was
found that ca. five equivalents of CO_2 were produced from VDopa before maximum
inactivation was achieved and ca. 18 equivalents were produced from EDopa. So
in the case of the unsaturated dopa analogs, CO_2 production occurs in competition with inactivation. This contrasts with the FMDopa case in which there was
no measurable partitioning between inactivation and other processes producing
CO_2.

At this point we proposed the following working hypothesis for the inactivation caused by VDopa (Scheme 3). (A similar scheme can be written for EDopa).
This scheme is based on the possibility of the decarboxylated intermediate 5
being protonated at any of three possible sites. Protonation a would lead after
hydrolysis to "normal" decarboxylation product. Protonation b would produce
the methyl analog of the intermediate proposed to account for the inactivation

SCHEME 3

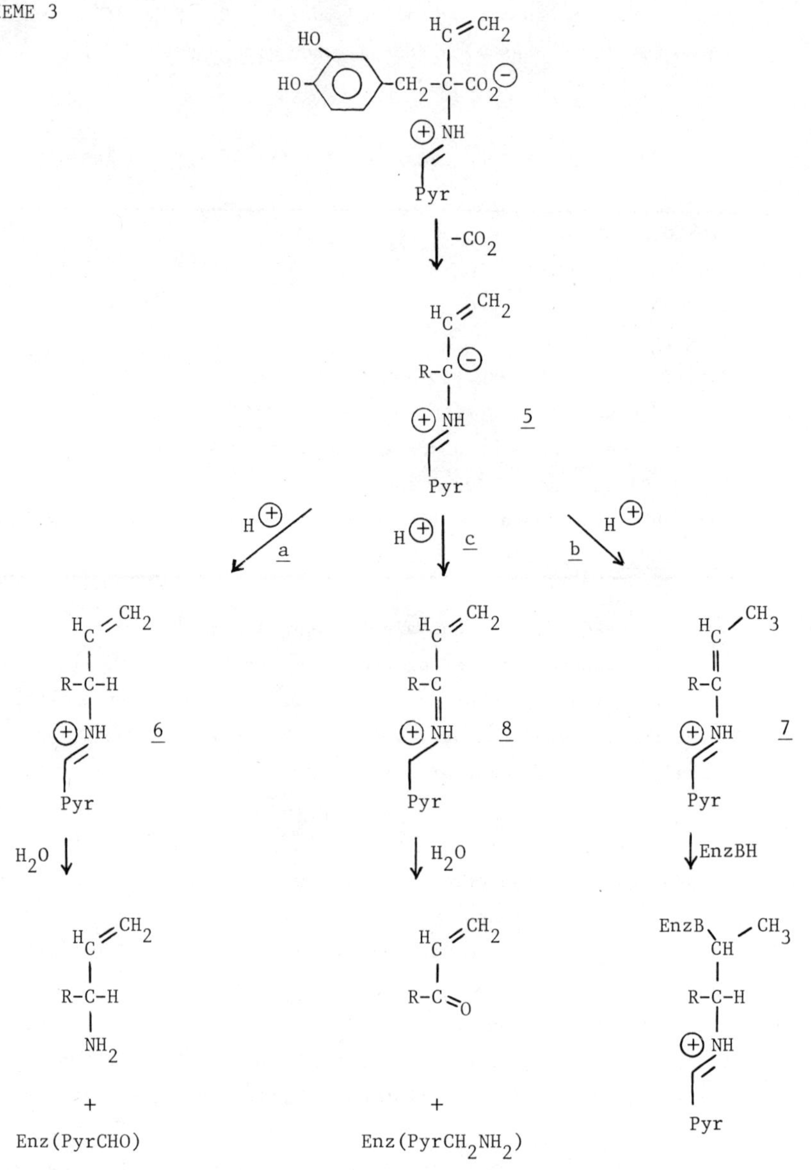

caused by FMDopa. Protonation <u>c</u> is the "abortive transamination" pathway, which is known to compete with "normal" protonation even during decarboxylation of substrates such as dopa or α-methyldopa.[26]

We suggest that the irreversible component of inactivation occurs from 7, which adds an enzyme nucleophile to form a stable covalent intermediate similar to that formed from FMDopa. The reversible component could be 8 which undergoes slow hydrolysis to produce dihydroxybenzylvinyl ketone and regenerate enzyme. Since the regenerated enzyme would contain cofactor in the wrong (pyridoxamine) oxidation state, reactivation by this route would require an additional step, namely transamination of cofactor to return it to the pyridoxal oxidation state. We have tested this hypothesis and found that, indeed, reactivation does not occur in the absence of exogenous pyridoxal phosphate.

We have been unable to detect any of the amine which would be expected (after hydrolysis) from protonation a. Hence the "normal" decarboxylation pathway does not seem to occur in competition with inactivation. We have also been unable to detect any α-vinyldopamine during reactivation of VDopa-treated enzyme, an observation which is consistent with the view that structure 6 is not the reactivatable form of inactivated enzyme.

We are presently attempting to identify the compound released during enzyme reactivation and the material which is produced along with the excess CO_2 during the course of inactivation.

In summary, the inactivation of dopa decarboxylase by FMDopa, VDopa and EDopa, is rapid at low concentrations, involves decarboxylation of the inhibitors and results in the formation of covalent enzyme inhibitor adducts. The processes differ, however, in that the inactivation caused by FMDopa is complete and irreversible, whereas that caused by VDopa and EDopa is incomplete and largely reversible.

Other mammalian decarboxylases. α-Fluoromethyl- and α-vinylamino acid analogs were also investigated as inhibitors of other decarboxylases. The results are collected in Table 4. As shown, all α-fluoromethylamino acids are time-dependent inhibitors of the respective amino acid decarboxylases. The inactivation rates, however, are seen to vary widely. No detailed mechanistic studies have been undertaken with these compounds, but it is reasonable to suppose that mechanisms similar to that shown in Scheme 1 obtain. The vinyl analogs of other amino acids were disappointing as inhibitors of the respective decarboxylases. α-Vinylhistidine was a competitive inhibitor of histidine decarboxylase, but caused no time-dependent inhibition, whereas α-vinylornithine produced time dependent but slow inhibition of ornithine decarboxylase. Neither of these compounds was studied further.

126

TABLE 4

EFFECTS OF POTENTIAL INACTIVATORS ON VARIOUS DECARBOXYLASES

Enzyme (source)	Inhibitor	Nature of Inhibition
Histidine decarboxylase (fetal rat liver)	α-Fluoromethyl-histidine	Time dependent, rapid
	α-Vinylhistidine	No time dependence
Ornithine decarboxylase (rat liver)	α-Fluoromethyl-ornithine	Time dependent, slow
	α-Vinylornithine	Time dependent, slow
Glutamic acid decarboxylase (rat brain)	α-Fluoromethyl-glutamic acid	Time dependent, slow

ACKNOWLEDGMENTS

The following people at Merck supplied generous portions of compounds, ideas, and enthusiasm in support of this work: G. Doldouras, D. Duggan, R. Ellsworth, W. Greenlee, R. Hoffsommer, S. Marburg, H. Meriwether, H. Mertel, L. Perkins, A. Rosegay, D. Taub, and M. Walsh.

REFERENCES

1. Morisaki, M. and Bloch, K. (1972) Biochemistry, 11, 309.
2. Rando, R.R. (1974) Science, 185, 320.
3. Abeles, R.H. and Maycock, A.L. (1976) Acc. Chem. Res., 9, 313.
4. Rando, R.R. (1978) Methods in Enzymology, 46, 28.
5. Walsh, C.T. (1977) in Horizons in Biochemistry and Biophysics, Quagliariello, E., Palmieri, F. and Singer, T.P. ed., Addison-Wesley Publishing Co., Reading, Mass., Vol. 3, p. 36.
6. Seiler, N., Jung, M. and Koch-Weser, J. ed., (1978) Enzyme-Activated Irreversible Inhibitors, Elsevier/North-Holland Biomedical Press, Amsterdam.
7. Boeker, E.A. and Snell, E.E. (1972) Enzymes, 3rd Ed. 6, 217.
8. Kahan, F.M. and Kropp, H. (1975) 15th Interscience Conference on Antimicrobial Agents and Chemotherapy, Abstract 100.
9. Kollonitsch, J., Barash, L., Kahan, F.M. and Kropp, H. (1973) Nature (London), 243, 346.
10. Kollonitsch, J. and Barash, L. (1976) J. Amer. Chem. Soc., 98, 5591.
11. Wang, E. and Walsh, C. (1978) Biochemistry, 17, 1313.
12. Kollonitsch, J. (1978) Isr. J. Chem., 17, 53.
13. Bey, P., Jung, M. and Metcalf, B. (1977) Medicinal Chem., 5, 115.
14. Kollonitsch, J. and Patchett, A.A. (1977) U.S. Patent Application 802,301.
15. Kollonitsch, J., Patchett, A.A., Marburg, S., Maycock, A.L., Perkins, L.M., Doldouras, G.A., Duggan, D.E. and Aster, S.D. (1978) Nature (London), 274, 906.
16. Taub, D. and Patchett, A.A. (1977) Tetrahedron Lett., 2745.
17. Greenlee, W.J., Taub, D. and Patchett, A.A. (1978) Tetrahedron Lett., 2745.

18. Maycock, A.L., Aster, S.D. and Patchett, A.A. (1978) in Enzyme-Activated Irreversible Inhibitors, Seiler, N., Jung, M. and Koch-Weser, J. ed., Elsevier/North-Holland Biomedical Press, Amsterdam, p. 211.
19. Maycock, A.L., Aster, S.D. and Patchett, A.A. (1979) Biochemistry (in preparation).
20. Bey, P. (1978) in Enzyme-Activated Irreversible Inhibitors, Seiler, N., Jung, M.J. and Koch-Weser, J. ed., Elsevier/North-Holland Biomedical Press, Amsterdam, p. 27.
21. Walsh, C., Johnston, M., Marcotte, P. and Wang, E. (1978) in Enzyme-Activated Irreversible Inhibitors, Seiler, N., Jung, M. and Koch-Weser, J. ed., Elsevier/North-Holland Biomedical Press, Amsterdam, p. 177.
22. Ulm, E.H., Sweet, C.S., Duggan, D.E. and Minsker, D.H. (1979) Fed. Proc., Fed. Am. Soc. Expl. Biol., 38, 1021 (Abstr.).
23. Jung, M.J., Palfreyman, M.G., Wagner, J., Bey, P., Ribereau-Gayon, G., Zraika, M. and Koch-Weser, J. (1979) Life Sciences, 24, 1037.
24. Day, M.D., Roach, A.G. and Whiting, R.L. (1973) Eur. J. Pharmacol., 21, 271.
25. Nickerson, M. and Ruedy, J. (1975) in the Pharmacological Basis of Therapeutics, 5th Ed., Goodman, L.S. and Gilman, A. ed., MacMillan, New York, p. 705.
26. O'Leary, M.H. and Baughn, R.L. (1977) J. Biol. Chem., 252, 7168.

DISCUSSION

JUNG: In view of the optical activity of fluoromethyldopamine, would you care to comment on the stereospecificity, in connection with what Brian Metcalf told us yesterday?

MAYCOCK: We looked at both isomers of fluoromethyldopamine, as inhibitors of the enzyme and we found that only the "expected" isomer was in fact an irrevisible inhibitor. "Expected" means based on the isomer of methyldopamine that one gets upon decarboxylation of methyldopa.

JUNG: So, you would assume that the active isomer of monofluoromethyldopamine is analogous to the product of the stereospecific decarboxylation of methyldopa, which occurs by retention of configuration?

MAYCOCK: That is correct.

JUNG: So, this truly proceeds via microscopic reversibility, by abstraction of the proton which is normally added during decarboxylation?

MAYCOCK: We are assuming that, based on your work. As I pointed out, we have not made the compound in which we have replaced the α-hydrogen with deuterium or tritium. Such an isotopically labelled compound should allow us to answer that question definitively.

JUNG: Still, at least on the basis of the stereochemistry of the inhibitor you could already have a hint as to the mechanism of the inactivation.

MAYCOCK: Right.

CHOWDHRY: In relation to your observation that 30% of the activity remains after treatment with vinyl- or ethinyldopa, I am curious, whether you tried the inactivation as a function of pH? I am wondering whether there is a slow exchange between an active form of the enzyme and a multimeric form, where the exchange is not rapid and between fluoromethyldopa and the vinyl- and ethinyldopa, that difference is manifested. You may notice that, if you let the reaction go for a very long time.

MAYCOCK: We have not tried any experiments like that. We did carry out a couple experiments in which we studied the inactivation rate as function of enzyme concentration. We found that the enzyme concentration made no difference.

CHOWDHRY: But you have not tried pH, have you?

MAYCOCK: No, that is correct.

CHOWDHRY: Is there any independent evidence in this enzyme for associated forms?

MAYCOCK: Not that I am aware of.

CHOWDHRY: Did you make tryptic maps of the inactivated enzyme in the case of the two classes of inhibitors, because that may tell you whether the sites are the same or not.

MAYCOCK: No, we have not.

WALSH: In connection with this 30% residual activity obtained with ethinyl- or vinyldopa; if you then treat the enzyme with α-fluoromethyldopa, do you get rid of the remaining 30%?

MAYCOCK: We think so. We have tried that experiment a couple of times, but we have had difficulty with the competing reactivation process. As the enzyme begins to reactivate, that portion which is reactivated also becomes susceptible to inactivation by fluoromethyldopa. However, the fact seems to be that the 30% residual activity *is* susceptible to fluoromethyldopa.

WALSH: Which would be consistent with a different isozyme, would it not?

MAYCOCK: Yes, I think so.

WALSH: Of course, this is not uniquely interpretable. Have you made α-fluoroethyldopa, which would presumably lead directly to your enamino intermediate, which should partition identically?

MAYCOCK: No we have talked about it, but we have not made it.

ONDETTI: In the case of the inhibition with your vinyl and ethinyl analogs, you quoted the incorporation of radioactive label as 0.8 to 1.1 per mole. Was that calculated on the basis of 70% inactivation?

MAYCOCK: No, that was calculated on the basis of total enzyme used in the experiment. We have to be careful when we interpret those incorporations, because the 30% residual activity does not necessarily correspond to 30% of the enzyme moleculecules. For instance, suppose we have a situation in which only one percent of enzyme molecules accounts for the residual enzyme activity. In such a case, when we have inactivated enzyme to this 30% level, we would expect to see essentially 1 equivalent of inhibitor incorporated. So, based on the incorporation we cannot make any firm conclusions relating the enzyme activity to the ratio of enzyme species that are present. Now, if the experiment had come out the other way around, such that we incorporated, say, only 0.1 equivalent of inactivator, but killed 70% enzyme, then we could say something about relative ratios of species that might be present.

SCHAEFFER: One of the aspects that you have not discussed is the abortive deamination yielding a vinyl ketone byproduct, which may account for the reversible phase of recovery of the inhibition. Have you looked at things like methyl vinyl ketone to see whether that initially inhibits irreversibly and does reverse?

MAYCOCK: No, we have not. We run all of our experiments in the presence of mercaptoethanol, so if we were actually going to look for the vinyl ketone, we would probably have to look for the adduct one would get by Michael-addition of mercaptoethanol to the vinyl ketone.

SCHAEFFER: That also depends on whether the vinyl ketone is indeed liberated.

MAYCOCK: Right. We assume that it would be liberated during the reactivation process.

EFFECTS OF ENZYME-ACTIVATED IRREVERSIBLE INHIBITORS OF AROMATIC AMINO ACID
DECARBOXYLASE ON ENDOGENOUS SYNTHESIS OF BIOGENIC AMINES

MICHEL J.JUNG, MICHAEL G.PALFREYMAN, GILLES RIBEREAU-GAYON, PHILIPPE BEY, BRIAN
W.METCALF, JAN KOCH-WESER AND ALBERT SJOERDSMA
Centre de Recherche Merrell International
16, rue d'Ankara, 67000 Strasbourg, FRANCE

INTRODUCTION

Aromatic amino acid decarboxylase is able to decarboxylate several aromatic
α-amino acids, namely dopa, 5-hydroxytryptophan and, to a lesser extent, histidine[1]. The enzyme is widely distributed in animal tissues and is found especially in the peripheral and central nervous systems[2]. Dopamine, the product of
dopa decarboxylation, is not only a neurotransmitter in the central nervous
system but also an intermediate in the synthesis of the catecholamines noradrenaline and adrenaline. 5-Hydroxytryptamine is also a neurotransmitter in the
central nervous system and is an autacoid in physiological processes such as
inflammation, anaphylaxis or platelet aggregation[3]. An imbalance in central or
peripheral biosynthesis of catecholamines may be associated with disease states
such as Parkinsonism[4], hypertension[5] and various neurological disorders[6].

The biosynthetic and main biodegradative pathways of dopamine, noradrenaline
and adrenaline are shown in figure 1. Those of 5-hydroxytryptamine are closely
related.

The rate-determining step in catecholamine synthesis is the hydroxylation of
tyrosine to dopa[7] catalyzed by pterine-dependent tyrosine hydroxylase. The actual mechanism of aromatic hydroxylation is poorly understood[8], hence the task
of designing enzyme-activated inhibitors for this class of enzymes is quite
difficult. Several competitive inhibitors are known for tyrosine hydroxylase,
such as α-methyl-para-tyrosine[9], benzimidazole-5(6)-alanine[10] and its α-methyl
analogue[11]. These compounds very effectively reduce tissue concentrations of
catecholamines in animals. However, the intricate endogenous regulation of tyrosine hydroxylase activity[12] and the competitive nature of the inhibitors
greatly complicate control of the depletion.

Aromatic amino acid decarboxylase, the second enzyme of the monoamine biosynthetic pathway is pyridoxal-dependent. The mechanism of action of α-amino
acid decarboxylases is well characterized[13] and, in addition, the activity of

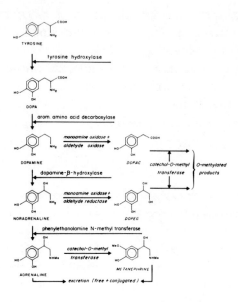

Fig. 1. Metabolic pathways of catecholamines.

aromatic amino acid decarboxylase is not as stringently controlled as that of tyrosine hydroxylase. Therefore, this enzyme is an ideal target for the design of enzyme-activated inhibitors. However, due to the overwhelming excess of aromatic amino acid decarboxylase activity over tyrosine hydroxylase activity, it was predictable that the regulation of biogenic amine synthesis by inhibition at the decarboxylation step would be very difficult[7]. In fact, competitive inhibitors such as α-methyl-hydrazinodopa (carbidopa)[14] or benserazide[15] effectively slowed the peripheral decarboxylation of administered dopa or 5-hydroxytryptophan but had little or no effect on concentrations of endogenous amines. More potent inhibitors were needed to make dopa decarboxylation the rate-limiting step and enzyme-activated inhibitors were likely candidates.

The mechanism of action of α-amino acid decarboxylases and the structure of potential or proven enzyme-activated inhibitors of this class of enzymes have been discussed in previous reviews[16,17] and also in this symposium (see the contributions of R. RANDO, B.W. METCALF, and A. MAYCOCK). In this presentation we shall summarize the biochemical and biological properties of α-vinyldopa, α-ethynyldopa, α-difluoromehtyldopa and α-monofluoromethyldopa. The structures of the four compounds are shown in figure 2.

133

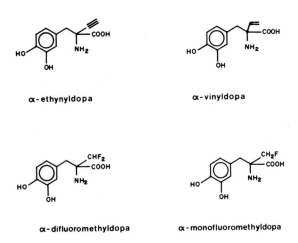

α-ethynyldopa

α-vinyldopa

α-difluoromethyldopa

α-monofluoromethyldopa

Fig. 2. Structures of four inhibitors of aromatic amino acid decarboxylase.

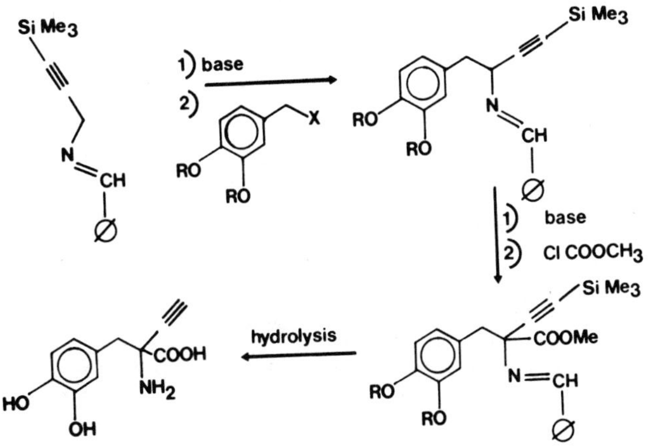

Fig. 3. Synthesis of α-ethynyldopa.

α-Ethynyldopa and α-vinyldopa

The synthesis of these compounds was described independently by two groups [18,19] following similar routes as summarized in figure 3 for α-ethynyldopa. When aromatic amino acid decarboxylase purified from hog kidney is incubated with eigher compound, there is an extremely rapid drop of enzyme activity followed by a much slower time-dependent decrease[20,21]. The initial drop of activity has been attributed by one group to a covalent binding of the inhibitor to the enzyme, partially reversable by dialysis[20] and by the second group to a strong competitive inhibition[21] (figure 4). Upon incubation of aromatic amino acid decarboxylase with 1-^{14}C labeled α-ethynyldopa, Maycock et al found that [14]CO_2 was released even after the enzyme had lost its ability to decarboxylate dopa [20]. This could not be confirmed by analysis of the reaction mixture by high pressure liquid chromatography[21] : the concentration of ethynyldopa did not decrease and, even more importantly, no other product was formed. More work is needed to explain the interaction between these β,α-unsaturated dopa analogues and aromatic amino acid decarboxylase.

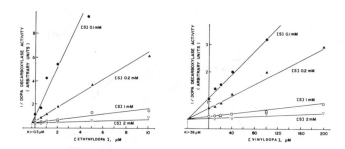

Fig. 4. "Competitive inhibition" of aromatic amino acid decarboxylase by α-ethynyldopa and α-vinyldopa. Purified aromatic amino acid decarboxylase was incubated for 5 min without adding pyridoxal-phosphates with 1-^{14}C-dopa and the inhibitors at the indicated concentrations added simultaneously. Radioactive CO_2 was trapped and measured.

Four hours after intraperitoneal injection of 100 or 500 mg/kg of ethynyldopa or vinyldopa into rats, the activity of aromatic amino acid decarboxylase was decreased by 50-60 % in kidney, 20-40 % in heart and 10-20 % in brain[21]. This level of inhibition would not be expected to affect monoamine synthesis in any of these organs. On the other hand, in animals injected with trace amounts of ring-tritiated dopa, ethynyldopa produced a dose-related increase of ^{3}H-dopa and ^{3}H-catecholamines in the brain. Similarly, more serotonin is found in the brain and less in the heart in mice given 5-hydroxytryptophan together with α-ethynyldopa than in those given 5-hydroxytryptophan alone. This indicates that the level of inhibition was sufficient to reduce the peripheral decarboxylation of exogenously supplied dopa or 5-hydroxytryptophan, allowing more of the amino acid to reach the brain where the corresponding amines can be formed.

α-Difluoromethyldopa

This compound was synthesized in our laboratories by the reaction sequence summarized in figure 5[22].

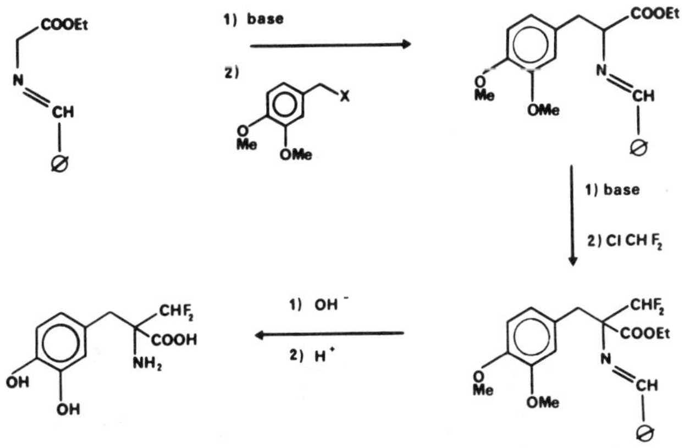

Fig. 5. Synthesis of α-difluoromethyldopa

Incubation of purified aromatic amino acid decarboxylase with difluoromethyl-dopa results in a time-dependent loss of enzyme activity. The rate of inhibition deviates markedly from pseudo-first-order kinetics (figure 6). The slowing of the inhibition does not correlate with disappearance of difluoromethyldopa or the appearance of a transformation product of the inhibitor. The existence of isoenzymes of aromatic amino acid decarboxylase has been postulated in a similar context [20]. The inhibition cannot be reversed by dialysis.

It had already been shown in model studies[16], that catalytic amounts of pyridoxal are able to induce decarboxylation of difluoromethylphenylalanine

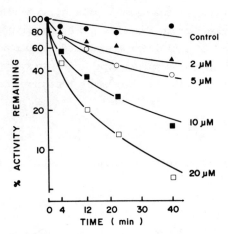

Fig. 6. Time-dependent inhibition of aromatic amino acid decarboxylase by di-fluoromethyldopa. Purified enzyme was incubated at pH 7.4 in 50 mM phosphate buffer with different concentrations of inhibitor. At given time intervals aliquots were withdrawn and assayed for remaining enzyme activity using 1-^{14}C dopa as substrate.

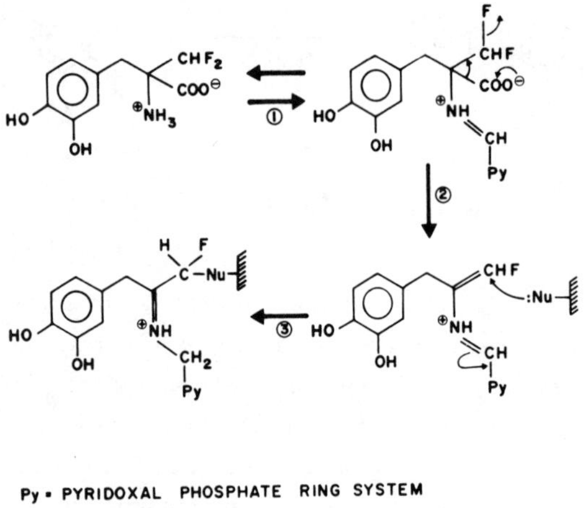

Py = PYRIDOXAL PHOSPHATE RING SYSTEM

Fig. 7. Mechanism of the time-dependent inhibition of aromatic amino acid decarboxylase by difluoromethyldopa.

accompanied by fluorine elimination at 80°C. When tritiated α-difluoromethyldopa (ring-labeled) is used, there is a stoichiometric incorporation of radioactivity into the inhibited protein (Ribereau-Gayon, to be published). All
these arguments are in favour of the mechanism of inhibition proposed in
figure 7[23] .

In vivo, difluoromethyldopa produces a rapid, time- and dose-dependent decrease of aromatic amino acid decarboxylase activity in heart and kidney and has
only a marginal effect on the brain enzyme[23]. For instance, 6 hours after a
dose of 25 mg/kg given intraperitoneally to mice, the remaining enzyme activity
is 15 % in kidney, 55 % in heart and 85 % in brain. Even after a dose of 500 mg/
kg, which almost completely blocks the enzyme in heart and kidney, the enzyme
activity is still 75-80 % in the brain. The inhibition achieved is not sufficient to affect the concentration of biogenic amines even after repeated administration[24] .

Like α-ethynyldopa, α-difluoromethyldopa prevents the peripheral decarboxylation of exogenously supplied dopa or 5-hydroxytryptophan so that more of the
amino acid reaches the brain and can be transformed to the corresponding amine.
The time course of the effect is in good agreement with the inhibition of the
enzyme in peripheral organs (figure 8).

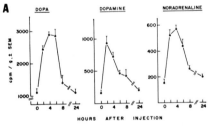

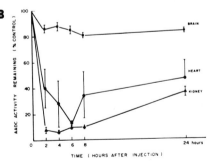

Fig. 8. Duration of aromatic amino acid decarboxylase inhibition
in peripheral organs after 100 mg/
kg of difluoromethyldopa given intraperitoneally to mice.
A) ^{3}H-Dopa was administrated i.p.
30 min before killing and at various times after the inhibitor.
Brains were homogenized in 0.2 M
$HClO_4$ and the radioactivity associated with dopa, dopamine and
noradrenaline was determined in
the supernatant.
B) Aromatic amino acid decarboxylase activity was determined by
the $^{14}CO_2$ trapping method using
1-^{14}C-dopa as substrate in homo-
genates of heart, brain and
kidney.

138

α-Monofluoromethyldopa

α-Monofluoromethyldopa was synthesized independently by Kollonitsch et all[25] and in our laboratories[26]. The compound is a very potent time-dependent inhibitor of aromatic amino acid decarboxylase. A binding constant of 4×10^{-8}M has been reported[25]. We found that the monofluoro analogue is about 10 times more active than α-difluoromethyldopa and that the inhibition does not follow pseudo-first-order kinetics as already discussed for the difluoromethyl analogue. The mechanism of action has been very convincingly demonstrated by Kollonitsch et al[25] and is similar to that described in figure 7. There is stoichiometric binding of inhibitor to the enzyme as determined with α-monofluoromethyldopa tritiated on the aromatic ring. No radioactivity is incorporated into the inhibited enzyme when $1-^{14}$C-monofluoromethyldopa is used, and during the inhibition there is a stoichiometric release of fluorine.

When administered to mice or rats by any systemic route, α-monofluoromethyldopa causes a rapid, dose-dependent decrease of decarboxylase activity in kidney, heart and brain[26] (figure 9). At doses lower than 2.5 mg/kg, the enzyme activity in brain is not markedly decreased, so that there is selectivity for the periphery at these doses. When the dose is increased to 100-250 mg/kg the enzyme is completely inhibited in the brain as well.

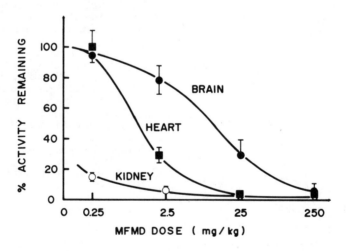

Fig. 9. Dose-dependent inhibition of aromatic amino acid decarboxylase activity in kidney, heart and brain of mice injected intraperitoneally with α-monofluoromethyldopa 4 hours before killing[26].

The inhibition is long-lasting in all three organs. After a dose of 100 mg/
kg, no enzyme activity is detectable for almost 24 hours. The slow increase
seen after one day is presumably due to new enzyme synthesis and can be used
to estimate the biological half-life of aromatic amino acid decarboxylase
(figure 10). This dose of monofluoromethyldopa also decreases concentrations
of catecholamines as illustrated in figure 10 for brain dopamine and noradrenaline. The effect is maximal at 24 h, but the decrease is still significant by
day 3-4.

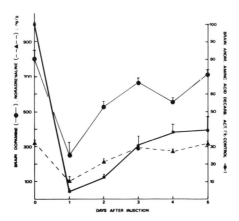

Fig. 10. Duration of the effects of a single dose of 100 mg/kg monofluoromethyldopa on catecholamine metabolism in mouse brain. Aromatic amino acid decarboxylase activity (■) dopamine (●) and noradrenaline (▲) concentrations. The
catecholamines were determined by high pressure liquid chromatography using
electrochemical detection[27].

In order to prove that the depleting effect of monofluoromethyldopa is due
only to inhibition of dopa decarboxylation, we compared the changes in concentration of dopa, dopamine, noradrenaline and dihydroxyphenylacetic acid, the
main metabolite of dopamine, in mouse brain after various treatments known to
affect catecholamine metabolism (figure 11).

140

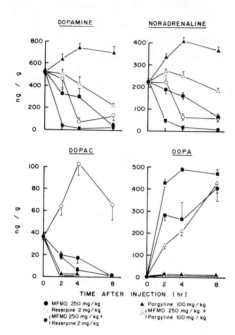

Fig. 11. Metabolism of brain catecholamines after administration of
monofluoromethyldopa, reserpine
and pargyline to mice.
Groups of 5 mice were injected intraperitoneally at time zero as
specified on the figure. They were
killed 2, 4, 8 hrs after treatment.
Brain catechols were determined as
previously[27]. Values are uncorrect-
ed for recovery and represent the
mean $\pm$ SEM of 5 animals.

A single dose of 250 mg/kg of monofluoromethyldopa causes a decrease of
dopamine, noradrenaline and dihydroxyphenylacetic acid. Dopa, which is normally
not detectable, is accumulated. Reserpine causes a depletion of biogenic amines
from their storage vesicles[28]. These amines become accessible to monoamine oxidase and are degraded. Therefore, there is a decrease of dopamine and noradrenaline and an increase of dihydroxyphenylacetic acid.

When reserpine and monofluoromethyldopa are combined the depletion of dopamine and noradrenaline is faster than when either is given alone. Dihydroxyphenylacetic acid is no longer accumulated and the increase of dopa concentration is even larger than with the decarboxylase inhibitor alone. Pargyline, an
irreversible inhibitor of monoamine oxidase[29], produces a transient increase of
dopamine and noradrenaline, a rapid decrease of dihydroxyphenylacetic acid and
no increase of dopa. When monofluoromethyldopa is given together with pargyline,
the amine concentrations no longer increase but decrease. The concentration of
dopa is smaller than after monofluoromethyldopa alone. The difference in dopa

accumulation, which represents an *in vivo* measurement of tyrosine hydroxylase activity, can be explained by the fact that dopamine and noradrenaline are feed-back inhibitors of that enzyme. During combined treatment with reserpine and monofluoromethyldopa the concentration of the amines is at its lowest, hence tyrosine is least inhibited, while in the case of the pargyline plus de-carboxylase inhibitor treatment the levels of dopamine and noradrenaline are initially maintained.

These results suggest that monofluoromethyldopa does not inhibit tyrosine hydroxylase and does not release the amines from their storage sites. From the return of the amine concentration to control values around day 4 shown in fig-ure 10, a nerve degenerating effect like that of 6-hydroxydopamine[30] can also be excluded.

Since aromatic amino acid decarboxylase is also responsible for the forma-tion of 5-hydroxytryptamine in serotonergic neurons, monofluoromethyldopa also decreases the concentration of the indole amine in heart and brain[31].

CONCLUSION

Based on mechanistic considerations, four potential enzyme-activated inhibi-tors of aromatic amino acid decarboxylase were synthesized. The mode of inter-action between this enzyme and the β,α-unsaturated analogues of dopa, α-ethynyl-dopa and α-vinyldopa, is still not totally clarified. These two compounds pro-duce only moderate inhibition of the decarboxylase *in vivo* and therefore have only a limited interest. α-Difluoromethyldopa is a relatively potent irreversi-ble inhibitor of the decarboxylase *in vitro* and *in vivo*. The degree of inhibi-tion achieved *in vivo* is not sufficient to reduce endogenous synthesis of bio-genic amines. Due to its selective inhibition of the enzyme in peripheral or-gans this compound can be used in combination with L-dopa to increase the syn-thesis of dopamine in the brain. α-Methylhydrazinodopa (carbidopa) is so used in the treatment of Parkinsonism[32]. The most potent of these four irreversible inhibitors is α-monofluoromethyldopa. At doses lower than 5 mg/kg, only the pe-ripheral enzyme is inhibited, so that when dopa is coadministrated more of this amino acid reaches the brain and more dopamine is formed there[33]. At higher doses, the degree of decarboxylase inhibition becomes sufficient to block cate-cholamine and serotonin biosynthesis both peripherally and centrally. α-Mono-fluoromethyldopa is the first compound potent enough to block the synthesis of monoamines by inhibiting aromatic amino acid decarboxylase in non-toxic doses. Preliminary pharmacological investigations show that inhibition of peripheral sympathetic function can be achieved with this compound[34]. The effects of mono-amine depletion centrally should be no less interesting.

The type of activity demonstrated for monofluoromethyldopa illustrates the great potential of enzyme-activated irreversible inhibitors as pharmacological agents. The lesser effectiveness of difluoromethyldopa, vinyldopa and ethynyl-dopa indicates that irreversible inhibitors even for the well-known α-amino acid decarboxylases cannot yet be designed on an entirely rational basis.

REFERENCES

1. Aures, D., Hakanson, R., Clark, W.G. (1970) in Handbook of Neurochemistry Lajtha, A., ed., Plenum New-York Vol IV, 165-196.
2. Lovenberg, W. (1970) in Methods in Enzymology, Tabor, H., and Tabor, C.W., eds., Academic Press, New-York Vol XVII B, 652-656.
3. Ersparmer, V. (1966) in Handbook of Experimental Pharmacology, Ersparmer, V., ed., Springer Verlag, New-York Vol XIX, 132-181.
4. Sandler, M. (1972) in Handbook of Experimental Pharmacology, Blaschko, H., and Muscholl, E., eds., Springer Verlag, New-York Vol XXXIII, 845-899 and references cited.
5. Versteeg, D.H.G., Tanaka, M., and de Kloet, E.R. (1978), Endocrinology, 103, 1654-1661.
6. Galzigna, L. (1973) Chem. Biol. Interactions, 7, 1-9.
7. Levitt, M., Spector, S., Sjoerdsma, A., and Udenfriend, S. (1965) J. Pharma-col. Exp. Ther. 148, 1-8.
8. (1972), Biological Hydroxylation Mechanisms, Boyd, G.S. and Smellic, R.M.S., eds., Academic Press, London-New-York.
9. Nagatsu, T., Levitt, M., and Udenfriend, S. (1964) J. Biol. Chem. 239, 2910-2917.
10. Johnson, E.M.Jr., Zenker, N., and Wright, J. (1972) Biochem. Pharmacol. 21, 1777-1783.
11. Zenker, N., Morgenroth, V.H. III and Wright, J. (1974) J. Med. Chem. 17, 1223-1225.
12. Costa, E., and Meek, J.L. (1974) Ann. Review Pharmacol. 14, 491-511.
13. Boeker, E.A. and Snell, E.E. (1972) in The Enzymes, Meister, A. ed., 6, 217-53.
14. Sletzinger, M., Chemerda, J.M., and Bollinger, F.W. (1963) J. Med. Chem. 6, 101-103.
15. Burkard, W., Gey, K.F. and Pletscher, A. (1963) Experientia, 18, 411-412.
16. Bey, P. (1978) in Enzyme-Activated Irreversible Inhibitors, Seiler, N., Jung, M.J., and Koch-Weser, J., eds., Elsevier, North-Holland, 27-41.
17. Jung, M.J., Koch-Weser, J., and Sjoerdsma, A. in Enzyme Inhibitors as Drugs, Sandler, M. ed., Butterworth, London, in press.
18. Taub, D., and Patchett, A.A. (1977), Tetrahedron Letters, 2745-2748.
19. Metcalf, B.W., and Jund, K. (1977), Tetrahedron Letters, 3689-3692.
20. Maycock, A.C., Aster, S.D. and Patchett, A.A., in Enzyme-Activated Irrever-sible Inhibitors, Seiler, N., Jung, M.J., and Koch-Weser, J., eds., Elsevier, North-Holland, 211-220.
21. Ribereau-Gayon, G., Danzin, C., Palfreyman, M.G., Aubry, M., Wagner, J., Metcalf, B.W., and Jung, M.J., Biochem. Pharmacol. in press.
22. Bey, P., Vevert, J.P., Van Dorsselaer, V., and Kolb, M., J. Org. Chem. in press.

23. Palfreyman, M.G., Danzin, C., Bey, P., Jung, M.J., Ribereau-Gayon, G., Aubry, M., Vevert, J.P., and Sjoerdsma, A. (1978), J. Néurochem. 31, 927-932.
24. Palfreyman, M.G., Danzin, C., Jung, M.J., Fozard, J.R., Wagner, J., Woodward, J.K., Aubry, M., Dage, R.C., and Koch-Weser, J. (1978) in Enzyme-Activated Irreversible Inhibitors, Seiler, N., Jung, M.J., and Koch-Weser, J., eds., Elsevier, North-Holland, 221-233.
25. Kollonitsch, J., Patchett, A.A., Marburg, S., Maycock, A.L., Perkins, L.M., Doldouras, G.A., Duggan, D.E. and Aster, S.D. (1978), Nature, 274, 906-908.
26. Jung, M.J., Palfreyman, M.G., Wagner, J., Bey, P., Ribereau-Gayon, G., Zraïka, M., and Koch-Weser, J. (1979), Life Sciences, 24, 1037-1042.
27. Wagner, J., Palfreyman, M.G., and Zraïka, M., J. Chromatography Biomed. Appl. in press.
28. Glowinski, J., Iversen, L.L., and Axelrod, J. (1966), J. Pharmacol. Exptl. Ther. 151, 385-399.
29. Swett, L.R., Martin, W.B., Taylor, J.D., Everett, G.M., Wykes, A.A., and Gladish, Y.D. (1963) Ann. N.Y. Acad. Sci. 103, 891-898.
30. (1971), 6-Hydroxydopamine and Catecholamine Neurons, Malmfors, T., and Thoenen, H., eds., Elsevier, North-Holland.
31. Jung, M.J., Palfreyman, M.G., Ribereau-Gayon, G., Wagner, J., and Zraïka, M., Brit. J. Pharmacol. in press.
32. Bianchine, J.R. (1976), New England J. Med. 295, 814.
33. Palfreyman, M.G., Jung, M.J., Danzin, C., Ribereau-Gayon, G., Bey, P., Zraïka, M., and Sjoerdsma, A., in Catecholamines Basic and Clinical Frontiers, Usdin, E. ed., Pergamon Press, Oxford, in press.
34. Fozard, J.R., Palfreyman, M.G., Spedding, M., Wagner, J. and Woodward, J.K., Brit. J. Pharmacol. in press.

DISCUSSION

YAU-KWAN HO: May I ask why the difluoromethyl-dopa is less active than the monofluoro analog?

JUNG: I have no complete answer to this question. It could be in the first place a matter of difference in affinity for the enzyme; secondly the rate of enzyme-catalyzed decarboxylation can be different. We have no idea which is the rate-limiting step of the inhibition process. We plan to study the mode of reaction of the corresponding α-substituted phenylalanines with pyridoxal-phosphate in the absence of enzyme. The identification of reaction products and the determination of activation energies should bring more information about the molecular events occurring in the enzyme's active site during the inhibition. It is also possible as suggested by Dr. Walsh's results that the enzyme alkylated with the difluoromethyl analogue can regenerate the native enzyme. This would explain why we see a much faster recovery of decarboxylase activity in rats or mice after administering difluoromethyldopa than after administering monofluoromethyldopa.

WALSH: In that same connection, really going on with the question you asked me yesterday; you show in Fig. 7 the initial product of nucleophilic attack on the monofluoroenamine yielding on ketonization the imine, with the alpha carbon substituted with a fluorine and the nucleophile - two hetero-atoms. Now, I wonder, why that is a stable adduct; because, if the nucleophile is oxygen, it is a fluorohydrin, if it is an amine, it should decompose. The question is, if it is sulfur, what is the stability of α-fluorothioethers? Maybe someone can tell me. If they are not very stable, then you have to suppose that that microenvironment is really doing something to keep that effectively dihetero-substituted carbon from reverting to the enamine. In general, one will have to worry about the stability of that difluoromethyl substituted carbon.

CHWANG: Can you reverse the activity of all those fluoro analogs with the natural substrate? If you have given dopa to an animal 1 hr before or 1 hr after you inject your drug, can you reverse the activity?

JUNG: *In vitro*, dopa slows down the rate of inhibiton of dopa decarboxy-lase by the fluoromethyl analogues. *In vivo* we did not study the effects of administering dopa prior to the inhibitor. However, giving dopa at the same time or after a 10 mg/kg dose of monofluoromethyldopa results a) in an accumulation of dopa in the periphery due to the blockage of decarboxylation in peripheral organs; b) in an increase of dopa and dopamine in the brain, as the brain enzyme is not yet affected at this dose. At doses of 100 mg/kg of monofluoromethyl dopa which cause catecholamine depletion, coadministration of dopa does not reverse the depleting effects.

ALLENIC AMINES AS INACTIVATORS OF MITOCHONDRIAL MONOAMINE OXIDASE

A. KRANTZ[+*], B. KOKEL[+], Y. P. SACHDEVA[+], J. SALACH[++], A. CLAESSON[+++], AND
C. SAHLBERG[+++]
Department of Chemistry, State University of New York, Stony Brook, NY, 11794[+],
Molecular Biology Division, VA Hospital, 4150 Clement Street, San Francisco, CA
94121[++], Uppsala University, Biomedical Center, Uppsala, Sweden[+++]

INTRODUCTION

Despite its infancy, the concept of enzyme suicide or k_{cat} inhibitors has
been a powerful stimulus for the synthesis of novel enzyme inactivators and is
a promising and intellectually appealing strategy for drug design.[1-5] The
simple expedient of placing a triple bond in proper juxtaposition to the re-
quisite substrate functionality has led to a number of highly specific and potent enzyme inactivators.[5,6] These acetylenic pro-inhibitors can be designed to
exploit the potential high reactivity to Michael addition[7,8] that is characteristic of a triple bond (or an allene) when it is brought into conjugation with
powerful electron withdrawing groups.

$$-C\equiv C-\underset{\underset{H}{|}}{C}-X=Y \longrightarrow \underset{H}{\overset{\diagdown}{}}C=C=\overset{\diagup}{C}-X=Y \qquad (1)$$

$$-C\equiv C-\underset{\underset{H}{|}\,\,\underset{H}{\diagdown}}{C}-X \longrightarrow -C\equiv C-\underset{|}{C}=X \qquad (2)$$

The allenic functionality may be enzymatically generated from acetylenic precursors via propargylic rearrangements[9] initiated by hydrogen transfers, eqtn
(1). Enzymatic oxidations, eqtn (2), can, in principle, provide access to
powerful α,β-acetylenic Michael acceptors.

Although a number of well-known drugs contain allenic functionality, explicit
use of the allenic moiety in the design of mechanism-based inhibitors had not
been reported until recently.[10] In many respects allenes parallel acetylenes
in their chemistry[11] and may represent useful alternatives to acetylenic inhibitors. As a first step towards the systematic development of allenic inactivators, we have intensively investigated the reaction of the enzyme mitochondrial
monoamine oxidase [EC 1.4.3.4, MAO] with allenic amines. This enzyme has been
a prime pharmacological target for almost thirty years, since its inhibition

---

* Author to whom inquiries should be addressed.

was understood to be relevant to controlling mood.[12] Its ability to oxidatively deaminate a wide variety of substances including 1°, 2° and 3° amines (eqtn 3) makes it an important testing ground for functionality potentially useful in the

$$RCH_2N\overset{R^1}{\underset{R''}{\diagdown}} + H_2O + O_2 \xrightarrow{MAO} \overset{R}{\underset{O}{\diagup}}C\overset{H}{\diagdown} + \overset{R^1}{\underset{H}{\diagup}}N\overset{R''}{\diagdown} + H_2O_2 \qquad (3)$$

design of mechanism-based inhibitors.

One interesting aspect of our study is a comparison of the action of the isomeric acetylenic and allenic amines, N-2-butynyl-N-benzylmentylamine[13] (1) and N-2, 3-butadienyl-N-benzylmethylamine,[14] (2), on the enzyme.

$$CH_3C{\equiv}C-CH_2N\overset{CH_3}{\underset{CH_2\phi}{\diagdown}} \qquad\qquad H_2C{=}C{=}CHCH_2N\overset{CH_3}{\underset{CH_2\phi}{\diagdown}}$$

$$1 \qquad\qquad\qquad\qquad 2$$

The fact that conjugated allenes are considerably more reactive than isolated ones[15,16] provides a rationale for the suitability of β,γ,δ-allenic amines as enzyme suicide inhibitors of MAO (eqtn 4).

$$\overset{|}{C}{=}C{=}\overset{|}{C}CH_2N\diagdown \xrightarrow[?]{MAO} C{=}C{=}C{-}\overset{|}{C}{=}\overset{+}{N}\diagup \qquad\qquad (4)$$
$$\underset{\delta\ \ \gamma\ \ \beta}{}$$

MATERIALS AND METHODS

Materials. Bovine liver mitochondrial monoamine oxidase was purified by the method of Salach.[17] Flavin peptides were prepared as reported by Edmondson et. al.[18] Allenic amines were synthesized according to the procedure of Claesson and Sahlberg,[19] or by condensing N-benzylmethylamine (Aldrich Chemical Co., Inc.) with the appropriate allenic mesylate. 3-Methyl-lumiflavin (3, 3-MLF) was prepared according to the prescription of Hemmerich.[20]

Analytical Procedures. MAO activity was measured as previously reported.[21] Radioactivity was determined in a Beckman Model LS-150 counter. Binding experiments utilizing Sephadex G-25 were performed by the procedure of Penefsky.[22] For identification of the coproduct, N-benzylmethyl amine, a Norelco Pye No. 104 gas chromatograph equipped with a 5 ft by 4 mm 10% 20 M Polyethylene glycol column containing 2% KOH on 80/90 mesh AnaKrom A was used. Electronic Spectra of the inhibited enzyme were recorded on a Cary 14 recording spectrophotometer. For studies involving the photochemistry of 3-MLF, infrared spectra were recorded on a Perkin-Elmer model 727 spectrophotometer, and NMR spectra were determined on either a Varian Associates EM 360 or HFT-80 Spectrometer. Optical

spectra were recorded on a Varian Techtron model 635 UV-visible spectrophotometer. Preparative photolyses were carried out according to Gartner[23] using a
450 W. Ace-Hanovia medium pressure quartz mercury-vapor lamp (Ace Glass, Inc.,
Vineland, N.J.), fitted with a Pyrex glass filter.

RESULTS

Spectral Change during the Inhibition. When micromolar samples of bovine
liver MAO are made 10^{-4}M in N-2-butynyl-N-benzylmethylamine $\underset{\sim}{1}$, loss of enzymatic
activity is accompanied by strong absorption centered at 391 nm ($\varepsilon \sim 2 \times 10^{4}$) with
simultaneous loss of the 455-nm band of the native flavoenzyme. (Fig. 1).

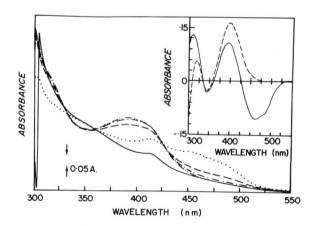

Fig.1. Absorption spectra of MAO and of the adduct formed with the acetylenic
amine $\underset{\sim}{1}$. Oxidized enzyme (·····); enzyme reduced anaerobically with benzylamine (———); adduct formed with a two-fold excess of compound $\underset{\sim}{1}$: 2 min after
mixing of reactants (- - -); same after 5 min (·−··−); Same after 15 min
(−··−··−). Inset, difference spectra. Solid line, adduct minus oxidized
enzyme; dashed line, adduct minus substrate reduced enzyme.

148

Incubation of purified bovine liver MAO (0.066 M phosphate buffer, pH 7.2, 25°), in solutions which are $\sim 10^{-5}$ M in N-2,3-butadienyl-N-benzyl-N-methylamine 2 results in bleaching of the 455 nm band of the enzyme, but in contrast to the action of 1, the electronic spectrum of the product from 2 exhibits no absorption characteristic of a flavocyanine, nor does it show any new maximal absorption in the region above 360 nm (Fig. 2). Normal substrates of MAO protect against the inhibition indicating that 2 is an active-site titrant.

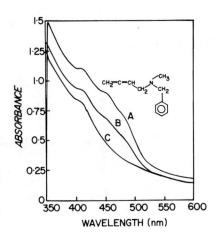

Fig. 2. Spectral changes accompanying inhibition of MAO by N-2,3-butadienyl-N-benzyl methyl amine (2). MAO, 3.1 mg (specific activity 3.6 µmol/min/mg) equivalent to 23.7 nmol, in 0.8 ml 50 mM HEPES buffer, pH 7.2, containing 10 mg/ml Triton X-100 was incubated with inhibitor for 3 to 5 min at 30°, then activity was measured and spectra were recorded. Curve A, native enzyme; B, enzyme inhibited 44% with 11.8 nmol of 2; C, enzyme completely inhibited with an additional 31.4 nmol of 2.

Incorporation of Radioactivity. The stoichiometry of the reaction between 2 and MAO was investigated by treating the enzyme with [1-^{14}C]-N-2,3-butadienyl-N-benzylmethyl amine (4). A plot of the ratio of nanomoles of inhibitor incubated with nanomoles of flavoenzyme, against (y axis left) the ratio of

nanomoles of inhibitor bound to nanomoles of flavoenzyme is displayed in figure
3. Approximately one equivalent of the amine becomes associated with the enzyme.
Even large excesses of the allenic amine do not lead to further uptake of the
inhibitor, demonstrating the specificity of attack for flavin as is suggested
from the spectral changes above. The incorporation of radioactivity is also
well-correlated with loss of activity of MAO. Enzymic activity is abolished by
1.1-1.2 equivalents of 4.

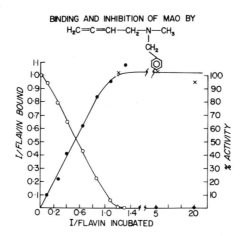

Fig. 3. Correlation between the loss of enzyme activity and the incorporation
of radioactivity upon incubation of bovine liver MAO with [1-^{14}C]-N-methyl-N-
benzyl-N-2,3-butadienamine (4). Open circles represent residual enzyme activity;
closed circles and X's indicate equivalents of radiolabelled inhibitor bound per
nmol of enzyme flavin. Enzyme 2.7 mg (specific activity 3.17) in 0.6 ml 50 mM
NaPi, pH 7.2 were incubated 20 min at 30° with varying amounts of inhibitor
(specific radiolabel, 0.38 μCi/μmol. Aliquots were treated and analyzed by the
procedure of Penefsky (1977).

Stability of the Adduct. Dialysis of the inhibited enzyme for 17 h against
several changes of phosphate buffer does not lead to restoration of the enzyme
activity or to any significant spectral changes, nor does exposure of the system
to molecular oxygen regenerate the spectrum of oxidized flavin. The nature of

the complex between allene and flavin prosthetic group is unambiguously demonstrated to be covalent, by challenging the enzyme with $[1-^{14}C]$-N-2,3-butadienyl-N-benzyl-N-methylamine $\underset{\sim}{4}$, denaturing the inhibited enzyme with trichloroacetic acid and then enzymatically degrading the precipitated flavoprotein with (a) chymotrypsin and trypsin, (b) nucleotide pyrophosphatase and (c) pronase (Table I). The flavin peptide-inhibitor complex, that results from this treatment is at the "FMN level" but still retains the radiochemical label and does not exhibit maximal absorption above 360 nm, vide infra. Clearly the label, and by inference the four carbon chain in $\underset{\sim}{2}$ is firmly associated with the flavin moiety at least up to the phosphocellulose chromatography. The spectrum of the flavin-inhibitor complex (Fig. 4) after standard florisil chromatography, or phosphocellulose chromatography (fraction 2) exhibits absorption at 343 and 327 nm.

TABLE I

ASSAY OF FLAVIN (A_{450nm}) AND RADIOACTIVITY DURING PURIFICATION OF MAO PEPTIDE-$[1-^{14}C]$-N-2,3-BUTADIENYL-N-BENZYL-N-METHYLAMINE ADDUCT.

STEP		nmol ^{14}C label	%	nmol Flavin (A450)	%
Enzyme		–	–	743	100
Enzyme + Inhibitor		821	110	–	–
Proteolytic Digest[a]		682.4	91.8	–	–
Nucleotide Pyrophosphatase & Further Proteolytic Digestion[b]		644.9	86.8	–	–
Florisil Chromatography		515.0	69.3	0.02	–
1st Phosphocellulose chromatography	Peak 1	47.2	6.4	30.33	4.1
	Peak 2	315.0	42.4	0.00	0.0
2nd Phosphocellulose chromatography	Peak 1	50.8	6.8	38.52	5.2
	Peak 2	127.2	17.1	0.00	0.0
	Peak 3	143.1	19.2	23.1	3.1

[a]Chymotrypsin and trypsin were utilized in the proteolytic digestion. [b]Further proteolytic digestion was carried out with pronase.

However the complex is unstable to conditions that have been previously employed in the purification of flavin peptides. Elution from phosphocellulose (using a linear gradient 0.45 M pyridinium acetate, pH 5.4 into an equal volume of 0.05 M pyridinium acetate pH 3.91) generates ^{14}C-containing fractions which fluoresce and absorb at values typical of flavoquinones. The instability of the complex has necessitated modification of the usual protocol.

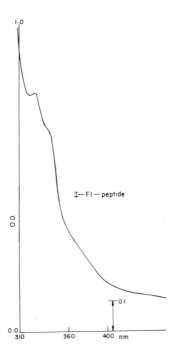

Fig. 4. Spectrum of the adduct peptide after Florisil and phosphocellulose chromatography (fraction 2, see Table 1 and text).

Kinetics. At large ratios of the inhibitor (2) to MAO, [I]/[E] > 22, the kinetics of the inhibition conform to a pseudo first-order reaction (Fig. 5). At 30°, the kinetics are indistinguishable from those of a bimolecular mechanism (Fig. 6). The bimolecular rate constants for 2 and $1-d_2-N-2,3$-butadienyl-N-benzyl-methylamine (5) are in the ratio of $5.18=k_H/k_D$. The deuterium isotope effect indicates that enzymatic attack on the allenic amine corresponds to the normal metabolic point of attack,[12] at a C-H bond adjacent to nitrogen in this case within the butadienyl residue.

At 2.5°, saturation kinetics are observed (Fig. 7) and it is possible to determine K_I.=0.0656 mM and k_{cat} = 0.0663 sec^{-1} for the inhibition. As in the

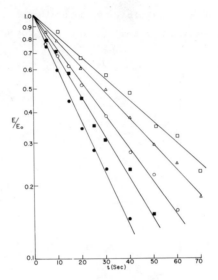

Fig. 5. Data indicating pseudo-first order inhibition of MAO by N-2,3-buta-
dienyl-N-benzyl-N-methylamine (2). Inhibitor concentrations were: open box,
4.07 μM; Δ 5.42 μM; 0, 6.78 μM; closed box, 8.13 μM; closed circle, 10.84 μM.
Enzyme, 0.079 mg (specific activity 3.3 μmol/min-mg) in 2.9 ml of 50 mM NaPi,
pH 7.2 was incubated at 30° with varying inhibitor concentrations. Flavin concentrations was determined to be 1.89×10^{-7}M.

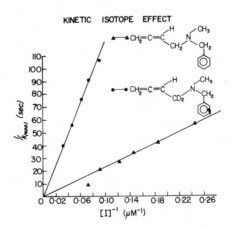

Fig. 6. Secondary plot rate constants derived from pseudo-first order reaction
of MAO with varying concentrations of N-2,3-butadienyl-N-benzylmethylamine (2)
(Fig. 5) and its 1,1-dideuterio analog (5). The deuterium isotope effect based
on the bimolecular rate constants of $k_H = 4.29 \times 10^3$ M^{-1} sec^{-1} and $k_D = 0.828 \times 10^3$ M^{-1}
sec^{-1}, is $k_H/k_D = 5.18$.

β,γ acetylenic amine series, the dimethylamino analog 6 (K_I = 0.158 mM, k_{cat} = 0.00266 sec^{-1} at 30°, Fig 8) is a much weaker inhibitor than the N-benzyl-N-methyl derivative.[24]

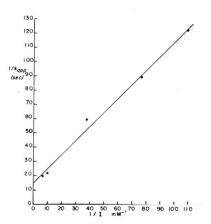

Fig. 7. Secondary plot of rate constants derived from pseudo first-order re-action of MAO with N-2,3-butadienyl-N-benzylmethylamine (2) at 2.5°. Enzyme, 0.037 mg (specific activity 3.6 μmol/min-mg) in 2.9 ml 50 mM NaPi, pH 7.2 was incubated with inhibitor concentrations of 0.0091 to 0.156 mM. All rates and intercepts were calculated by linear regression analyses. (K_I = 0.0656 mM, k_{cat} = 0.0663 sec^{-1}, at 2.5°).

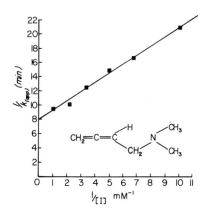

Fig. 8. The dependence of k_{app} upon the concentration of the inhibitor, N-2,3-butadienyl-N,N-dimethylamine (6), plotted as reciprocals.

Structure vs Activity Correlations. Preliminary studies to determine the essential structural unit for facile inhibition of MAO by allenic amines are indicated in Table II. Although we have not as yet determined turnover rates for many of these allenic amines, and have not determined the overall affinity of allenic amines for MAO it is still possible to obtain a qualitative ranking of their effectiveness as MAO inhibitors.

TABLE II

RELATIONSHIP BETWEEN STRUCTURE OF β,γ,δ-ALLENIC AMINES AND THEIR INHIBITORY ABILITY[a]

Structure	Conc (M)	$t_{1/2}$ (min)
$CH_2=C=CH-CH_2-NH_2$	0.7×10^{-5}	3.5
$CH_3-CH=C=CH-CH_2-NH_2$	10^{-6}	33.0
$CH_3-CH=C=C(CH_3)-CH_2-NH_2$	0.85×10^{-5}	9.5
$CH_2=C=C(CH_2-NH_2)(CH_2-C_6H_5)$ (7)	10^{-5}	8
$CH_2=C=CH-CH_2-NH-CH_2-C_6H_5$	0.8×10^{-5}	4.8
$CH_2=C=CH-CH_2-N(CH_3)(CH_3)$ (6)	1.1×10^{-3}	15.5
$CH_2=C=CH-CH_2-N(CH_3)(CH_2-C_6H_5)$ (2)	10^{-5}	1.5
$CH_2=C=C(CH_3)-CH_2-N(CH_3)(CH_2-C_6H_5)$	1.2×10^{-4}	9.9
$CH_2=C=C(CH_2-N(CH_3)(CH_3))(CH_2-C_6H_5)$	0.78×10^{-2}	25.0
$CH_2=C=CH-CH_2-N(CH(CH_2-C_6H_5)(CH_3))(CH_3)$	1.1×10^{-4}	7.2
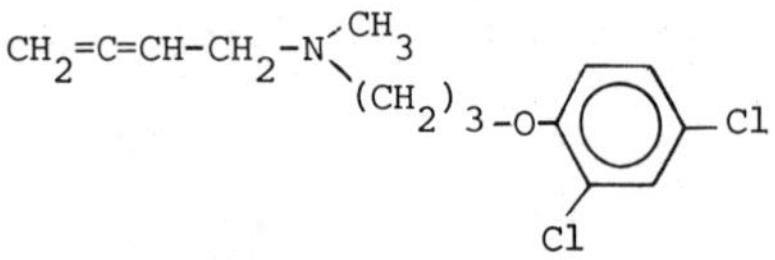 $CH_2=C=CH-CH_2-N(CH_3)((CH_2)_3-O-C_6H_3Cl_2)$	10^{-4}	4

TABLE II (Con't)

$CH_3-CH=C=CH-CH_2-N\overset{CH_3}{\underset{CH_2-C_6H_5}{}}$	10^{-3}	6.1
$\overset{CH_3}{\underset{CH_3}{}}C=C=CH-CH_2-N\overset{CH_3}{\underset{CH_2-C_6H_5}{}}$	$>10^{-3}M$	-

[a]MAO (0.2-0.3 units) in 0.5 ml of 0.067 M NaPi, pH 7.2 containing 0.6% glycerol were incubated with appropriate concentrations of allenic amines at 26°.

The reactivity profile for inhibition resembles the pattern observed for substrates of MAO; primary, secondary and tertiary amines inhibit MAO and methylation at nitrogen retards inhibition.[12] The rate of inhibition is apparently more sensitive to substitution at the terminal allenic position than at the internal allenic carbon. Each methyl group at C_δ slows the inhibition by a factor of 10^2, at 25°C. The effect of substituents at C_β is more subtle. But the observation that the enzyme can tolerate substitution at C_β is an important one which may allow extensive variation of the structure of allenic amines to optimize biological activity and specificity towards isoenzymes of MAO. Inhibition of MAO by most of the β,γ,δ-allenic amines is accompanied by bleaching of the 455 nm band and gives spectra characteristic of reduced flavins. 2-Benzyl-2,3-butadienylamine (7) is an exception. When the enzyme is inhibited by 7 the spectrum of the mixture displays residual (30-40%) flavin-like (455 nm) absorption. (Fig. 9). The possibility of inhibition owing to covalent linkage of an active-site residue other than flavin is suggested and is currently under investigation.

Treatment of MAO with N-2,3-Butadienyl-N-benzyl-N-[14C-] methyl Amine (8).The fate of the N-benzyl-N-methyl group in 2 was explored using N-2,3-butadienyl-N-benzyl-N-[14C] methyl amine (8). The results of treating MAO with 8 are compared to those obtained with 4 in Table III. The excluded volume from Sephadex G-25 filtration of the incubated medium contained only a small fraction (12%) of the original counts. After precipitation with TCA and enzymatic degradation no more than 4% of the label is associated with inhibitor-flavin peptide complex. Analysis with gas chromatography of the included fraction from the gel filtration reveals N-benzylmethyl amine 9. Apparently 9 is a coproduct of the adduct and serves as a carrier of the radiochemical label.

156

TABLE III

STABILITY OF THE ADDUCT FROM N-2,3-BUTADIENYL-N-BENZYL-N-METHYLAMINE WITH MAO.

Treatment	Nature and Position of Radiolabel in Inhibitor			
	[14]C in butadienyl residue		[14]C in N-methyl residue	
	nmols	%	nmols	%
Enzyme (flavin)	89.3	(100)	94.9	(100)
Radiolabel retained after:				
Sephadex G-25	76.1	85.2	12.1	12.8
5% TCA, Acetone ppt. & washes & proteolytic digestion	76.1	85.2	4.0	4.2

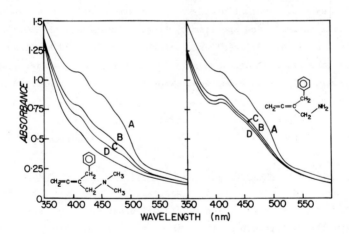

Fig. 9. Spectral changes upon treatment of MAO with 2-benzyl-2,3-butadienamine (7). Curve A, corresponds to native enzyme; in B, MAO is 56% inhibited; C, 83.3% inhibited; D, 99.4% inhibited (right panel).

Photolyses of 3-Methyllumiflavin with Amines 6 and 10. When millimolar quan-
tities of 3-methyllumiflavin were irradiated with Pyrex-filtered light in the
presence of a ten-fold excess of N-2,3-butadienyl-N,N-dimethylamine (6) in 20%
acetonitrile-80% (0.1M) phosphate buffer, pH 7.2, and the reaction mixture worked up according to Gärtner,[23] we obtained >90% yields of a yellow brown powder
which was characterized as 5-[3'-(dimethylamino-imino)-1'-methyl)-3-methyl-1,5-
dihydrolumiflavin betain (11): m.p.207-210° (dec); NMR(CDCl$_3$) δ 2.22 (3H,s),
2.28 (3H,s) ([7,8]-CH$_3$), 2.36 (3H,s,1' CH$_3$), 2.94 (3H,s,10-N-CH$_3$), 3.28 (3H,s,
3-N-CH$_3$), 3.34 (3H,b.s.), 3.39 (3H,s), [N(CH$_3$)$_2$] (5.27-5.42), 5.75-5.89) [broad,
2'-H] two olefinic resonances split in ratio of 2:1, 6.82 (1H, br. s, 9-H),
6.97 (1H, br. 6-H) 7.53 (1H, d, J$_{2,3}$12Hz, 3'-H); λ$_{max}$ (ε mM) CHCl$_3$ 413 (13.0),
313 (12.6); CH$_3$OH: 387 (16.6), 301 (15.3); pH 7.2 (phosphate buffer): 374
(17.3), 299 (15.8); pH 2.0 (HCl) 368 (19.0), 299 (12.7); in CF$_3$CO$_2$H: 368
(19.0), 299 (12.7); ν$_{max}^{CHCl_3}$ 1640 cm^{-1} ([2,4]-C=O); pK$_a$=4.9.

The solvent dependence of the electronic spectrum of 11 is very typical of
flavocyanines,[23] as is the value of the pK$_a$. Whereas 6 gives almost exclusively
the flavocyanine 11, isosbestic point 402 nm [80% aq. acetonitrile, pH 7.2, 0.1M
phosphate buffer), Fig. 10], the irradiation of 3-MLF with the isomeric acetylenic amine N-2-butynyl-N-N-dimethylamine (10) under essentially identical conditions gives two major isolable photochemical products: the flavocyanine 11 in
20% yield, and 1-hydroxy-3,5,8,10,11-pentamethyl-1H, 8H-benzo [g]-pyrrolo[2,1-e]
-pteridine-4,6-dione (12), 32%, yellow crystals (ether), m.p. 194°; NMR (C^{2}HCl$_3$)
NMR (C^{2}HCl$_3$): 1.79 (3H,s, 3-CH$_3$),2.19([6H,s, [10,11]-CH$_3$]), 3.27 (3H,s, 8-NCH$_3$)
3.57 (3H,s, 5-NCH$_3$), 4.47 (1H disappears in D$_2$O,d, J$_{1,OH}$=11.6 Hz, 1-OH), 5.60
(1H, d (collapses with D$_2$O), 1-H), 5.84 (1H, s, 2-H), 6.72, 6.99 (2s, 2H [9,12]-
H; ν$_{max}$ (CHCl$_3$, cm^{-1}) 1665 (6-C=O), 1705 (4-C=O), 3450 (1-OH); λ$_{max}$ CH$_3$OH, 368
(4.0), 300 sh (5.7), 2.79 (13.0), 234 (17.3) 214 (20.0) nm (ε mM^{-1}cm^{-1}).

DISCUSSION

Our interest in allenic amine inhibitors of MAO was stimulated by the report
of Maycock et. al,[25] that the drug pargyline 13, an antidepressant and antihypertensive agent long known to be an inhibitor of MAO, became irreversibly linked to the flavin prosthetic group in the form of a flavocyanine 14 (Fig. 11).
The characterization of this adduct was aided considerably by the fact that a
photoproduct between 3-methyllumiflavin and pargyline (or its dimethyl analog,
15) which exhibited strong absorption similar in position and intensity to that
of the enzymatic adduct, proved to be a flavocyanine.[23,26,27]
Three mechanisms have been advanced[25] to rationalize the formation of

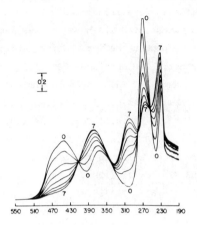

Fig. 10. Time course of the Pyrex-filtered photoreaction between 3-MLF (0.5 x 10^{-4}M) with N-2,3-butadienyl-N,N-dimethylamine (6) hydrochloride (0.5x10^{-3}M) in 0.1M phosphate buffer (pH 7.2) containing 20% acetonitrile. Reaction was conducted in a 3 ml cuvette irradiating through a Pyrex-filter with a 450 watt mercury lamp. Spectra were recorded at 0, 0.25, 1, 2, 4, 8, 12 and 20 min. 0 and 7, correspond to the starting mixture and the 20 min. irradiation, respectively. Note isosbestic point at 402 nm (x-axis scale is in nm).

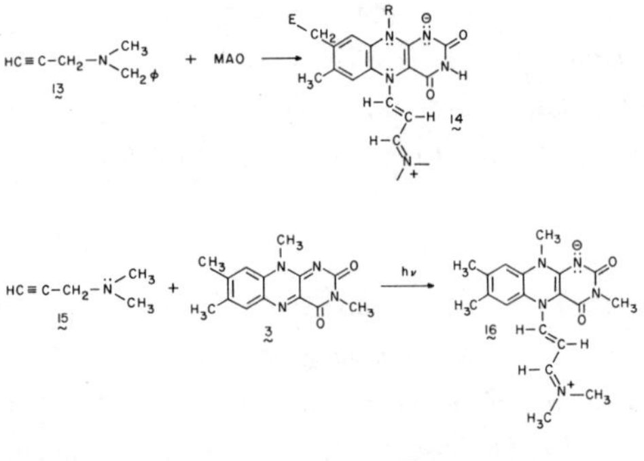

Fig. 11. Similarity in the structure of flavin adducts from the photoreaction of 3-MLF with N,N-dimethyl propargylamine (15), and the inhibition of MAO by pargyline (13).

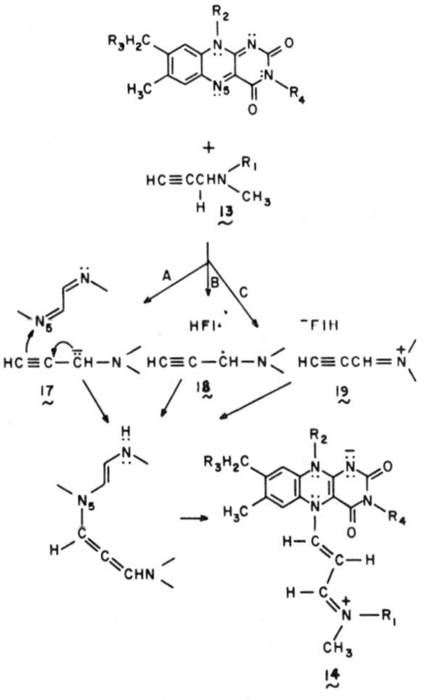

Fig. 12. Proposed mechanisms for the action of pargyline, $R_1=CH_2\phi$ on mono-amine oxidase. R_2=adenine dinucleotide, R_3=apoprotein, R_4=H.

flavocyanine from MAO (Fig. 12). Path A features attack on the oxidized form of the flavin by a resonance stabilized, formally carbanionic species. Activation of the substrate is by proton removal, the incipient carbanion becoming linked at its γ-terminus to N_5 of the flavin. The formation of such a carbanion by non-enzymatic proton removal proceeds with great difficulty as evidenced by the need for very strong basic conditions, (potassium t-butoxide/100°, alumina-potassium amide and their ilk), to effect isomerization of propargyl amines.[28,29] Judging from the half-life for exchange ($t_{1/2}$ = 5 min, 1 M NaOD/D_2O, 25°) of propargyl protons of the quaternary ammonium ion $HC\equiv CCH_2N^+$ $(CH_3)_3Br^-$ at 0.48 N, a substantial reduction in activation energy for removal of the propargylic hydrogen can be achieved if the substrate amine is effectively quaternized by protonation at the active site.[10] Ambiguities concerning the microenvironment at the active site, the disposition of appropriate bases, and the synchrony of hydrogen removal with attack on flavin, make this qualitatively improbable alternative, difficult to assess rigorously. Precedent does exist, however, for the genera-tion of carbanions from unnatural substrates (the chlorolactate-lactate oxidase system),[30] and for carbanionic attack on N_5 of the flavin moiety in D-amine acid oxidase.[31]

In path B covalent union is regarded as a consequence of radical formation and subsequent coupling. Bruice, by resort to kinetic and thermodynamic data, has argued persuasively in favor of radical intermediates in the reduction of carbonyls by dihydroflavins[32] (the microscopic reverse of alcohol oxidation by flavins). If Bruice's model reactions are relevant to the enzymatic case, it is likely true that radicals intervene in amine oxidation by MAO.

A third possibility (C in Fig. 12) correlates flavocyanine with the Michael addition of reduced flavin and a putative immonium ion 19. This path is dis-tinguished by two electron oxidation of the substrate. It is easy to see why irreversible covalent bond formation would be favorable in the case of 19, but not in the case of natural substrates. Intuitively, condensation of a nucleo-phile with 19 should be orders of magnitude faster than with simple unconjugated immonium ions, and considerably more exothermic. Note that combinations of these mechanisms may apply; all three intermediates 17, 18, and 19 in Fig. 12 would intervene prior to linkage with flavin, if proton removal from 13 trig-gered successive one-electron transfers.

Relevant to these hypotheses, are the observations that the isomers N-2-butynyl-N-benzylmethylamine 1, a homolog of pargyline,[13] and N-2,3-butadienyl-N-benzylmethylamine 2 are reported to be MAO inhibitors. The mode of action of the allene and its structural requirements for MAO inhibition is unknown. If any of the above mechanistic hypotheses is applicable, current theory would predict the flavocyanine to be a product from both isomers 1 and 2. This point is illustrated for path A (Fig. 13), and is based on the assumptions that inter-mediate enamines 20 and 21 would rapidly convert by proton transfer to a common flavocyanine, that no metal atoms participate in catalysis, and that site selec-tive attack on the flavin is not determined by the apoprotein.

We fully anticipated that the acetylenic amine 1 in the manner of pargyline, would yield a flavocyanine 22 which could serve as an independent synthesis of the potential allenic amine-MAO adduct. The observation of strong absorption centered at 391 nm ($\varepsilon \sim 2 \times 10^4$, isosbestic point at 426 nm) with concomitant loss of the 455 nm band of the native flavoenzyme, when MAO is treated with 1, signals the formation of an adduct between the flavin prosthetic group and the

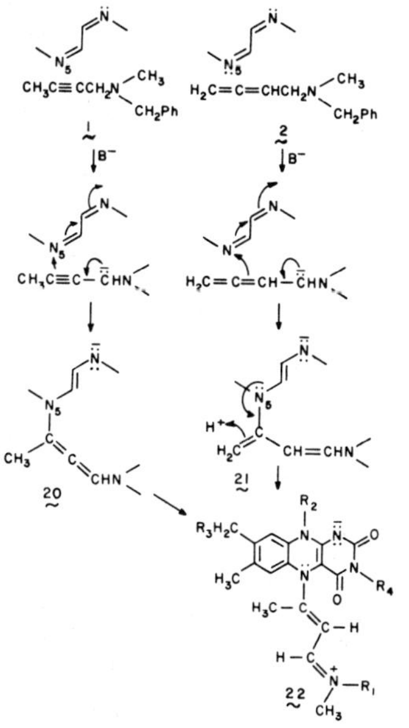

Fig. 13. A hypothetical pathway predicting a common flavocyanine product (22) from isomeric β,γ,δ-allenic and β,γ-acetylenic amines.

acetylenic amine. The position and intensity of the new band are similar to
values observed for the corresponding inhibitions with pargyline and its analogs
and are typical values for flavocyanines.[23]

In fact, we have prepared a model flavocyanine 11 which closely matches the
spectral properties of the inactivated enzyme. Thus it appears likely that the
action of compound 1 is closely related to that of pargyline.

In contrast to the action of 1, the electronic spectrum of the product of
MAO and the allenic amine 2 shows no absorption characteristic of a flavocyanine, nor does it show any maximum at wavelengths longer than 360 nm (Fig. 2).
Featureless absorption from the protein obscures the spectrum of the adduct.
Bleaching of the flavoquinone spectrum, shifting maximal absorption significantly below 400 nm, are symptoms usually associated with the production of reduced
flavins.

The adduct has been unequivocally demonstrated to be covalent by treating the
enzyme with the radiochemically labelled $N(1-^{14}C)$-2,3-butadienyl-N-benzylmethyl-
amine (4). If the inactivated enzyme is denatured by precipiting it with
trichloroacetic acid, then enzymatically digesting the precipitate with chymotrypsin amd trypsin, and applying the resulting mixture of peptides to a florisil column, the radioactive eluent contains a peptide which absorbs at 327 and
343 nm as distinct shoulders on a diffuse spectral band. The firm association
of the radiochemical label with the flavin up to this point, establishes that
the enzyme-allene adduct is indeed covalent and essentially irreversible.

One equivalent of 2 (Fig. 3) suffices to abolish MAO activity completely and
to bleach the spectrum of the oxidized flavin. The reaction terminated after
one equivalent of radiochemical label was bound to the flavin. A large excess
of inactivator did not result in further binding to the flavoprotein, as determined by gel filtration on Sephadex G-25. This point was substantiated by the
observation that even after enzymatic degradation of the denatured enzyme-inhibitor complex, one equivalent of the radiochemical label per flavin was still associated with the flavin peptides. Apparently the enzyme does not complete a
full cycle of catalysis.

The efficiency of inactivation could be interpreted in two ways. The conventional view is that an intermediary modification of the amine is generated by
the enzyme, and trapped with 100% efficiency by the flavin.

$$E + I \rightleftarrows E \cdot I \rightleftarrows E' \cdot I' \xrightarrow{k_e} E + I'$$

$$\downarrow k_c$$

$$E' - I'$$

The escape versus capture ratio (k_e/k_c) is thus zero. In the design of a drug this ratio would be most favorable, because it is undesirable to "litter" the cell or plasma with such reactive particles.

In view of the tendency of allenes[33-35] to engage in condensation with multiple bonds another possibility must be considered. Allenes are known to undergo two types of cycloadditions with multiple bonds, a $[_\pi 2 + _\pi 2]$ - and a $[_\pi 2 + _\pi 4]$ - reaction. For simple allenes elevated temperatures are generally

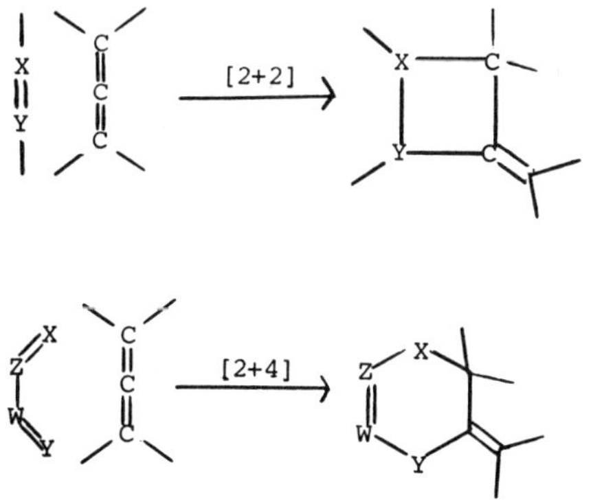

required for cycloaddition, but the possibility exists, a priori, that binding to the enzyme activates the allenic amine for condensation at the imine linkages of the flavin. The mere presence of an allene is not a sufficient condition for inactivation since buta-2,3-dienol 23 and N-3,4-pentadienyl-N-benzylmethylamine 24 do not inactivate MAO. If cycloaddition preempts inactivation stemming from

$$H_2C=C=CHCH_2OH$$
23

$$H_2C=C=CHCH_2CH_2\overset{\overset{\displaystyle CH_3}{|}}{N}\diagdown CH_2\phi$$
24

enzyme catalysis, it would have to be the result of a precisely defined orientation between the allene and the flavin.

To distinguish between the possibilities, we compared the rate of inactivation of MAO by compound 2 with its 1,1-dideutero analog 5 (Fig. 6). A deuterium isotope effect $k_H/k_D \sim 5.18$ was measured from kinetic studies of the reaction of MAO with 2 and 5. Clearly, hydrogen abstraction from the butadienyl chain, corresponding to the metabolic point of attack must be occurring. This result proves that the enzyme regards 2 as a substrate, because the key step of its normal catalytic sequence is required for inactivation. From the stoichiometry of the reaction, the profound spectral change, and the observation that normal substrates protect against the inhibition, we conclude that 2 is a titrant of the active-site flavin prosthetic group. Saturation, time-dependent, pseudo-first order kinetics as well as the deuterium-isotope effect convincingly demonstrate that the allenic amine 2 qualifies as an enzyme-suicide inhibitor. The substrate-like reactivity profile of the allenic amine inhibitors in Table II is also consistent with our claim.

Structural Aspects of the Inactivation of MAO by Allenic Amines. Since neither compound 23 nor 24 is an inactivator of MAO, it follows that the critical allenic element must be linked directly to a nitrogen-bound methylene unit $(C_\alpha H_2)$ in order for inactivation to take place. Although it had previously been reported that substituents at the internal allenic position (C_β) abolish the inhibitory activity of allenic amines, our own recent investigations show, quite the contrary, that compounds with benzyl and methyl substituents at (C_β), still retain considerable inhibitory ability (Table II). This finding is important because it broadens the scope of synthesis of potential allenic amine inhibitors of MAO. On the basis of the above qualitative observations and the well-known inability of MAO to oxidize amines lacking an α-CH$_2$ group, the essential structural unit for allenic amine inactivation must be $\begin{matrix}\diagdown \\ \diagup\end{matrix}C=C=C-CH_2N\begin{matrix}\cdots \diagup \\ \diagdown\end{matrix}$

Substitution of the terminal allenic hydrogens of compound 2 alters its inhibitory power. The rate of inactivation of MAO is reduced by approximately two orders of magnitude by a single methyl substituent at the terminal allenic position. The compound with two methyl groups at the terminus was a poor inhibitor.

Despite the very large number of compounds known to inhibit MAO, for only a few examples[25,36] has the structure of an adduct between MAO and the inhibitor been elucidated. Until a few years ago, lack of progress in this field may have been due to the absence of a satisfactory procedure for isolating the covalently bound flavin peptide, the probable target of most of these inhibitors. This difficulty was overcome by the studies of Kearney et al.,[37] and Walker et al.[38] who devised the procedure for isolating a pentapeptide containing the cysteinyl flavin core of the enzyme. This flavin peptide is short enough so that characterization can be focused primarily on the flavin-inhibitor adduct.

The characterization of pargyline-inactivated MAO was aided by several circumstances. The very dramatic absorption of the enzymatic adduct sharply limited the number of structures which could be reasonably assigned to the product. The photoadduct (16) between compound 15 and 3-methyllumiflavin possessed a highly characteristic flavocyanine spectrum and properties which were congruent with the flavin-peptide derived from the enzymatic adduct. The flavin-inhibitor adduct was also of sufficient stability to survive the procedures of denaturation, enzymatic degradation, and purification by chromatography and electrophoresis.

Our experience with the adduct of allenic amine and MAO contrasts with those characteristic of the adduct of the β,γ-acetylenic amine case. The electronic spectrum provides no specific structural information, although it is suggestive of a reduced flavin. Regeneration of the flavin spectrum from a fraction of the peptide during purification on phosphocellulose implies that the isoalloxazine ring remains intact in the inactivated enzyme. There are only a limited number of substitutive patterns of the isoalloxazine framework which could shift absorption of the native enzyme from 450 nm to below 360 nm in the adduct.

Attack at the benzene ring at either the C_6 or C_8 positions is unlikely to cause such a hypsochromic shift, unless deep-seated rearrangements take place. The most sterically accessible and reactive positions of the flavin tend to be the C_{4a} and N_5 positions and C_{4a}, N_5-adducts absorb at relatively short wavelength (325-360 nm) with modest extinction coefficients (ε 5000-10,000).[39,40] Although we have no direct structural evidence in support of a C_{4a}, N_5-adduct, it represents a plausible working hypothesis. We therefore considered structure 25 as a possible adduct, one which could be derived from 26 (Fig. 14) by hydrolysis, and which should be unstable at the flavin-peptide level.

To test this hypothesis the enzyme was incubated with N-2,3-butadienyl-N-^{14}C-methyl-N-benzylamine 8 until inactivation was essentially complete (98.4%). When

26 → 25

the mixture was applied to a column containing Sephadex G-25, almost 90% of the radioactivity was recovered in the included volume, whereas the excluded volume contained protein which could be enzymatically degraded to a small flavin peptide containing less than 5% of the original counts. A parallel experiment using 1-^{14}C-N-buta-2,3-dienyl-N-benzylmethylamine (4) showed the eluted protein

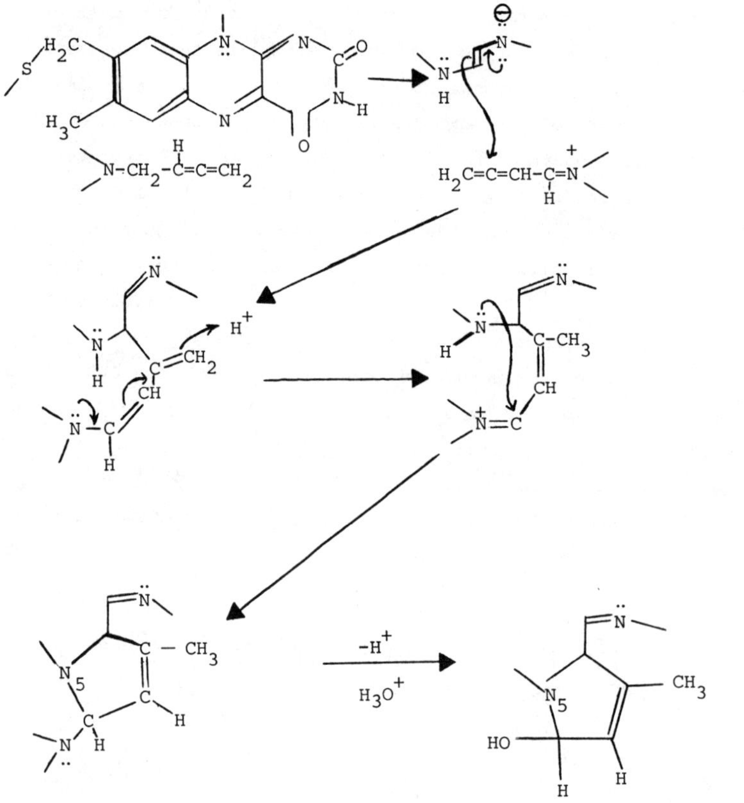

Fig. 14. A hypothetical pathway illustrating the formation of the potential C_{4a},N_5 adduct 25 from union of MAO with the allenic amine 2.

and the flavin peptide derived from it, to retain nearly an equivalent of the label. Significantly, gas chromatographic analysis of the included fraction revealed the presence of N-benzyl-N-methylamine 9.

When the inactivated enzyme was worked up in the manner previously described by Maycock and coworkers,[25] and the flavin peptide purified on Florisil and phosphocellulose, the ratio of absorbance at 343 and 327 nm to radioactivity was reasonably constant in all the fractions containing the inhibitor-flavin peptide adduct. The adduct appeared to be stable to chromatography on Florisil, but underwent considerable reorganization on phosphocellulose (pH gradient from 2.5 to 4.0). Experiments are in progress to determine the ultimate fate of the allenic amine fragments. Although no firm conclusions can as yet be drawn regarding the structure of the adduct of compound 2 with MAO, the detection of N-benzyl-N-methylamine as a coproduct of the reaction, places severe constraints on speculations regarding the structure of the adduct.

A tentative mechanism which takes into account the low wavelength absorption of the adduct signifying a reduced flavin, the loss of the methyl label in the form of N-benzylmethylamine, the retention of the ^{14}C-label in the butadienyl moiety, and the instability of the flavin peptides is formulated in figure 14. The foregoing observations are compatible with the notorious instability and spectral properties of C_{4_a}, N_5-substituted flavins,[23,41] but may not be unique to them.

Determinants of the Enzymatic Adduct. Why does the action of the acetylenic amine 1 on MAO form a flavocyanine while that of the allenic amine, compound 2 does not?

The reasons for product discrimination by the enzyme between acetylene and allene are unclear, but are unlikely to be the result of the action of mutually distinct reactive intermediates on the flavin, i.e., radicals in one case, carbanions in the other. Subtle electronic factors may favor attack at the C_{4_a} position in the case of the allene, but for the acetylene the N_5 position may be preferred. There is a structural distinction between the bis-enamines 20 and 21 (Fig. 13) but since these molecules are closely related tautomers, it is difficult to imagine the formation of flavocyanine in one case and not the other unless, a potentially reactive arrangement, imposed by the protein, promotes condensation between the flavin (or amino acid residues) and the butadienyl moiety of compound 21.

.A major determinant of site specific attack should be the geometrical relation between the flavin and the inhibitor at the active site. The local symmetry of the propynyl group ($CH_3C{\equiv}C-$) differs from the allenic moiety ($H_2C=C=CH$). This factor could be decisive, if the acetylenic and allenic moieties are positioned differently relative to flavin upon binding of compounds 1 and 2 to MAO, and these positions are held during covalent bond formation. More specific speculations must await concrete evidence for the structure of the adduct.

Photoadducts. Photoreductive alkylation of 3-methyllumiflavin by acetylenic amines, has been a covenient route to model flavin compounds, whose structures are relevant to the products of flavoenzymes with acetylenic inactivators.[23] Besides providing important clues to the structure of these adducts, a point of potentially deeper significance is the relation between the photochemical and enzymatic reaction pathways, and whether they involve similar intermediates.

One scenario that seems plausible to us, which rationalizes the formation of the similar flavin adducts 14 and 16, features the intermediary immonium ion 27, and is formulated in Figure 15. For the enzymatic reaction the adduct is generated _via_ a path initiated by hydrogen atom transfer to flavin, followed by electron transfer leading to the reduced flavin and the immonium ion 27.

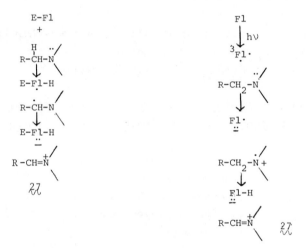

Fig. 15. Hypothetical scheme illustrating how similar reactive intermediates could be generated _via_ enzymatic and photochemical pathways.

The same immonium ion could be formed photochemically by a similar sequence initiated by triplet flavin, or by an inverted sequence, in which hydrogen atom transfer is preceded by electron transfer. The latter scheme is particularly attractive because it involves individual steps which have firm chemical precedents. The generation of intermediates of the same type in nonenzymatic and enzymatic reactions would provide a means of evaluating the influence of the

apoprotein in directing product formation, as well as make available useful
flavin compounds that are otherwise difficultly accessible. Our interest was
thus focused on the photoreactions of allenic amines with 3-methyllumiflavin in
the hope of obtaining a substance whose properties could be related to the enzymatic adduct.

Clearly, the allenic amine 6 does not give a major photoproduct whose electronic spectrum matches that of the enzymatic adduct. Unlike the example of
propargylamines, the photochemical reaction of 3-MLF with 6 (or 7) does not
lead to a major photoproduct of obvious relevance to the corresponding enzymatic (MAO) reaction. In fact the photoproduct of 3-MLF and the allenic amine
6 (or 7) corresponds in structure to the butynyl-MAO adduct! Even the photochemical reactions of 6 and 10 with 3-MLF must differ in important mechanistic
aspects. At least that segment of the reaction path leading to 12 is not an
important one for the allenic amine - (3-MLF) system (Fig. 16). The forces that
determine binding at the active site of the enzyme are certain to be different
from those that determine the structure of charge transfer complexes (or exciplexes) between amines and excited flavins.

The discrepancy in the structure of the flavin adducts from the photochemical
and enzymatic reactions of allenic amines could be a consequence of mutually
distinct reactive intermediates (radical vs. immonium ions?). Or it may simply
be due to the influence of the protein on the flavin and/or the catalytically
modified inactivator. The structural properties of flavin-inactivator complexes
at the enzyme active site, and potential exciplexes of the photochemical reaction
are likely to be important structural determinants of the products. If the
regiospecificity of attack on flavin in the photochemical reaction, is governed by
the structure of charge transfer complexes (or exciplexes), differences in the
structure of such molecular complexes could be translated into differences in
site-specific attack on flavin. Mutually exclusive molecular complexes, as a
consequence of distinct donor components, are anticipated for the interaction
of amines 6 and 10 with triplet 3-MLF.

Hemmerich has made extensive contributions in the area of flavin photochemistry[42] and regards the reaction of 3-MLF with β,γ-acetylenic amines as one
of a group of photoreactions involving "group transfers," which include decarboxylative alkylation of flavin by β,γ-unsaturated carboxylic acids,[43] and alkylation of flavins of propylene and other olefins.[44] In the case of
propargylamines, a propargylic carbanion has been proposed as a viable intermediate for attack on triplet flavin (or its conjugate acid) in the photochemical reactions.[23] However, the pK_a of a propargyl hydrogen must be greater than 25 and thus the carbanion is an unlikely candidate for initiating covalent bond formation at a flavin site.

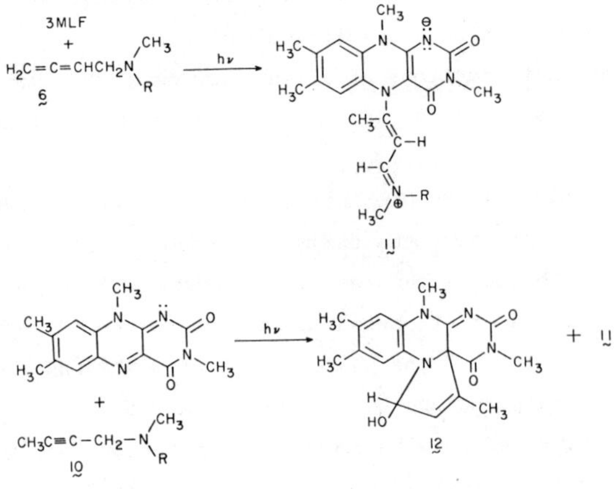

Fig. 16. Photoadducts of 3-methyllumiflavin with isomeric allenic and acetylenic amines, $R_1 = CH_3$.

A more physically reasonable picture (Fig. 17) stems from the observation
that tertiary alkyl amines are known to form complexes with the excited states
of organic molecules, which may lead to electron transfer, hydrogen abstraction,
and linkage of the acceptor molecule to the carbon atom adjacent to the amine
nitrogen.[45,48] Reduction by amines appears to proceed generally, by rapid initial interaction at the non-bonding electrons of the amines, leading to a
charge transfer complex.[49,50] Thus it is not uncommon for amines to play the
role of electron transfer agents. Examples of such reactions, which include
the photoreduction of triplet carbonyl species, are legion.[51] The work of
Loutfy[52], Weller[53] and Cohen[51] support the view that amines assume the donor
role and transfer one electron at a time to photochemically excited species.
Our proposal for the photochemical reaction of amines with 3-MLF is further
strengthened by a calculation of the energetics for the electron transfer step.
(Table IV). The energetics are favorable for one electron transfer to the
neutral flavin triplet and highly exothermic (12 kcal/mole) for transfer to its
conjugate acid (pK$_a$ 5.5) a few percent of which should be present at pH 7.2.
Our scheme (Fig. 17) is made even more credible since we have unequivocally
established that the photoreactions of 6 and 10 involve triplet flavin[54] and
that the reduced flavin anion[55] is produced during the photoreactions.

A sequence involving hydrogen obstraction is also energetically feasible
and may apply in some cases, particularly in the alkylation of flavin by
propylene and other olefins.

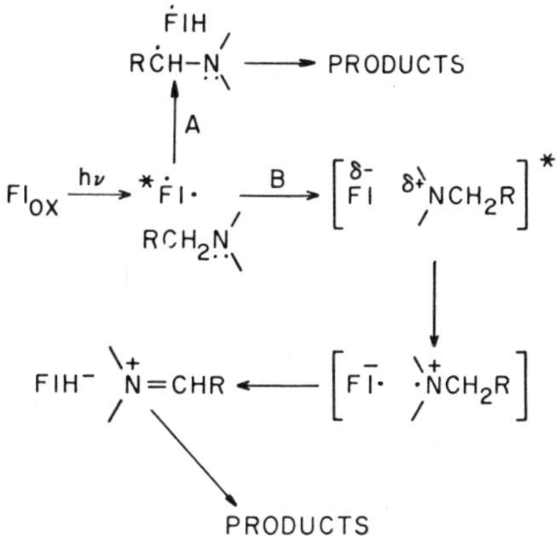

Fig. 17. Proposed mechanism for photoalkylation of 3-methyllumiflavin by amines
(Path B). A sequence involving hydrogen abstraction is also energetically
feasible and may apply in some cases (Path A).

TABLE IV

ENERGETICS OF ELECTRON TRANSFER FROM 3^O AMINES TO TRIPLET 3-MLF

$R-CH_2N\begin{smallmatrix}R\\ \\R_2\end{smallmatrix}:$	$\longrightarrow$	$R-CH_2-\overset{+}{N}\begin{smallmatrix}R_1\\ \\R_2\end{smallmatrix} + e$	$+1.32^a$
$^3Fl\cdot$	$\longrightarrow$	$Fl + h\nu$	-2.06^b
$H^+ + Fl + e$	$\longrightarrow$	$FlH\cdot$	$+0.24^c$
$HFl\cdot$	$\longrightarrow$	$Fl\cdot^- + H^+$	$+0.44^c$
$^3Fl\cdot + R-CH_2N\begin{smallmatrix}R_1\\ \\R_2\end{smallmatrix}:$	$\longrightarrow$	$Fl\cdot^- + R-CH_2-\overset{+}{N}\begin{smallmatrix}R_1\\ \\R_2\end{smallmatrix}$	~ 0

[a]Guttenplan, J. B. and Cohen, S. G. (1972) J. Am. Chem. Soc. 94, 4040. [b]Sun, M.,
Moore, T. A. and Song, P.-S. ibid., 1730. [c]Bruice, T. C., (1976) in Prog. Biorg.
Chem., Kaiser, E. T. and Kezdy, F. J., ed., John Wiley and Sons, Inc., N.Y.,
N.Y., p. 1.

For alkylation of flavins by carboxylate salts the electron transfer mechanism may also apply. Indeed, the fact that the carboxylic acid form cannot serve in the stead of carboxylate[43] to alkylate flavin is consistent with such a mechanism. Electron transfer from the carboxylate to flavin followed by decarboxylation of the carboxyl radical are reasonable chemicals events; the particularly favorable cases of decarboxylative alkylation which have been reported, are those in which the driving force is the formation of resonance stabilized allylic or benzylic radicals, steps which should proceed exceptionally rapidly.

The essential feature of our proposal, electron transfer (perhaps following charge transfer or exciplex formation) between donor substrate and acceptor flavin, has the virtue of explaining the pH dependence of this set of flavin photoalkylations.[43,44] The "photo pK" effect is nicely rationalized by involking a protonated flavin excited state,[56] better able to act as one electron acceptor than its conjugate base.

SUMMARY

We have shown that β,γ,δ-allenic amines are potent mechanism-based inhibitors of MAO. The essential structural unit for facile inhibition is $\ce{>C=C=C-CH_2-N<}$. Generally the adduct is a reduced flavin. The photochemical adduct of 3-MLF with N-2,3-butadienyl-N,N-dimethylamine (6), or 2 does not correspond in structure to the enzymatic adduct of MAO with 2. The photochemical adducts are derived from triplet flavin probably by a path involving electron transfer from 3° amines.

ACKNOWLEDGMENTS

Acknowledgment is made to Professor K. Bloch (Harvard University) for his hospitality to A. Krantz during the initial stages of this work. This work was supported by Research Service Award No. 1-F32-NS05401-01 and grant no. 1 R01 NS13220-01 from the National Institutes of Health to A. Krantz; by a stipend from the donors of the Petroleum Research Fund administered by the American Chemical Society to B. Kokel; by the Friends Medical Science Research Center, Inc. and National Institutes of Health grant no. 1 R01 NS14222-01 to J. Salach. Support (to A.C.) from the following sources: IF:s Stiftelse för farmaceutisk forskning, Apotekare C.D. Carlssons stiftelse, and Lennanders fond is also gratefully acknowledged. We wish to thank Kristina Detmer for expert technical assistance.

REFERENCES

1. Rando, R.R. (1974) Science 185, 320.
2. Rando, R.R. (1975) Accts. Chem. Res. 8, 281.
3. Abeles, R.H. and Maycock, A.L. (1976) Accts. Chem. Res. 9, 313.
4. Walsh, C.T. (1977) in Horiz. Biochem. Biophys. (Quagliarello, E.,
   Palmieri, F., and Singer, T.P., eds.), Vol. 3, p. 36, Addison-Wesley,
   Reading, Massachusetts.
5. Walsh, C., Cromartie, T., Marcotte, P. and Spencer, R. (1978) in Methods of
   Enzymology (Fleischer, S., and Packer, L., eds.), Vol. 53, Part D., p. 437,
   Academic Press, N.Y.
6. Rando, R.R. (1977) in Methods of Enzymology (Jakoby, W.B. and Wilchek, M.,
   eds.), Vol. 46, p. 158, Academic Press, New York.
7. Winterfeldt, E. (1969) in Chemistry of Acetylenes (Viehe, H.G.), p. 366,
   Marcel Dekker, Inc., New York.
8. Dickstein, J.I., and Miller, S.I. (1978) in The Chemistry of the Carbon-
   Carbon Triple Bond (Patai, S., ed.), p. 813, John Wiley & Sons, Ltd., London.
9. Theron, F., Verny, M., and Vessiere, R., ibid., p. 381.
10. Krantz, A. and Lipkowitz, G.S. (1977) J. Am. Chem. Soc. 99, 4156.
11. Rutledge, T.F., Acetylenes and Allenes (1969) Rheinhold Book Corp., NY.
12. Kapeller-Adler, R. (1970) Amine Oxidases and Methods for their Study, John
    Wiley and Sons, Inc., New York, NY.
13. Swett, L.R., Martin, W.B., Taylor, J.D., Everett, G.M., Wykes, A.A., and
    Gladish, Y.C. (1963) Ann. NY Acad. Sci. 107, 891.
14. Halliday, R.P., Davis, C.S., Heotis, J.P., Pals, D.T., Watson, E.J., and
    Bickerton, R.K. (1968) J. Pharm. Sci. 57, 430.
15. Taylor, D.R. (1967) Chem. Rev. 67, 317.
16. Ghosez, L. and O'Donnell, M.S. in Pericyclic Reactions (Marchand, A.P. and
    Lehr, R.E., eds.), Vol. 2, p. 109, Academic Press.
17. Salach, J.I., Jr. (1978) in Methods of Enzymology (Fleischer, S. and
    Packer, L., eds.), Vol. 53, Part D., p. 495, Academic Press, New York.
18. Edmonson, D.E., Kenney, W.C. and Singer, T.P., ibid., p. 449.
19. Claesson, A. and Sahlberg, C. (1978) Tetrahedron Lett., 1319.
20. Hemmerich, P., Prijs, B. and Erlenmeyer, H. (1960) Helv. Chim. Acta, 43, 372.
21. Tabor, C.W., Tabor, H. and Rosenthal, S.M. (1954) J. Biol. Chem., 208, 645.
22. Penefsky, H.S. (1977) J. Biol. Chem. 252, 2891.
23. Gärtner, B., Hemmerich, P. and Zeller, E.A. (1976) Eur. J. Biochem. 63, 211.
24. McEwen, C.M., Jr., Sasaki, G. and Jones, D.C. (1969) Biochemistry 8, 3963.
25. Maycock, A.L., Abeles, R.H., Salach, J.I., and Singer, T.P. (1976) Biochem-
    istry 15, 114.
26. Gärtner, B. and Hemmerich, P. (1975) Angew. Chem. Int. Ed. 14, 110.
27. Maycock, A.L. (1975) J. Am. Chem. Soc. 97, 2270.
28. Ben-Efraim, D.A. (1973) Tetrahedron 29, 4111.
29. Hubert, A.J. and Viehe, H.G. (1968) J. Chem. Soc. (C), 228.
30. Walsh, C., Lockridge, O., Massey, V. and Abeles, R. (1973) J. Biol. Chem.
    248, 7049.
31. Porter, D.J.T., Voet, J.G. and Bright, H.J. (1973) J. Biol. Chem. 248, 4400.
32. Williams, R.F., Shinkai, S.S. and Bruice, T.C. (1977) J. Am. Chem. Soc. 99,
    921.
33. Huisgen, R., Grashey, R. and Sauer, J. (1964) in The Chemistry Alkenes,
    (Patai, S., ed.), p. 78, John Wiley & Sons, Ltd., London.
34. Lee, C.B., Newman, J.J. and Taylor, D.R. (1978) J.C.S. Perkin I, 1161.
35. Brady, W.T., Stockton, J.D. and Patel, A.D. (1974) J. Org. Chem. 39, 236.
36. Nagy, J., Kenney, W.C. and Singer, T.P. (1979) J. Biol. Chem. 254, 2684.
37. Kearney, E.B., Salach, J.I., Walker, W.H., Seng, R.L., Kenney, W.C.,
    Zeszotek, E. and Singer, T.P. (1971) Eur. J. Biochem. 24, 321.

38. Walker, W.H., Kearney, E.B., Seng, R.L. and Singer, T.P. (1971) Eur. J. Biochem. 24, 328.
39. Ghisla, S., Massey, V.,Lhoste, J.-M., Mayhew, S.G. (1974) Biochemistry 13, 589.
40. Ghisla, S., Hartmann, U., Hemmerich, P. and Müller, F. (1973) Justus Liebig's Ann. Chem., 1388.
41. Schonbrunn, A., Abeles, R.H., Walsh, C.T., Ghisla, S., Ogata, H. and Massey, V. (1976) Biochemistry 15, 1798.
42. Hemmerich, P. (1976) Fortsch. Chem. Forsch. 33, 512.
43. Haas, W. and Hemmerich, P. (1972) Z. Naturforsch. 27b, 1035.
44. Knappe, W.R. and Hemmerich, P. (1972) ibid., 27b, 1032.
45. Lewis, F.D. and Ho, T.-I. (1977) J. Am. Chem. Soc. 99, 7991.
46. Dalton, J.C. and Snyder, J.J. (1975) ibid., 97, 5192.
47. Van, S.-P. and Hammond, G. (1978) ibid., 100, 3895.
48. Aloisi, G.G., Mazzucato, U., Birks, J.B. and Minuti, L. (1977) 99, 6340.
49. Cohen, S.G. and Cohen, J.I. (1967) J. Am. Chem. Soc. 89, 164.
50. Cohen, S.G. and Cohen, J.I. (1968) J. Phys. Chem. 72, 3782.
51. Cohen, S.G., Parola, A. and Parsons, G.H., Jr. (1973) Chem. Rev. 73, 141.
52. Loutfy, R.O. and Loutfy, R.O. (1972) Can. J. Chem. 50, 4052.
53. Knibbe, H., Rehm, D. and Weller, A. (1968) Ber. Bunsenges. Phys. Chem. 72, 257.
54. Krantz, A., Kokel, B., Lewis, F. D. and J. T. Simpson, to be published.
55. Roth, H. D. and Krantz, A., unpublished results.
56. Schreiner, S., Steiner, U. and Kramer, H.E.A. (1975) Photochem. Photobiol. 21, 81.

DISCUSSION

MAYCOCK: Could your adduct be the compound formally derived from normal oxidation of your allenic amine, followed by hydrolysis of the imminium salt, followed by Michael addition of reduced flavine (at the N_5 position) to the resulting allenic aldehyde?

KRANTZ: We have not seen intense absorption in the region of 360 nm which would be anticipated for a molecule of that structure.

METCALF: Have you looked at the allenic amines in other types of enzymes, e.g., plasma amine oxidase?

KRANTZ: Yes, we have looked at diamine oxidase, and it turns out there are some very interesting results with the primary amines. Obviously the secondary and tertiary amines do not work and we certainly checked that just to make sure, because it would have been interesting, had they done so. But the primary amines, particularly the 2,3-butadienylamine is a very very good inhibitor in micromolar concentrations. It seems to be irreversible. Now, we have not investigated it as vigorously as we did the pargyline analog with MAO, but dialysis does not reverse. However, when you take internally substituted allenes that are primary amines, they seem to be reversible, even though they inhibit in a time dependent manner.

METCALF: Can you comment on any possible selectivity between inhibition of monoamine oxidase A and B with allenic amines?

KRANTZ: Well, that is in the works. That is something we are doing now. So, we have a deprenyl analog, and a chlorgyline analog for these studies.

MECHANISM OF INACTIVATION OF MITOCHONDRIAL MONOAMINE OXIDASE BY N-CYCLOPROPYL-
N-ARYLALKYL AMINES

RICHARD B. SILVERMAN AND STEPHEN J. HOFFMAN
Department of Chemistry, Northwestern University, Evanston, Illinois 60201,
USA

Mitochondrial monoamine oxidase (MAO) [EC 1.4.3.4] is a flavin-dependent
enzyme which catalyzes the first step in the catabolism of certain biogenic
amines. Compounds that inhibit this enzyme have been found to be antidepressant and antihypertensive agents.[1] MAO inhibitors were the principal antidepressant drugs used in the late 1950's and early 1960's.[2] Then, undesirable side effects were observed, notably the "cheese effect,"[3] a toxic reaction in patients taking MAO inhibitors who had ingested foods (e.g., sharp
cheeses) containing a high concentration of tyramine. The increased tyramine
concentration triggered the release of another biogenic amine, norepinephrine,
which is responsible for vasoconstriction, thus leading to increased blood
pressure. Since these people were taking MAO inhibitor drugs, they did not
have the capability of degrading the excess norepinephrine and were, therefore,
unable to control the rise in blood pressure. A hypertensive crisis, the
"cheese effect," resulted. MAO inhibitors were then restricted to use with
institutionalized patients where diets could be strictly regulated.

In 1968 it was reported that there were two distinct forms of MAO in humans,
termed MAO A and MAO B.[4] Specific inhibitors of these separate forms were
realized and there is now a host of such specific inhibitors. The two most
prevalent classes of compounds which have been synthesized as specific
inhibitors are the propargyl amines and the N-cyclopropyl-N-arylalkyl amines.
Dr. Krantz has discussed the mechanism of action of the propargyl amines
which leads to a stable covalent adduct with the N-5 position of the flavin
coenzyme of MAO. In this paper a proposed mechanism of inactivation of MAO
by the N-cyclopropyl-N-arylalkyl amines is discussed. We have chosen to study
this mechanism using N-cyclopropylbenzylamine and N-cyclopropyltryptamine as
model compounds. Although neither of these compounds is specific for MAO A or
MAO B, we believe that the specificity of certain inhibitors arises from binding interactions in the E·I complex and that the chemistry of the inactivations
is fundamentally the same for all of the compounds. Therefore, the chemistry
of inactivation with the selected compounds can be generalized to all of the
members of this class of MAO inhibitors.

176

We have found that N-cyclopropylbenzylamine and N-cyclopropyltryptamine
are suicide (or mechanism-based) inactivators of purified mitochondrial MAO
from pig liver. This conclusion was reached from the following data:
Incubation of MAO with 50μM N-cyclopropylbenzylamine at 25° resulted in a
pseudo first-order time-dependent loss of enzyme activity (Figure 1). The
loss of activity was considerably slower at pH 7.0 than at pH 9.0, the pH
optimum of the enzyme (Figure 1). This suggests that the mechanism of the
inactivation is enzyme dependent. The enzyme was protected and the rate of
inactivation diminished by the presence of benzylamine, a substrate for the
enzyme (Figure 1). Therefore, inactivation occurs as a result of an active

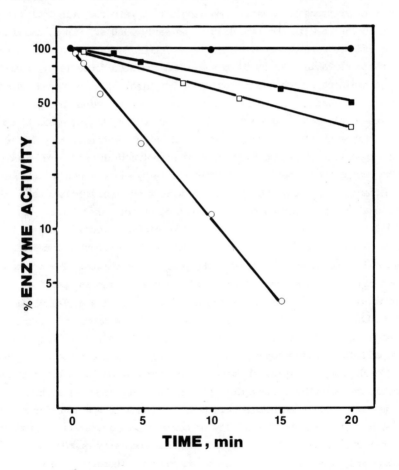

Figure 1. Irreversible inactivation of MAO by N-cyclopropylbenzylamine (50μM)
at 25°. ○—○, pH 9.0; □—□, pH 7.0; ■—■, pH 9.0 containing 450μM
benzylamine; ●—●, no inactivator.

site interaction. Similar results were obtained using N-cyclopropyltryptamine
(50μM, 25°, t½=1.5 min.). Dialysis at pH 7.0 of either of the N-cyclopropyl-
N-arylalkyl amine-inactivated MAO mixtures resulted in little or no return of
enzyme activity. Incubation of MAO with [phenyl-^{14}C]-N-cyclopropylbenzylamine,
followed by dialysis at pH 7.0 led to association of the radioactivity with
the protein to the extent of 1.1-1.4 mole of inactivator per mole of enzyme.
These data suggest an irreversible (covalent) inactivation of the enzyme.

The mechanism of this inactivation is based on the reaction catalyzed by
mitochondrial MAO, shown in scheme 1, which is the oxidative deamination of
certain monoamines.

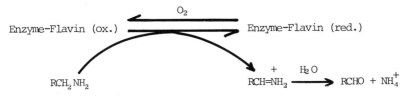

Scheme 1. Reaction catalyzed by mitochondrial monoamine oxidase.

Concomitant with substrate oxidation, the enzyme-bound oxidized flavin coenzyme
is converted to enzyme-bound reduced flavin which is non-enzymatically reoxidized by O_2. We propose the mechanism shown in scheme 2 as a possibility to
explain our findings that N-cyclopropyl-N-arylalkyl amines are inactivators
of MAO. According to this mechanism, the enzyme catalyzes the oxidation of the
cyclopropyl carbon to yield the highly electrophilic cyclopropanone imine
species. This, then, is attacked by the incipient reduced flavin by analogy
to the well-established reaction of propargyl amines with mitochondrial MAO[5].
Recently, Wiseman and Abeles[6] have proposed that the mechanism of inactivation
of aldehyde dehydrogenase by coprine and cyclopropanone hydrate involves the
generation of cyclopropanone as the reactive intermediate. In their study
the inactivators already were in the same oxidation state as cyclopropanone.
N-Cyclopropyl-N-arylalkyl amines, however, must be oxidized to cyclopropanone
imines in order for the analogous reaction to occur. Since N-cyclopropyl-N-
arylalkyl amines are not particularly reactive, this suggests that a mechanism-
based inactivation via oxidation to the cyclopropanone imine is more likely
than an affinity labeling mechanism.

The mechanism described in scheme 2 was deduced from the experiments described below. Since the species proposed to be responsible for the inactivation is the highly electrophilic cyclopropanone imine, modifications at the

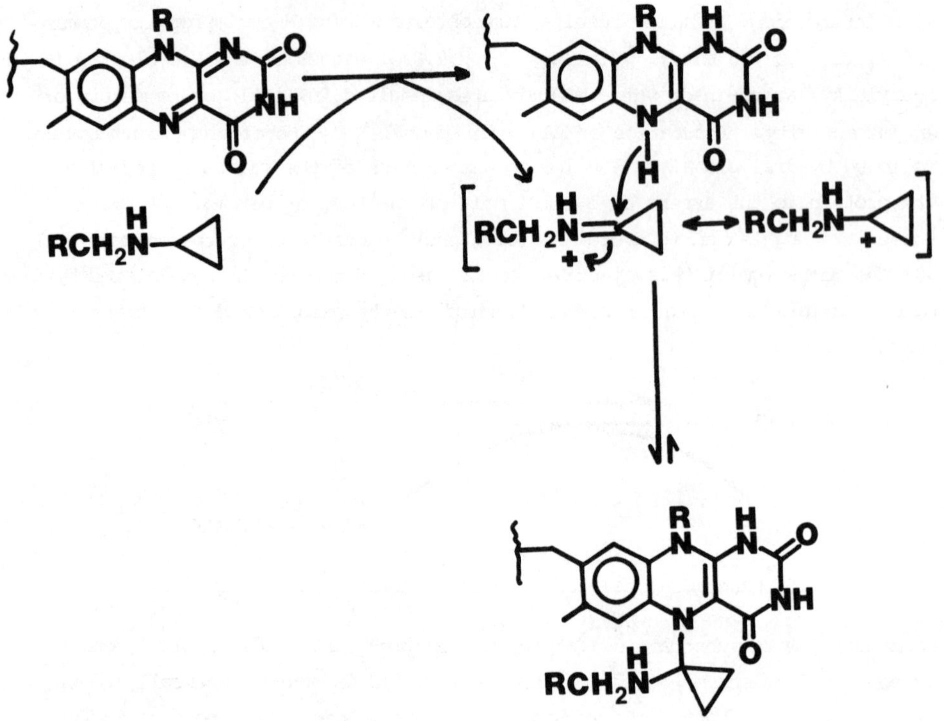

Scheme 2. Proposed mechanism of inactivation of mitochondrial
MAO by N-cyclopropyl-N-arylalkyl amines.

N-cyclopropyl moiety were made in order to test this. N-Isopropylbenzylamine
was found to be a competitive, reversible inhibitor of MAO. If the secondary
carbon of the isopropyl group were oxidized, this would lead to an acetone
imine which is not exceptionally electrophilic and, therefore, a covalent
interaction would not be expected. Likewise, N-cyclobutylbenzylamine is a
reversible inhibitor. Cyclobutanone also is not highly reactive. Insertion
of a methylene between the nitrogen and the cyclopropyl also would prevent a
cyclopropanone imine from being generated. Thus, N-cyclopropylmethyltryptamine was found to be a competitive, reversible inhibitor of MAO. It
appears that only N-alkyl derivatives which would lead to a reactive imine
upon oxidation produce irreversible inactivation of the enzyme. How about
oxidation of the benzyl methylene carbon instead of the cyclopropyl carbon?

When benzylamine is used as the substrate, it is the benzyl methylene carbon
which is oxidized, so we tested the product of methylene oxidation of N-
cyclopropylbenzylamine, namely, N-benzylidenecyclopropylamine. If N-benzylidenecyclopropylamine is the active species, it would be generated concomitant with the formation of reduced flavin. Therefore, MAO was converted
anaerobically to the reduced form, then incubated with N-benzylidenecyclopropylamine at pH 9.0. The half-life of hydrolysis of this compound at
pH 9.0 and 25[0] is about 35 minutes and under the conditions of the experiment the enzyme should have been completely inactivated in 20 minutes if
N-benzylidinecyclopropylamine were the active species. No inactivation
occurred. This compound also is a non-competitive, reversible inhibitor
of the oxidized form of the enzyme. Preliminary results indicate that little
or none of the methylene carbon is oxidized during inactivation of MAO by
N-cyclopropylbenzylamine. Thus, oxidation of the methylene carbon is not
responsible for irreversible inactivation.

According to the mechanism shown in scheme 2, the oxidized coenzyme is
converted into an alkylated reduced coenzyme. This should result in a
change in the flavin spectrum during inactivation. As shown in Figure 2,
there is a decrease in the absorbance between 430 and 510 nm concomitant
with inactivation of the enzyme. This is reminiscent of the behavior of
the flavin spectrum during inactivation of MAO by propargyl amines[7] and by
allyl amine[8]. Although scheme 2 describes the interaction as a bond between
the flavin N-5 and the inactivator, this may not necessarily be the case.
A similar flavin spectrum change could arise from interaction of the inactivator with the protein which then blocks the entrance of O_2 to the active
site and prevents the flavin from being reoxidized.

The coenzyme-inactivator complex in scheme 2 is shown as being in equilibrium with the cyclopropanone imine and the reduced flavin. Precedence for
this equilibrium comes from the work of Wasserman and Clagett[9]. They found
that cyclopropanone reacted rapidly with ethanol to give the ethyl hemiacetal
of cyclopropanone. Treatment of the ethyl hemiacetal with methanol gave the
methyl hemiacetal. The mechanism proposed for this interconversion was a pre-
equilibrium between the hemiacetals and cyclopropanone followed by a rapid
trapping of cyclopropanone by the solvent. The ethyl hemiacetal also was
converted to the dianilino ketal of cyclopropanone by treatment with aniline.
This compound is directly analogous to the coenzyme-inactivator complex
proposed in scheme 2. If this equilibrium exists with the enzyme-inactivator
complex, then it should be possible to trap the cyclopropanone imine as it is

180

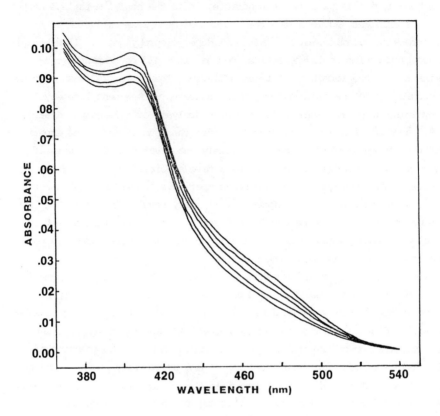

Figure 2. Flavin spectrum change during inactivation of MAO by
N-cyclopropylbenzylamine. The five tracings in order
of decreasing ε value correspond to enzyme activity
of 100% (control), 72%, 47%, 23%, and 4%, respectively.

released from the flavin. This trapping reaction is shown in scheme 3 using
benzylamine as the nucleophile. When MAO which was inactivated by either
N-cyclopropylbenzylamine or N-cyclopropyltryptamine and then dialyzed at
pH 7.0 was treated with 1mM benzylamine, the results shown in Figure 3
were obtained. In both cases, a time-dependent return of enzyme activity
to 100% was observed. The two different rates reflect the different substituents, benzyl and indolylmethyl, of the inactivators. These substituents
either have different steric properties or affect the rate of the back reaction in the equilibrium to the cyclopropanone imine. When this experiment was

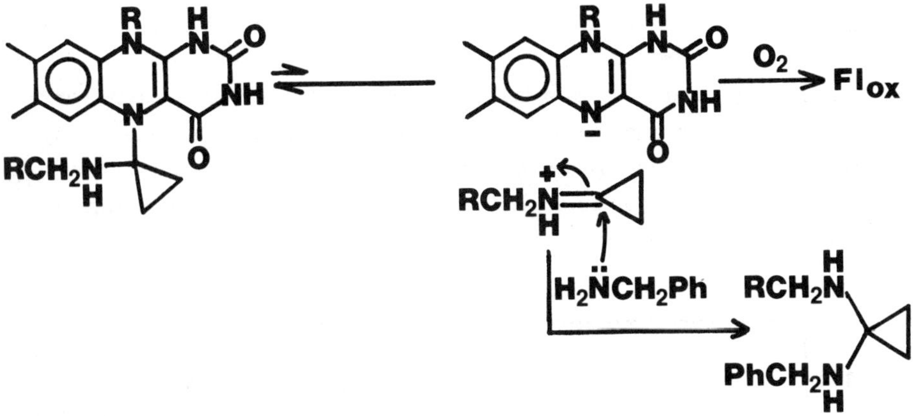

181

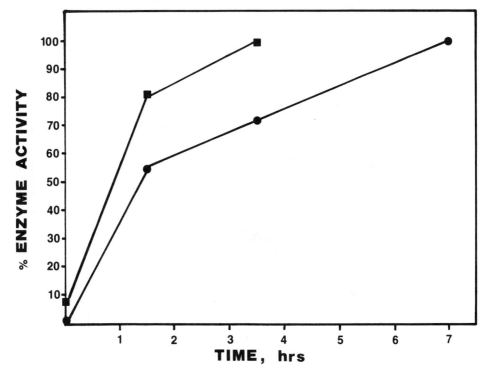

Scheme 3. Proposed mechanism for reactivation of N-cyclopropyl-
N-arylalkyl amine-inactivated MAO by benzylamine.

Figure 3. Reactivation of N-cyclopropyl-N-arylalkyl amine-inactivated MAO
by benzylamine (1mM, 25⁰). ●—●, N-cyclopropylbenzylamine-
inactivated; ■—■, N-cyclopropyltryptamine-inactivated.

carried out with MAO which was inactivated with ^{14}C-labeled N-cyclopropyl-benzylamine, all of the radioactivity was released when the enzyme activity was 100% of the control.

The question of whether this trapping reaction was enzyme-catalyzed or simply a chemical interaction was investigated by comparing the rate of the return of enzyme activity by benzylamine to that using methylamine, a compound which is a very poor substrate of MAO. Figure 4 shows that methylamine is not an effective trapping reagent. Since methylamine should be more

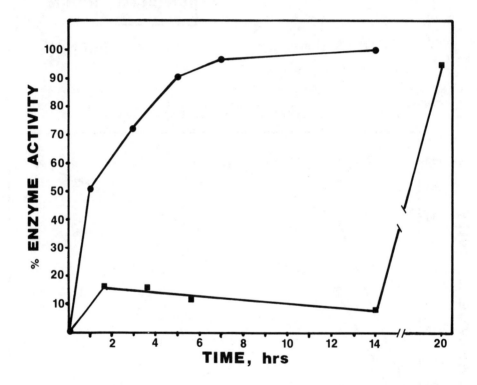

Figure 4. Reactivation of N-cyclopropylbenzylamine-inactivated MAO by 1mM benzylamine and 1mM methylamine. ●—●, benzylamine; ■—■, methylamine. At 14 hr, benzylamine (to 1mM) was added to the methylamine incubation mixture.

nucleophilic than benzylamine, this appears to be an enzyme-catalyzed process. However, the pK_a of benzylammonium ion (9.35) is 1.3 units lower than that of methylammonium ion[10]. Possibly the difference in the effectiveness of

these two amines is the concentration of free base present at pH 7.0 , the
pH at which the trapping experiment was done. Other amines are being studied.

We were interested in isolating the enzyme-inactivator adduct, but because
of the lability of this adduct it has not been possible. Not only is the
adduct unstable to benzylamine, but if the dialysis of the inactivated enzyme
is carried out at pH 9.0 instead of pH 7.0, all of the enzyme activity
returns. Also, if ^{14}C-labeled MAO is applied to a column of Sephadex G-25
at pH 7.0, all of the radioactivity is released and the enzyme activity is
regenerated. The return of enzyme activity after pH 9.0 dialysis may be the
result of the higher concentration of hydroxide ion than at pH 7.0. Gel
filtration is a much more efficient means of separating molecules because of
its larger number of theoretical plates than dialysis. Also, the structure
of the gel beads may catalyze trapping of the adduct. Denaturation of the
enzyme-(^{14}C)-inactivator complex by heat or urea led to complete release of
the radioactivity. It appears that the approach to the understanding of
the mechanism of the inactivation will have to be by isolation and structure
determination of the compounds released from the enzyme under different
conditions. At this point we have established that the compound released
from the enzyme which is inactivated by N-cyclopropylbenzylamine is not
N-cyclopropylbenzylamine. Thus, MAO was inactivated with ^{14}C-labeled
N-cyclopropylbenzylamine followed by dialysis, and the labeled enzyme was
either applied to Sephadex G-25 directly or first treated with benzylamine
then applied to Sephadex. In both cases, no N-cyclopropylbenzylamine was
found. Therefore, the inactivator is transformed into something else during inactivation. We are currently investigating the structures of the
labeled compounds released from the enzyme.

The N-cyclopropyl-N-arylalkyl amines, although just as potent MAO
inhibitors, are very different than the propargyl amines. Whereas the
propargyl amines form very stable covalent linkages with the flavin, the
N-cyclopropyl-N-arylalkyl amines form labile adducts with MAO. Which is
pharmacologically more effective? At first, it may seem that lability
would be pharmacologically undesirable, but the labile adducts have one
advantage that the stable ones do not have. Consider the people taking
MAO inhibitors who ingested high tyramine-containing foods. Since they
were unable to degrade the excess norepinephrine that was released, a
hypertensive crisis resulted. Had these patients been using labile MAO
inactivators, it could be speculated that the increased concentration of
active amines would have reactivated their MAO, as we have shown in vitro,

consequently averting the hypertensive crisis. Thus, the labile inactivators could hypothetically act as "fail-safe" drugs.

In summary, it appears that a possible mechanism of inactivation of
mitochondrial MAO by N-cyclopropyl-N-arylalkyl amines is a suicide inactivation in which these compounds are oxidized by the enzyme to highly electrophilic cyclopropanone imines, which then form weak covalent bonds with the
coenzyme or protein.

ACKNOWLEDGMENTS

The authors sincerely wish to thank Professor Lars Oreland for his kind
donation of purified pig liver mitochondrial MAO and Dr. Martin Winn for
samples of N-cyclopropyltryptamine and N-cyclopropylmethyltryptamine.

REFERENCES

1 a. Dunlop, E. (1963) Ann. N.Y. Acad. Sci., 107, 1107-1116.
  b. Bryant, J.M., Schvartz, N., Torosdag, S., Fertig, H., Fletcher, L.,
      Schwartz, M., and Quan, R.B.F., (1963) Ann. N.Y. Acad. Sci., 107,
      1123-1132.
2 a. Ho, B.T. (1972) J. Pharm. Sci., 61, 821-837.
  b. Berger, P.A. and Barchas, J.D. (1977) in Psychotherapeutic Drugs,
      Part II, Usdin, E. and Forrest, I.S., ed., Marcel Dekker, Inc.,
      N.Y.
3.   Blackwell, B. (1963) Lancet, ii, 849-851.
4.   Johnston, J.P. (1968) Biochem. Pharmacol., 17, 1285-1287.
5.   Maycock, A.L., Abeles, R.H., Salach, J.E., Singer, T.P. (1976)
      Biochemistry, 15, 114-125.
6.   Wiseman, J.W. and Abeles, R.H. (1979) Biochemistry, 18, 427-435.
7.   Hellerman, L. and Ewing, V.G. (1968) J. Biol. Chem., 243,
      5234-5243.
8.   Rando, R.R. and Eigner, A. (1977) Molecular Pharmacol., 13,
      1005-1013.
9.   Wasserman, H.H. and Clagett, D.C. (1966) J. Am. Chem. Soc., 88,
      5368-5369.
10.   CRC Handbook of Biochemistry 2nd Edit., Sober, H.A., ed.,
      Chemical Rubber Co., Cleveland, 1970.

DISCUSSION

P. BARTLETT: What pH did you use in the reactivation experiments with
methylamine?

SILVERMAN: That experiment was done at pH 7, because the incaticated
enzyme is stable at that pH.

CHOWDHRY: Have you tried to trap your postulated imine with borohydride?

SILVERMAN: No, we have not yet done that, but we are planning experiments of that sort.

CHOWDHRY: Presumably, you could look for incorporation of tritium into your starting material, couldn't you?

SILVERMAN: Yes. Also, we are getting ready to synthesize the dibenzyl-amino aminal of cyclopropanone to see if, in fact, that it is the species which is released from the enzyme after trapping with benzylamine.

CHOUDHRY: You showed that isopropylbenzylamine is a competitive reversible inhibitor and suggested that, if it got oxidized, it would not generate a reactive imine. Why can it not just be an inhibitor that binds but is not oxidized?

SILVERMAN: It could, but I was just trying to make a non-functional analogue of the N-cyclopropyl derivatives. The structure of the isopropyl analogue is similar enough to the cyclopropyl analogue that even if it did get oxidized rather than just bind, you would not expect inactivation to occur. We have not yet looked at this interaction to see if the isopropyl analogue is metabolized or if it just sits there.

KRANTZ: The cyclopropylamines are very unusual. They are one of the only type of amine that is oxidized by, or at least react with, monoamine oxidase and does not have a CH_2 next to the nitrogen. Would you care to speculate on the mechanistic implications of this unique situation and why it happens with cyclopropylamines?

SILVERMAN: I think that the oxidation could be a one-electron transfer mechanism where an electron from the amine is transferred to the flavin to generate a radical cation. This would be followed by α-proton abstraction to give a carbon radical which can either transfer another electron to the flavin or the two radicals can combine. Our results suggest that, if this mechanism is operative, for some reason, proton abstraction occurs almost exclusively from the cyclopropyl side. We are not sure why this is so, but we plan to do electrochemical model studies with cyclopropylbenzylamine to see what happens chemically after the radical cation is generated. The N-cyclopropyl-N-arylalkylamines could be the key to the understanding of the mechanism of substrate oxidation by MAO.

WALSH: I agree that given the precedent of Wiseman and Abeles[1], one should look for and expect cyclopropanone hydrates or hemiaminals. But if you have radical mechanism, don't you worry about rapid ring opening? Is it not a possibility?

SILVERMAN: To date I am aware of no mechanistic studies of cyclopropylamine radical cations so it is not known how facile this process is. Certainly with cyclopropylmethyl cations rearrangements occur rapidly, but this is still an equilibrium mixture which contains unrearranged intermediate. Carbonium ions only have a sextet of electrons, though. Cyclopropylmethyl radicals also rearrange, but not by a ring expansion route, rather by an elimination to the butenyl radicals. Again, though, much, and sometimes, most[2] of the product is derived from unrearranged intermediate. The equilibrium depends on the substituents attached to the cyclopropylmethyl radical[3]. When the radicals are unable to diffuse, as in more viscous solvents, the major products, by far, are the cyclopropylmethyl analogues rather than the 3-butenyl compounds[4].

It is known from electrochemical[5] as well as chemical[6] oxidation studies of alkyl amines that the first step is a slow one-electron transfer to generate the amine radical cation. This followed by a fast α-proton abstraction to give the α-carbon radical. In the case of cyclopropyl amines, if the proton loss is faster than rearrangement, thereby generating the cyclopropyl amine carbon radical, then either the flavin radical and the inactivator radical can combine (more likely) or the second electron from the inactivator radical can be transferred to the flavin, generating the flavin anion and the inactivator cation, which is the resonance structure of the protonated cyclopropanone imine. Since I know of no studies of cyclopropylamine radical cations, which probably act more like radicals than cations, this question cannot be answered at this time. As I mentioned before, we are beginning electrochemical and photochemical model studies to gain information in this regard.

WALSH: I am sure you are aware that phenylhydrazine compounds have recently been shown[7] to inactivate a flavoenzyme by covalent adducts a C4a, not at N5, forming a possible phenyldiazine and then presumably a phenyl anion equivalent, although that is unclear. So, I think one should be careful, as I know you are, but it is worth pointing out that N5 of the flavin is not the only site of likely combination. Certainly C4a, I do not think can be excluded on the basis of what you have shown.

SILVERMAN: True.

REFERENCES

1. Wiseman, J.W. and Abeles, R.H. (1979) Biochemistry, 18, 427.
2. Renk, E., Shafer, P.R., Graham, W.H., Mazur, R.H., and Roberts, J.D. (1961) J. Am. Chem. Soc. 83, 1987.
3. Halgren, T.A., Howden, M.E.H., Medof, M.E., and Roberts, J.D. (1967) J. Am. Chem. Soc. 89, 3051.
4. Sheldon, R.A. and Koch, J.K. (1970) J. Am. Chem. Soc. 92, 5175.
5. Mann, C.K. and Barnes, K.K. (1970) Electrochemical Reactions in Non-aqueous Systems,Marcel Dekker, Inc., New York.
6. Lindsay Smith, J.R. and Mead, L.A.V. (1973) JCS Perkin II, 206.
7. Nagy, J., Kenney, W.C., and Singer, T.P. (1979) J. Biol. Chem. 254, 2684.

CYCLOPROPYLAMINES AS NOVEL INACTIVATORS OF CYTOCHROME P-450

ROBERT H. TULLMAN AND ROBERT P. HANZLIK[*]
Department of Medicinal Chemistry, School of Pharmacy,
University of Kansas, Lawrence, Kansas, 66045, USA

The biotransformation of drugs and other chemicals usually has important consequences for the biological activity of the parent compound. For example, biotransformation of many compounds results in their "detoxification" and prepares
them for more rapid elimination from the body. Many examples of the converse,
i.e. "bioactivation" of toxins, are also now known. In the case of most drugs,
biotransformation is the event which terminates their pharmacological action.
While this situation is not undesirable per se, it is a two-edged sword, because
in some cases rapid biotransformation becomes a limiting factor in the overall
biological effectiveness and practical utility of the drug. Included in this
group are compounds such as acetylcholine, the natural prostaglandins, and other
agents for which enzymes catalyzing their biotransformation are widely distributed and highly active; such compounds have very short half-lives in vivo, and
are used by continuous infusion if at all. Another general situation in which
biotransformation limits the practical utility of a drug is the so-called
"first-pass effect". This is usually defined in terms of reduced bioavailability for orally as compared to intravenously administered drug.

Orally administered compounds must generally pass through the intestinal wall
to reach the bloodstream. Before reaching the general systemic circulation,
compounds so absorbed must travel via the hepatic portal vein and pass through
the liver. Both the intestinal mucosa and liver have high activity for bio-
transformations of certain kinds, and drugs which are suitable substrates for
these pathways may be largely or even completely inactivated by biotransformation prior to reaching the systemic circulation. For some drugs first pass
effects render the oral route of administration totally useless. In other cases
inter-individual variability in the degree of first pass effect can account
for wide variations in dose needed to acheive comparable effects in different
individuals.

A pathway of particular importance in the first-pass biotransformation of
amines is N-dealkylation. Examples of drugs whose oral bioavailability is
significantly reduced in this way include nalorphine(1), propoxyphene(2-5),
lidocaine(5,6), propranolol(7,8), diphenhydramine(9), nortriptyline(10) and
perhaps imipramine(11,12). A wide variety of substituents can be removed in

this pathway, including methyl and higher n-alkyl homologs, allyl, propargyl, benzyl, and cyclopropylcarbinyl(13). The N-dealkylation of tertiary amines involves α-hydroxylation, catalyzed by cytochrome P-450 type mixed function oxygenase enzymes(14). The intermediate carbinolamine generally decomposes spontaneously to the dealkylated amine and a carbonyl compound. Tertiary amine N-oxides have been considered as intermediates in this process, but in general they appear not to play a major role(15,16). However, with many secondary amines, N-oxides, as their hydroxylamine tautomers, are involved in the major pathway of dealkylation(17). Thus while P-450 catalyzed carbinolamine formation can occur, an alternate pathway, often quantitatively more important involves two sequential flavoprotein monooxygenase-mediated oxidations as shown in Figure 1.

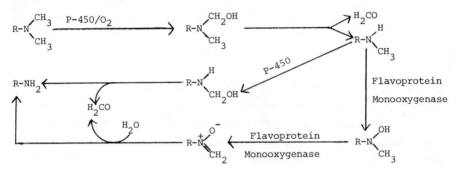

Fig.1. Pathways for N-dealkylation.

The mechanism of cytochrome P-450 mediated hydroxylations has been a major interest of a number of laboratories including our own. Several years ago this interest lead us into a collaborative program aimed at obtaining a better under-standing of the first-pass phenomenon on a biochemical level. One aspect of this program was to involve the rational design of specific inhibitors of N-dealkylation for use in in vivo studies. Previous work had established the importance of lipophilicity and pKa considerations in governing the affinity of substrates for cytochrome P-450(18,19). In our approach to the "design" of inhibitors of N-dealkylation we focussed attention on the catalytic aspects of the pathway, i.e. mechanism and turnover. In this light cyclopropylamines appeared especially intriguing. It was felt that the unique electronic struc-ture of the cyclopropane ring might pose an unusual challenge to the enzyme at a mechanistic level. If that were so, a cyclopropylamine with other N- and/or ring-substituents tailored to achieve high affinity for P-450 might lead to a unique group of inhibitors for this class of enzymes.

The literature on cyclopropylamines revealed a wealth of information on the

inhibition of monoamine oxidase by these compounds(20-23), but only a single
report of their effect on a cytochrome P-450-mediated process. McMahon et al.
(24) investigated the effects of the tricyclic amines 1a and 1b, as well as
several other related compounds as inhibitors of cytochrome P-450-mediated
dealkylations. The cyclopropyl compound 1a was always a more potent inhibitor
than any of about eight others. It was speculated that steric or pKa effects

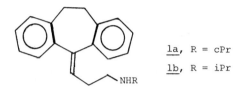

1a, R = cPr

1b, R = iPr

were too small to account for their unique potency, but no other mechanistic
studies were reported. Encouraged by this singular observation we initially
prepared a series of N-benzyl cyclopropylamines(2a-6a) and their corresponding
isopropyl analogs(2b-6b), and evaluated them as inhibitors of aminopyrine
N-demethylation in vitro. The results of this study clearly showed that the
cyclopropyl compounds were significantly more inhibitory than their isopropyl
analogs (Table 1 and ref. 25). However, our initial satisfaction over the
apparent generality of this effect was temporarily diminished when we determined
the pKa's of 2a-6a and 2b-6b (Table 1).

Table 1. Inhibition of Aminopyrine Demethylation (at pH 7.6)
as a Function Inhibitor pKa.[a]

Inhibitor (1 mM)	pKa	%-Inhibition
p-XC$_6$H$_4$CH$_2$NHcPr		
2a, x=CH$_3$O	8.48	54 $\pm$ 1
3a, x=CH$_3$	8.45	77 $\pm$ 2
4a, x=H	8.30	60 $\pm$ 1
5a, x=Cl	7.96	80 $\pm$ 4
6a, x=Br	7.86	78 $\pm$ 1
p-XC$_6$H$_4$CH$_2$NHiPr		
2b, x=CH$_3$O	9.90	0 $\pm$ 2
3b, x=CH$_3$	9.85	2 $\pm$ 4
4b, x=H	9.65	9 $\pm$ 6
5b, x=Cl	9.45	25 $\pm$ 3
6b, x=Br	9.25	27 $\pm$ 4

[a] Aminopyrine demethylation was assayed at 33° on one-third
the scale but otherwise as described in "Fundamentals of
Drug Metabolism and Drug Disposition", B.N. LaDu, H.G.
Mandel, and E.L. Way, Eds., Williams and Wilkins, Baltimore, 1972, pp 546-550.

It appeared at first that most of the greater potency of the cyclopropylamines could simply be due to their smaller degree of ionization at the pH of the incubations(7.6). This issue was soon resolved, however, by the observation that the inhibition due to the cyclopropyl compounds(3a and 4a)was time-dependent whereas that due to the isopropyl compounds(3b and 4b) was time-independent. Further studies showed that in the presence of NADPH 3a and 4a caused a progressive loss of demethylase activity which followed first order kinetics. A plot of log%(remaining activity) vs. time gave a straight line indicating a half-life of 6-8 minutes for 1mM 4a.

Catalytic turnover of cytochrome P-450 depends on electrons supplied principally from NADPH via a flavoprotein, NADPH-cytochrome c reductase, which also functions as a P-450 reductase. The supply of NADPH in turn depends on the activity of a regenerating system, based in these studies on glucose-6-phosphate dehydrogenase. Neither the cyclopropylamines nor their isopropyl analogs were

Table 2. Effect of N-Cyclopropyl- and N-Isopropyl-
Benzylamines on NADPH-Cytochrome c Reductase.[a]

Amine (1 mM)	μmole Cytc reduced/min/mg protein
none	38.1 ± 2.9
5a	36.4 ± 4.6
5b	43.5 ± 3.5
6a	41.5 ± 3.6
6b	39.8 ± 1.3

[a] Assays performed at 37° as described in "Fundamentals of Drug Metabolism and Drug Disposition," B.N. La Du, H.G. Mandel, and E.L. Way, Eds., Williams and Wilkins, Baltimore, 1971, pp 575-577. Data given are the mean $\pm$ S.D. for 3 determinations.

Table 3. Dependence of Aminopyrine Demethylation and its
Inhibition on Cofactor Source.[a]

Cofactor Source	Inhibitor (1 mM)	μmole CH_2O/10 min	Percent Inhibition
NADPH-GS[b]	none	75.0 ± 0.4	–
"	6a	15.2 ± 0.8	80 ± 4
"	6b	55.5 ± 2.2	26 ± 3
NADPH[c]	none	75.0 ± 0.8	–
"	6a	12.8 ± 0.2	83 ± 1
"	6b	60.8 ± 1.1	18 ± 2

[a] Assays conducted as in Table 1. Data given are means $\pm$ S.D. for 3 determinations. [b] NADPH-generating system was used. [c] NADPH was added at 5.5 mg/ml.

found to inhibit NADPH-cytochrome c reductase (Table 2). Replacement of the
NADPH did not change the pattern of inhibition (Table 3). These results suggest
that the cyclopropylamines were acting on cytochrome P-450 per se and not the
ancillary proteins connected with supplying reducing equivalents.

Data presented in Table 4 further characterizes the nature of the interaction
between cytochrome P-450 and cyclopropylamines and related compounds. It is
readily apparent that the inhibition due to 4a increases rapidly with time,
while that due to 4b and two other low pKa amines, N-benzylmorpholine and
N-benzyl-N-trifluoroethylamine, does not change significantly as a function of
preincubation with the microsomes and cofactor. Inhibition due to the tranyl-

Table 4. Dependence of Loss of Aminopyrine Demethylase
Activity on Preincubation Time and Conditions.[a]

| Preincubation Conditions[c] | Percent Inhibition Observed[b] | |
	Without Preincubation	After 12 min Preincubation
Control	0	0[d]
+4a	29	70
+4b	9	9
+ N-benzylmorpholine	27	34
+ PhCH$_2$NHCH$_2$CF$_3$	32	31
+ Tranylcypramine (0.5mM)[f]	52	57
+ 4a, omit cofactor	–	13
+ 4a, CO/O$_2$ (80:20)[e]	–	24
+ cyclopropylamine	0	4
+ benzylamine	22	22
+ PhCH=N(cPr)	17	8
+ 4a, MMI[g]	25	57
+ 4a, GSH	17	62

[a]General incubation conditions and assay procedures are
as described for Table 1. [b]Average of 3-6 determinations
with several different microsome preparations. [c]Preincu-
bation conditions also obtain during the subsequent 5 min
assay period, except for a slight volume change upon addition of aminopyrine (3.0 mM) and a second aliquot of cofactor generating system. Glutathione (GSH) or other compounds (1.0 mM) were added at the start of the preincubation. [d]Loss of activity due to preincubation of microsomes and NADPH alone was variable but always less than
7-8%. [e]CO was replaced by air at the start of the assay
period. Separate controls showed that CO inhibition was
readily reversed by this procedure. [f]trans-2-Phenylcyclo-
propylamine. [g]2-Mercapto-N-methylimidazole.

cypramine was similarly time-invariant.

The time-dependent inactivation of cytochrome P-450 is also seen in Table 4 to require NADPH cofactor and to be inhibited by CO but not by MMI, an inhibitor of the microsomal flavin-containing amine oxidase which has little effect on cytochrome P-450 mediated reactions(17). Thus the secondary cyclopropylamines appear to be true suicide inactivators for cytochrome P-450. However, the lack of any inhibition of inactivation by GSH or semicarbazide (present in nearly all incubations at 10 mg/ml for the Nash formaldehyde assay) suggests that if a reactive electrophilic metabolite derived by oxidative attack on the cyclopropyl moiety is being formed, it probably does not leave the lipid environment of the microsomes before inactivating cytochrome P-450. The time dependence of inhibition due to 4a is unlikely to result simply from time-dependent formation of cyclopropylamine and/or benzylamine by metabolism of 4a. The former was found to have negligible activity as an inhibitor of aminopyrine demethylation, and while the latter (a lipophilic primary amine) was a good inhibitor, it would also be expected to accumulate from metabolism of 4b, yet inhibition due to the latter was time-independent. Finally, synthetic N-benzylidenecyclopropylamine was found to have relatively little activity as an inhibitor.

On the basis of information discussed above, and a wealth of precedent presented during this symposium and elsewhere, it is reasonable to speculate that we are dealing with a situation involving enzyme-mediated production of a self-inactivating metabolite. Such a process may be involved in the destruction of cytochrome P-450 by allylisopropylacetamide. This process is enzyme-mediated (26), and leads in vivo to formation of a covalent adduct between AIA and the heme moiety of cytochrome P-450, although the identity of the AIA metabolite and the structure of the heme adduct have not been reported(27). For the secondary N-benzyl cyclopropylamines 2a-6a one plausible reactive electrophilic metabolite would be N-cyclopropylidene benzylamine 8, or its protonated form 8-H$^+$, which might be derived from carbinolamine 7. Iminium salts are known to be formed concurrent with N-dealkylation of tertiary amines, and they are trapped efficiently by nucleophiles such as cyanide(28). N-Benzylcyclopropylamine(i.e.4a) covalently inactivates monoamine oxidase (R.B. Silverman, this Symposium), apparently by alkylating the flavin moiety after undergoing enzymatic conversion to 8 or 8-H$^+$. Similar chemistry is involved in the inactivation of aldehyde oxidase by 9, 10, or the mushroom toxin coprine 11, probably through formation of a stable (but reversible) hemithioketal linkage with the active site sulfhydryl group of this enzyme(29-31).

In this regard, preliminary experiments in our laboratory have shown that incubation of **4a** (labeled with tritium at the benzylic position) with microsomes plus cofactor leads to covalent labeling of protein if the protein is analyzed after denaturation with detergent. However, no covalent binding can be detected when the protein is precipitated with trichoroacetic acid prior to analysis. While these observations would be consistent with alkylation of a nucleophile in cytochrome P-450 by a metabolite such as **8**, further work will be needed to clarify this point, and such studies are now in progress. We are also investigating the generality of this property of cyclopropane derivatives, as well as their potential for selective inhibition among the diverse oxidations effected by cytochrome P-450 enzymes.

ACKNOWLEDGEMENT

The authors wish to thank the National Institute of General Medical Sciences for financial support of this work through a research grant (GM-22357) and a predoctoral training grant (GM-07775).

REFERENCES

1. K. Iwamoto and C.D. Klaussen, J. Pharmacol. Exp. Ther., 203, 365 (1977).
2. R.L. Wolen, C.M. Gruber, G.F. Kiplinger, and N.E. Scholz, Toxicol. Appl. Pharmacol., 19, 480 (1971).
3. D. Perrier and M. Gibaldi, J. Clin. Pharmacol. J. New Drugs, 12, 449 (1972).
4. P.J. Murphy, R.C. Nickander, G.M. Bellamy, and W. Kurtz, J. Pharmacol. Exp. Ther., 199, 415 (1976).
5. R.A. Branch, D.G. Shand, G.R. Wilkinson and A.S. Nies, J. Pharmacol. Exp. Ther. 184, 515 (1973).
6. W.W. Lautt and F.S. Skelton, Can. J. Physiol. Pharmacol., 55, 7 (1976).
7. D.G. Shand and R.E. Rangno, Pharmacology, 7, 159 (1972).
8. J.H. Anderson, R.C. Anderson, and L.S. Iben, J. Pharmacol. Exp. Ther., 206, 172 (1978).
9. K.S. Albert, M.R. Hallmark, E. Sakmar, D.J. Weidler, J.G. Wagner, J. Pharmacok Biopharm, 3, 159 (1975).
10. M. Gibaldi, J. Pharm. Sci., 64, 1036 (1975).
11. L.F. Gram and J. Christiansen, Clin. Pharmacol. Ther. 17, 555 (1975).
12. R. Stegmann and M.G. Bickel, Xenobiotica, 7, 737 (1977).
13. Th.E. Gram, Handbook of Experimental Pharmacology, 28, 334 (1975).

14. B. Testa and P. Jenner, "Drug Metabolism: Chemical and Biochemical Aspects," Dekker, New York, 1976, pp. 82-95.
15. J.W. Gorrod, in "Mechanisms of Oxidizing Enzymes," T.P. Singer and R.N. Ondarza, eds., Elsevier/North Holland, New York, 1978, pp. 189-97.
16. R.E. McMahon and H.E. Sullivan, Xenobiotica, 7, 377 (1977).
17. R.A. Prough and D.M. Ziegler, Arch. Biochem. Biophy., 180, 363 (1977).
18. R.E. McMahon and N.R. Easton, J. Med. Pharm. Chem., 4, 437 (1961).
19. A.K. Cho and G.T. Mirva, Drug. Metab. Disp., 2, 477 (1973).
20. R.W. Fuller and S.K. Hemrick, Proc. Soc. Exp. Biol. Med., 158, 323 (1978).
21. D.L. Murphy, C.H. Donnelly, E. Richelson, and R.W. Fuller, Biochem. Pharmacol. 27, 1767 (1978).
22. R.W. Fuller, S.K. Hemrick, and J. Mills, Biochem. Pharmacol., 27, 2255 (1978).
23. B.T. Ho, J. Pharm. Sci., 61, 821 (1972).
24. R.E. McMahon, H.W. Culp, and J. Mills, J. Med. Chem., 13, 986 (1970).
25. R.P. Hanzlik, V. Kishore, and R.H. Tullman, J. Med. Chem. (in press).
26. W. Levin, M. Jacobson, E. Sernatinger, and R. Kuntzman, Druf. Metab. Disp., 1, 275 (1973).
27. P.R. Ortiz de Montellano, B.A. Mico, and G.S. Yost, Biochem. Biophys. Res. Comm., 83, 132 (1978).
28. T.-L. Nguyen, L.D. Gruenke, and N. Castagnoli, J. Med. Chem., 19, 1168 (1976).
29. J.S. Wiseman and R.H. Abeles, Biochemistry, 18, 427 (1979).
30. O. Tottmar and P. Lindberg. Acta Pharmacol. et. Toxicol., 40, 476 (1977).
31. B. Wickberg, Acta Pharm. Suecica, 14 Suppl., 30 (1977).

DISCUSSION

SILVERMAN: A couple of years ago it was found[1] that administration of an N-cyclopropyl-N-arylalkylamine to mice resulted in reduced alcohol preference and caused elevated acetaldehyde levels. If we put together the work of Tullman and Hanzlik[2] with that recently reported by Wiseman and Abeles[3], this ethanol toxicity in mice pretreated with an N-cyclopropyl-N-arylalkylamine may be understood. Possibly these compounds may get oxidized by P-450 to the cyclopropanone imines which get hydrolyzed to cyclopropanone hydrate. This then could inactivate aldehyde dehydrogenase, resulting in elevated acetaldehyde levels and the reduced alcohol preference by the mice.

REFERENCES

1. Sanders, B., Collins, A.C., Petersen, D.R., and Fish, B.S. (1977) Pharmacol. Biochem. Behavior, 6, 319.
2. Tullman, R. and Hanzlik, R.P. (1979) this volume.
3. Wiseman, J.W. and Abeles, R.H. (1979) Biochemistry, 18, 427.
4. White, I.N.H. and Muller-Eberhard, U. (1977) Biochem. J. 166, 57.
5. Ortiz de Montellano, P.R., Kunze, K.L., Yost, G.S. and Mico, B.A. (1979) Proc. Natl. Acad. Sci. U.S.A., 76, 746.

Editor's note: Suicide inactivation of cytochrome P-450 by the oral contraceptive ethynyl sterols, e.g., norethisterone has recently been described[4,5], involving covalent linkage of the sterol to the heme prosthetic group through the activated acetylenic moiety[5].

III
β-Lactam Mechanisms

Published 1979 by Elsevier North Holland, Inc.
Kalman, ed. Drug Action and Design: Mechanism-Based Enzyme Inhibitors

VARIATIONS IN THE MECHANISM OF ANTIBACTERIAL EFFECTS OF BETA LACTAMS

ALEXANDER TOMASZ, KAZUAKI KITANO, RUBEN LOPEZ AND CICERO DE FREITAS
The Rockefeller University, New York, N.Y. 10021

INTRODUCTION

Inhibited enzyme, inhibited cell, inhibited parasite. Although much in-
genuity in drug design is aimed at the selective inhibition of "target" enzymes
studied and examined in a pure state, one should not forget that the long range
purpose is most often the selective inhibition of a living cell or pathogenic
microorganism. Furthermore, under the conditions of an ultimate practical use,
these living cells or organisms will be encountered by the drug molecules in a
complex environment (e.g., an infected host) that contains other living cells.
Drugs must retain their selectivity even under these conditions. The moving of
the drug target from the test tube into a live cell and the transfer of the
live cell from a culture medium into an infected host introduce vast degrees of
complexity into the mechanism of drug action and the purpose of my presentation
is to illustrate this in the case of beta lactam antibiotics, compounds of un-
surpassed selectivity and inhibitory power against bacteria. My presentation
will have three parts. First I shall briefly review the nature of beta lactam
sensitive bacterial proteins. Next, I shall describe in more detail experimental findings and ideas on how inhibition of these target proteins might
bring about reversible or irreversible inhibition of the bacterial cell. Finally, I shall describe observations that should illustrate the novel factors that
modulate the antibacterial effects of beta lactams if the bacterium is in an
environment containing host factors. This structure of the presentation should
illustrate the gradually increasing complexity of drug action as one moves from
target enzyme to a target cell and from the target cell in pure culture to the
target pathogen in the complex environment of the infected host.

From inhibited target enzyme to inhibited target cell

Even when the nature of the drug-sensitive reaction is well understood (and this is certainly not the case with beta lactams), the question of how and why specific interference with a metabolic reaction leads to inhibition of cellular growth or division is far from obvious. Neither is it self evident why even a complete and irreversible inhibition of an essential enzyme should cause irreversible inactivation of the whole cell since during the test for bacterial survival (i.e., after removal of the excess drug), cells might be expected to resynthesize new molecules of the inhibited enzyme (unless, of course, protein synthesis is also inhibited). The pathway from inhibited target enzyme to inhibited (non-growing or non-dividing) bacterium varies tremendously in "length" and complexity, and a few examples may illustrate this variation. In a bacterium treated with a sulfa drug inhibition of the folic acid synthetase may cause a complete halt in the production of this essential cofactor (co-enzyme) and growth of such a culture stops when the supply of this vitamin is diluted (by the increase in cell number) below the minimum required for continued bacterial proliferation. One may think that such a culture eventually stops growing literally because it runs out of fuel. Removal of the inhibitor within a reasonable time usually results in the resumption of growth.

In contrast, the actual mechanism gearing the whole cell to a transient halt may be remote from the site of inhibition. For instance, in a stringently controlled (Rel+) bacterium removal of the essential aminoacid does not cause inhibition of growth by the cell running out of an essential building block. Instead, the drop in the internal concentration of the aminoacid activates a complex regulatory circuit: a multifunctional nucleotide derivative (guanosine tetraphosphate) accumulates and triggers the inhibition of several key synthetic enzymes in RNA, lipid and cell wall syntheses.[1] Such high-level control mechanisms may have evolved to prevent the occurrence of potentially lethal (unbalanced) chemical composition in the cells. Indeed, bacteria defective in this control system (Rel-) have prolonged lag before resumption of growth after the readdition of the missing aminoacid. A similar variation exists in the mechanism of action of irreversible antimicrobial agents. Examples of a more <u>direct</u> irreversible mechanism would be the irrepairable structural damage to the plasma membrane of bacteria caused by polymyxin , ionophores or complement. In contrast, interference with DNA synthesis often initiates more complex and indirect antimicrobial mechanisms. For instance, thymidine starvation may cause loss of viability by triggering the lytic cycle of defective lysogenic prophage. In bacteria "cured" of prophage thymidine starvation is still lethal provided that the bacterium has the genetic constitution of rec A+. Studies with rec A⁻ mutants have shown that the dramatically reduced lethality of thymidine starvation in such bacterial mutants is <u>not</u> due to the leakiness of the primary mutation but rather, it seems to be related to the low levels of protein X (the rec A gene product).[2] In the rec A⁺ cells a halt in DNA synthesis stimulates the production of protein X, which, in turn, is known to interfere with several complex membrane functions and it appears plausible that the phenomenon of "thymine less death"[3] is caused by a change in the energized state of the plasma membrane induced by protein X.[4] Thus, whether or not thymidine starvation causes irreversible loss of viability would depend entirely on secondary processes coupled to the primary interference with DNA synthesis.

These examples are described in order to help to set the stage for the discussion of the extraordinarily complex antimicrobial mechanisms of beta lactams. Structurally different beta lactams may cause distinctly different inhibitory effects in the same bacterium. In addition, the same beta lactam can provoke reversible growth inhibition (e.g., in <u>Str. sanguis</u>[5] or in some penicillin tolerant mutants[6]); loss of viability (which may occur with a variety of rates, suggesting several different mechanisms), and loss of viability accompanied by rapid lysis (e.g., in <u>E. coli</u> or in pneumococci) - all depending on the nature of the bacterium and even depending on the conditions of growth.[7,8] The extraordinary mechanistic complexity of beta lactam effects is only beginning to be recognized now.

At least two types of factors seem to contribute to this complexity. First, beta lactam antibiotics can inhibit not one but a whole number of functionally different targets (penicillin binding proteins, PBPs) in bacteria and the nature and/or number of targets inhibited may depend on both the chemical structure of the beta lactam and the species of the bacterium as well.[9]

A second factor contributing to complexity of mechanism (and also contributing to the superior inhibitory effectiveness of beta lactams) is that, in some bacteria, beta lactams can induce a secondary regulatory defect in the cellular control of a group of hydrolytic enzymes (murein hydrolases).[10] In E. coli, beta lactams with special affinity for PBP 1b (e.g., cephaloridine or higher concentrations of benzylpenicillin) are particularly effective in this respect. In these cases, the suicidal activity of murein hydrolases (autolysins) appears to be responsible both for the death and for the destruction (lysis) of the cells.

Variation in the mechanism of antibacterial activity with beta lactam structure - The presence of multiple functional targets for beta lactams in the bacterial cell. All bacteria so far examined seem to contain a number (4 to 9) of proteins capable of binding radioactive penicillin. Most, if not all, of these proteins are probably enzymes involved with cell wall metabolism. Mutants of E. coli that lack the penicillin binding proteins 4, 5 or 6 showed normal growth patterns and unaltered sensitivities to various beta lactams; thus, PBPs 4, 5 and 6 are not likely to be involved with the antibacterial activities of beta lactams. On the other hand, inhibition of PBPs 1, 2 and 3 each causes selective morphological effects.[11-13] More or less selective inhibition of these proteins is possible either by the use of specific beta lactams[14] or by the use of E. coli mutants lacking one or the other of the PBPs. While the precise biochemical nature of reactions catalyzed by PBP 1, 2 or 3 are not yet

understood, the morphological consequences of inhibition suggest that these proteins perform functions in complex areas of cell physiology such as maintenance
of structural integrity (PBP 1), shape (PBP 2) and cell division (PBP 3).[14]
Furthermore, several lines of evidence suggest that beyond the distinct morphological effects, selective inhibition of PBP 1, 2 and, possibly even PBP 3, may
initiate antibacterial effects that occur via distinct mechanisms. This conclusion is suggested by several observations.

Beta lactams with special affinities for the E. coli protein(s) in PBP group
1 (e.g., cephaloridine, ampicillin, benzylpenicillin) are unique in causing extremely rapid loss of viability, culture lysis and (in the presence of osmotic
stabilizers) rapid formation of spheroplasts near the MIC concentration of the
antibiotics.[14,15] E. coli mutants defective in PBP 1b are hypersensitive to
these antibacterial effects of benzylpenicillin[16] while they exhibit normal
sensitivity to some other beta lactams (e.g., mecillinam). In addition, double
mutants defective in PBP 1b and also carrying a temperature sensitive mutation
in PBP 1a, were found to lyse upon shift to the higher temperature in a manner
characteristic of the penicillin treated parental strain.[11] The lytic effect
of benzylpenicillin and cephaloridine may be suppressed by growth of the E. coli
cultures at a relatively low pH value.[7] Nevertheless, the typical morphological
effects of other beta lactams (e.g., mecillinam or cephalexin) still occur under
these conditions.

Studies on the mode of action of mecillinam (a beta lactam that seems to
react with PBP 2 only)[17] suggest that this compound elicits its antibacterial
effects by a mechanism distinct from that of the PBP 1 reactive beta lactams.
Treatment of E. coli with mecillinam at or somewhat above the minimal inhibitory
concentration does not have prompt bactericidal or bacteriolytic effect. Instead, the drug causes conversion of the bacilli to a unique ovoid morphology
via growth.[18,19] Mutants lacking PBP 2 also have this morphology; they are
relatively resistant to mecillinam (but have normal sensitivities to other

lactams).[20] Prolonged exposure of wild type cells to mecillinam results in the gradual enlargement and eventual lysis of the ovoid-shaped cells. These latter phenomena appear to require relatively low cell concentration and cyclic AMP as well.[21] Synergistic growth inhibition by mecillinam and other beta lactams have been reported.[22]

One should add to this list another apparent difference between mecillinam and most of the other beta lactams: in contrast to the latter group, mecillinam does not seem to have any effect on the transpeptidase or murein carboxypeptidase reaction nor on any of a number of other reactions in cell wall synthesis.[23,24]

Beta lactams with special affinity for the E. coli PBP 3 may cause their inhibitory effects by still another mechanism,[15] although the distinction here is less clear than in the case of mecillinam versus benzylpenicillin since beta lactams preferentially attaching to PBP 3 still retain considerable affinities for the components of PBP 1 and the other binding proteins as well.[17,25] Nevertheless, this group of beta lactams (examplified by cephalexin, piperacillin and by low concentrations of benzylpenicillin) seem to interfere primarily with cell septation. Cephalexin-treated wild type cells or mutants with a thermosensitive defect in PBP 3 cultured at the higher temperature, grow as nonseptate filaments and the mutants at the higher temperature show a somewhat increased resistance to the inhibitory effects of cephalexin.[25]

Species to species variation in the mechanism of antimicrobial effects. The findings briefly reviewed in the previous section indicate that structurally different beta lactams added to the same bacterium (E. coli) may elicit their antibacterial effects by different mechanisms. The converse also seems to be true: the same beta lactam may produce different antimicrobial effects in different species of bacteria. This may be illustrated by the observations of Dr. Horne in our laboratory concerning the case of three species of streptococci treated with benzylpenicillin.[5] Group H, group A streptococci and pneumococci

each have about the same MIC values for benzylpenicillin. In each one of these
bacteria treatment with penicillin causes interference with cell wall synthesis,
secretion of lipids, lipoteichoic acids and other surface polymers. On the
other hand, the three species differ greatly in the eventual effects of the
antibiotic treatment: in group H streptococci penicillin is primarily a reversible growth inhibitor; group A streptococci rapidly lose viability (in the
absence of any observable structural defect) during penicillin treatment; pneumococci are both killed and lysed by penicillin (Fig. 1).

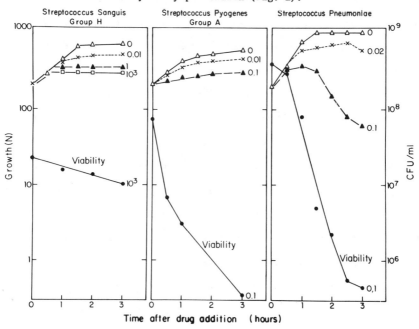

Fig. 1. Effects of benzylpenicillin on three species of Streptococci. Numbers
by each curve indicate concentration of drug (μg/ml). Closed circles indicate
viability of bacteria (CFU/ml) All other symbols indicate turbidity. Dashed
lines indicate MIC of drug. Reprinted with permission from Antimicrobial Agents
and Chemotherapy.[5]

In view of what has already been learned in the E. coli system, it is conceivable that this species variation in penicillin response may reflect the
presence or absence of unique penicillin binding proteins (corresponding to the

growth inhibitory, bactericidal or lytic "target" proteins). This possibility
has already been tested (with negative results) in pneumococci showing either
the bactericidal-bacteriolytic (wild type) or the growth inhibitory (penicillin
tolerant) responses to penicillin. An examination of the penicillin binding
proteins of wild type and tolerant pneumococci yielded identical patterns.

The basic difference between the group H, group A and pneumococcal penicillin
response concerns the reversibility of the antibiotic effect and one can imagine
that the inhibition of the same type of enzymatic target reaction may be modu-
lated to produce either a reversible or an irreversible growth inhibition. The
best candidate for such an enzyme seems to be the murein transpeptidase. The
fundamental importance and general occurrence of this reaction has been amply
confirmed in all bacterial systems[26-29] and the sensitivity of this reaction to
beta lactam antibiotics has been the focus of intensive studies in several laboratories.[27,30,31] Genetic studies in E. coli suggest that transpeptidation is
essential for the survival of cells and this is likely to be true for most bacteria. Thus, an irreversible inhibition of this enzyme system by the appropriate beta lactams should cause irreversible inhibition of bacterial growth provided that biosynthesis of new enzyme molecules (that might occur after the
removal of excess drug) is also inhibited. Such a mechanism (i.e., irreversible
inactivation of transpeptidase plus inhibition of protein synthesis) might possibly be the basis of the rapid bactericidal effect of benzylpenicillin on group
A streptococci. As of now, studies on the effect of penicillin treatment have
not revealed any signs of structural damage in these bacteria.

In principle, this model could be modified to explain the two other major
types of penicillin responses as typified by Str. sanguis and pneumococci respectively. In the first case, the primarily bacteriostatic effect of beta
lactams in S. sanguis would be caused by reversibility of the inhibition of target enzyme (either by regeneration of active enzyme from the penicilloyl form[27]
or by resynthesis of new target enzyme molecules[32]). In the case of pneumococci

one may argue that lysis is a side-effect that occurs (for unknown reasons) after the irreversible inactivation of the transpeptidase has already been completed (causing irreversible loss of viability). Lysis may be a useful side-effect that prevents resynthesis of enzyme molecules and thus contributes to the irreversibility of inhibition. In a popular hypothesis (unbalanced growth) penicillin induced lysis of bacteria was explained as a combination of two factors: the inhibited activity of murein transpeptidase and the uninhibited (continued) expansion of cytoplasmic mass in the penicillin treated cells. It was assumed that in the presence of penicillin, bacteria continue to add new units to the preexisting cell wall (via transglycosylation); however, these would not be crosslinked to neighboring peptides because of the inhibition of the transpeptidase. These mechanically weak poorly crosslinked zones would then be ruptured under the osmotic and mechanical pressure of the cytoplasmic mass.

However, two key assumptions of this model may not hold true for all bacteria that lyse when treated with penicillin. First, it has been shown in several species including pneumococci,[6] Bacillus subtilis,[33] B. licheniformis[34] and E. coli (Kitano and Tomasz, manuscript in preparation), that the penicillin-induced lysis of cells requires the activity of autolytic enzymes and the well-known dependence of penicillin-induced lysis on the active growth of the bacteria is most likely an aspect of autolysin activity (rather than representing the unbalanced growth of cytoplasmic mass). A second difficulty is that in several species of bacteria, the penicillin-sensitive transpeptidation seems to be the very reaction by which new disaccharide-peptides are attached to the old cell wall. In such bacteria, penicillin can actually inhibit the attachment reaction and uncrosslinked oligomers of wall material may accumulate or may be secreted into the surrounding medium.[35,36] It is difficult to see how in such cases inhibition of transpeptidation would provide a mechanism for the generation of "weak" spots in the cell wall surrounding the bacterium.

Thus, at the present time it is not clear exactly how the inhibition of the ubiquitous murein transpeptidases is linked to the induction of bacterial lysis. Nevertheless, a large number of observations strongly suggest a biochemical link between inhibition of transpeptidation and induction of lysis. Some of these observations will be discussed in more detail next.

Induction of murein hydrolase activity during penicillin treatment of E. coli and pneumococci.

The superior efficiency of certain beta lactams to cause rapid lysis of E. coli cultures has been known for some time and it is also known that antibiotics with high affinity for proteins in PBP group 1 are particularly effective in this respect. We have performed experiments to clarify the biochemical basis of this lytic phenomenon. The general design of the experiments was as follows. E. coli requiring diaminopimelic acid (dmp) was grown in radioactive dpm to label the cell walls. After subsequent culturing in isotope-free medium (in order to "chase" all the radioactive precursors into the cell wall) portions of the culture were exposed to various concentrations of beta lactams for a short time period (10 min). The treated bacteria were washed free of excess drugs, resuspended in simple buffer solutions and the rate of release of cell wall material was monitored during incubation. Some typical results are illustrated in Figure 2. It may be seen that benzylpenicillin (as well as a number of other beta lactams that exhibit selective affinities for PBP 1) induced rapid degradation of cell wall material even after the relatively short exposure to drug concentrations in the vicinity of the MIC values. In contrast, wall degradation was minimal even after high doses of mecillinam exposure; beta lactams with preferential affinities for PBP 3 showed autolysis-triggering efficiencies intermediate between the former two groups. These findings suggest that lysis of E. coli cultures during treatment with inhibitors of PBP 1 is caused by the triggering of uncontrolled autolysin activity.[37] The finding also corroborates the differences in the mode of action of beta lactams with preferential

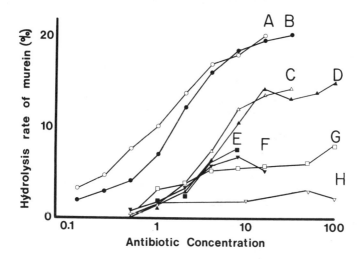

Fig. 2. Autolysin triggering efficiency of various beta lactams. The activity
of triggered autolysin is shown as the degradation rate (per cent) of murein
after 2 h incubation. Antibiotics: cephaloridine (A), cephalothin (B), benzylpenicillin (C), ampicillin (D), dicloxacillin (E), cephalexin (F), 6-APA (G)
and mecillinam (H).

affinities for PBPs 1, 2 and 3.

In experiments similar in design to the ones described for E. coli, the autolysis triggering efficiency of beta lactams was also determined in pneumococci.
Both wild type (lysis-prone) and mutant (autolysin defective) pneumococci were
grown, labeled with specific cell wall label and were subsequently exposed to
short treatment with various beta lactams. After transfer of the cells to buffer, the rate of cell wall degradation was followed. In the wild type cells,
wall degradation occurred, catalyzed by the endogenous autolysin. In the mutant
cells, no wall degradation was apparent unless wild type autolysin was also
added to the lysis buffer. Comparison of the effectiveness of different lactams
(at different multiples of their minimal growth inhibitory concentrations) again

indicated that beta lactams with selective affinity for PBP 1 in E. coli were
the most efficient, both as agents triggering the endogenous autolysin of wild
type cells as well as agents sensitizing the mutant bacteria to exogenous autolysin (Fig. 3).

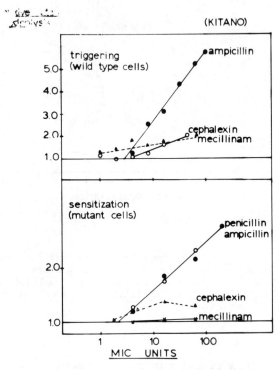

Fig. 3.   Relative rate of hydrolysis.

These experiments once again strongly imply a special target (analogous to
that of the PBP 1 of E. coli) for the induction of bacterial cell wall degradation in pneumococci. These Gram positive cocci contain a single major murein
hydrolase activity, an N-acetyl muramic acid-L-alanine amidase (in contrast to
E. coli which have been reported to contain a number of cell wall hydrolyzing
enzymes.[38] Genetic and physiological studies have shown that the suppression
of the activity of this enzyme (by any one of a number of means) results in a
striking, and, at first sight, paradoxical change in the response of pneumococci

to beta lactams (and other lytic agents). Such bacteria would exhibit normal sensitivity to beta lactams (as indicated by unchanged minimal inhibitory concentrations and normal dose response); on the other hand, such cells would no longer lyse during beta lactam treatment and, in some cases, the rate of loss of viability is also substantially decreased.[6] Examples of this penicillin "tolerant" response are illustrated in Figures 4 and 5 for the case of pneumococci in which the autolytic system has been suppressed by growing the bacteria in a medium containing ethanolamine in place of choline (the usual aminoalcohol component of pneumococcal cell walls).[39]

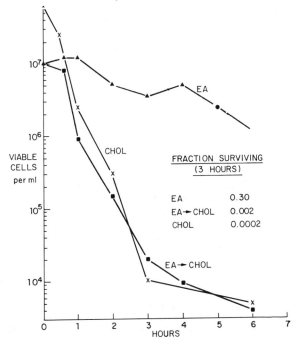

Fig. 4. Penicillin tolerance of <u>Streptococcus pneumoniae</u> grown in a medium containing ethanolamine (EA). Pneumococci grown in a growth medium containing choline (CHOL) have an active autolytic system, in contrast to those bacteria grown in EA. Benzylpenicillin (at five times the MIC) was added to cultures at time 0, and the decline in the titer of viable bacteria was monitored. Choline was added with the penicillin to one of the cultures grown in EA. (EA → CHOL) in order to reactivate the autolytic system. Reprinted with permission from <u>Nature</u>.[6]

210

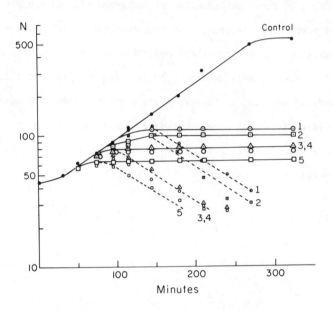

Fig. 5. The dose response to penicillin of lysis-prone and lysis-defective pneumococci. Five cultures of pneumococci were grown in choline-containing medium in which they are capable of lysis (-----). Another five cultures were grown in ethanolamine-containing medium, in which they are lysis-defective (————). At time 0, the cultures received benzylpenicillin at the following concentrations (μg/ml): 0.02 (1), 0.03 (2), 0.05 (3), 0.07 (4), and 0.1 (5). Growth and/or lysis were monitored by following the light scattering of cultures (N). Reprinted with permission from the Annals of the New York Academy of Sciences.[39]

It is known that these growth conditions force the bacteria to synthesize ethanolamine-containing cell walls that are resistant to the hydrolytic action of the pneumococcal autolysin.[40] An additional, related, biochemical defect of the ethanolamine-grown pneumococci is the absence of catalytically active auto-lysin.[41] The lack of autolytic activity of these bacteria does not seem to in-fluence their ability to grow with normal exponential rates. However, the cells are resistant to the lytic effects (and, to a considerable degree, to the bac-tericidal effects) of beta lactams.

Penicillin tolerance was also demonstrated in pneumococcal mutants defective in the autolysin[6] and certain growth conditions can amplify the beta lactam tolerance of these mutants. Mutants grown in the usual medium in which the phosphate content is low (1/20th of the normal concentration) and the buffer component is Tris-hydroxymethylamino methane (TRIS) exhibit a greatly amplified tolerance to penicillins: lysis is suppressed (measured both by optical methods and by the escape of intracellular protein markers during penicillin treatment) and loss of viability becomes very slow (Fig. 6).

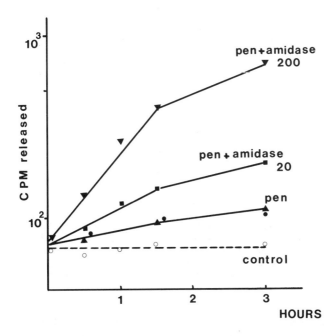

Fig. 6. Lysis of a penicillin tolerant pneumococcal mutant during treatment with penicillin plus wild type autolysin added to the growth medium. An autolysin-defective pneumococcal mutant was grown in Tris-containing medium and was labeled biosynthetically by radioactive phenylalanine. After several hours of growth in the isotope-containing medium (to label cellular proteins) the bacteria were transferred to fresh isotope-free medium, grown for 2 more cell generations and then portions were treated with benzylpenicillin (0.1 µg per ml) or a combination of penicillin plus purified wild type pneumococcal autolysin (amidase) and the release of radioactive proteins into the medium was determined in order to quantitate the degree of cell lysis. Symbols: control culture (○); cultures treated with penicillin alone (●) or with a combination of penicillin plus amidase, 20 µl per ml (■) or 200 µl per ml (▼). A control culture grown on high phosphate-containing medium was also compared (▲).

Furthermore, culture lysis and loss of viability may both be induced by the

addition of electrophoretically homogeneous wild type pneumococcal autolysin

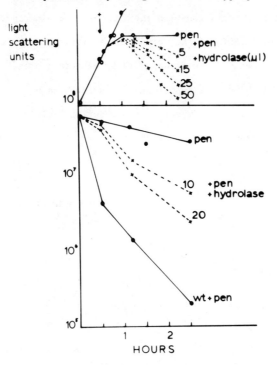

Fig. 7. Induction of culture lysis and loss of viability by treatment of penicillin tolerant pneumococci with penicillin plus wild type autolysin. An
autolysin defective pneumococcal culture was treated with penicillin (0.1 µg per
ml) with or without the addition of purified pneumococcal autolysin (murein
hydrolase) lysis was measured as decrease in the light scattering of cultures;
viability was assayed by plating.

Interestingly, increasing the concentration of penicillin in these experiments

causes a gradual shortening of the time of onset of autolysin-induced lysis

while an increase in autolysin concentration increases the rate of lysis and

death.

These experiments clearly imply the pneumococcal autolysin as the agent re-

sponsible for penicillin-induced lysis and, at least in part, in the loss of

bacterial viability as well. In the case of autolysis defective pneumococci,

inhibition of the penicillin sensitive primary target reactions alone seem to cause only a transient inhibition of growth, and the irreversible (bactericidal and bacteriolytic) effects of beta lactams are brought about by the uncontrolled (suicidal) activity of cellular factors (murein hydrolase) that do not directly react with the beta lactam molecule. The tolerant response of Streptococcus sanguis to penicillins (already discussed in some detail above) may also be related to the apparent lack of autolytic activity in these organisms.

The essential role of murein hydrolases in penicillin-induced lysis of bacteria is not restricted to pneumococci. Autolysis defective mutants of B. licheniformis and B. subtilis are also resistant to the lytic effects of beta lactams and recent reports in the medical literature indicate that penicillin tolerant bacteria may be isolated with surprisingly high frequency from clinical samples from certain types of relapsing infections.[42-44] Some of the penicillin tolerant staphylococci were reported to have a defective autolytic system.[43] Recently, Kitano has isolated penicillin tolerant mutants of E. coli. These mutants were resistant to both the lytic and bactericidal effects of moderate doses of penicillin and the cells had lowered autolysin activity (Kitano and Tomasz; manuscript in preparation).

The main conclusion emerging from this analysis of the penicillin induced lysis of pneumococci and E. coli is that cellular lysis requires the activity of bacterial murein hydrolases (autolysins). Since these enzymes do not seem to react directly with the beta lactam molecule, one has to provide an explanation as to why and how the activity of these hydrolases becomes "suicidal" in the penicillin treated bacterium.

Two different types of general mechanisms have been proposed to explain the degradation of murein in penicillin-treated bacteria. The first model which one may refer to as the "constitutive" model[45-48] assumes that murein hydrolases acting in concert with wall synthetic enzymes are part of the mechanism of cell wall enlargement, the "nicks" in the cell wall (created by a hydrolase) serving as growing points at which new cell wall elements are added to the preexisting wall by the synthetic enzymes. Inhibition of the synthetic reactions (by wall inhibitors) without a parallel inhibition of the hydrolases, would then automatically lead to cell wall rupture and lysis. Indeed, the penicillin tolerance of autolysin-defective pneumococci has first been interpreted as an experimental verification of this model.

It is conceivable that in some bacteria a murein hydrolase activity coupled to wall synthesis is indeed responsible for cellular lysis during inhibition of wall synthesis, as predicted by this model. However, in the case of pneumococci subsequent studies have encountered difficulties with this interpretation. In short, while the lytic agent "provoked" during penicillin treatment was clearly the amidase, it was difficult to see how this type of activity could be coupled to a synthetic reaction. Also, if this enzyme activity were needed for wall expansion, constitutive amidase-defective mutations would be expected to be lethal. Furthermore, indirect evidence indicated that the pneumococcal amidase may only be active at the end of the cell cycle catalysing the separation of daughter cells. In the view of these findings, it has become a mystery again why interference with cell wall synthesis should provoke the suicidal activity of the pneumococcal murein hydrolases.

Natural inhibitors of murein hydrolases. In 1975, Joachim Holtje, in our laboratory, demonstrated the powerful and specific autolysin inhibitory effect of the pneumococcal Forssman antigen and suggested that regulation of autolysin activity may be one of the physiological functions of lipoteichoic acids.[49] A collaborative study has extended the validity of the pneumococcal findings by demonstrating the autolysin inhibitory properties of polyglycerophosphate type lipoteichoic acids in several other bacterial systems.[50] Subsequently, certain phospholipids were also shown to inhibit the autolysis of Streptococcus faecalis.[51]

The existence of such potential autolysin regulatory substances in bacteria has turned our attention to the metabolism of these substances during penicillin treatment of pneumococci. It was found that autolysin-defective mutants (and wild type cells as well) have rapidly released an autolysin inhibitor into the growth medium upon addition of penicillin and other cell wall inhibitors to the cultures.[10,52] The inhibitor was subsequently identified as a complex of the Forssman antigen and some as yet unidentified macromolecules.[53] Rapid and massive release of acylated polyglycerophosphate-type lipoteichoic acids as well as cellular lipids was also documented during treatment of Str. sanguis and other bacteria with cell wall inhibitors.[5,54,55]

On the basis of these and other observations, another model ("autolysin triggering") was suggested to explain the mechanism by which a hydrolase-catalysed cell wall degradation may be provoked during penicillin treatment of pneumococci.[10,56] In essence, this model proposes that the pneumococcal amidase is inhibited during most of the cell cycle by inhibitor(s) containing the Forssman antigen. Penicillin treatment causes a dissociation of the enzyme-inhibitor complex and the inhibitor is actually lost to the medium by a mechanism that is not fully understood at the present time. Inhibitors of protein, RNA and lipid synthesis (i.e., agents that are known to antagonize the irreversible effects of penicillin) were all found to suppress the penicillin-induced release of lipids and lipid-teichoic acid complexes.[10,54,55] At the present time, the only known physiological function of the pneumococcal autolysin has to do with the separation of daughter cells.[57] It is conceivable that the physiological activity of this enzyme is also triggered at the end of the cell cycle by a transient genetically programmed halt or perturbation of murein synthesis by a mechanism similar to the premature antibiotic-induced triggering, except that the physiological activity would be localized, transient and properly timed.

It should be emphasized that even in the case of pneumococci this is a working hypothesis rather than an established mechanism. The evidence is strong for the involvement of unique PBPs (similar in lactam specificity to those of the PBP 1 of E. coli) and also for the essential nature of the N-acetyl-muramic acid-L-alanine amidase. However, the mechanism of triggering, i.e., the lethal "pathway" leading from these PBPs to the suicidal activity of the hydrolase is hypothetical.

It is possible that poorly crosslinked murein (either in soluble form or within the cell wall proper) may play some role as part of a triggering mechanism. It is remarkable indeed that triggering of lysis (by endogenous autolysin) and sensitization to lysis (by autolysin added to the medium of mutant cells [see Fig. 7]) are both caused most efficiently by the same group of beta lactams: penicillin, ampicillin, cephaloridine. This is the same group of antibiotics that is most effective in causing lysis of E. coli also and these beta lactams are known to have high affinity for PBP 1 which is supposed to contain the major murein transpeptidase of E. coli. It is possible that normal murein is essential for the retention or proper spatial arrangement of nonmurein components of the envelope (e.g., Forssman antigen) which function as autolysin inhibitors or protective groups blocking critical sites of the murein from autolytic attack. Poorly crosslinked murein may be defective in these respects and/or it may also be hypersensitive to autolysins.

Factors modulating the antibacterial effects of beta lactams in complex environments.

A still higher degree of complexity has to be considered if one were to account for the mechanisms that contribute to the inhibition or destruction of a beta lactam-treated bacterium inside an infected mammalian host. Observations in several laboratories indicate that pretreatment with beta lactams may sensitize bacteria to components of the immune system and that host factors and beta lactams may act in synergy in the inactivation of the infecting bacteria. Extensive studies of George Warren and his associates have been producing evidence since the early 1960s that indicate the sensitizing effects of certain beta lactams (applied at subinhibitory concentrations) to the lytic action of lysozyme,[58] to phagocytosis[59] or to the antibody-mediated cytocidal effect of comple-

ment.[60] The sensitizing effects were highly specific for certain beta lactams
(nafcillin in the case of staphylococci and cyclocillin in the case of E. coli)
and these studies represent some of the earliest documented cases suggesting
multiple beta lactam sensitive targets in bacteria.[58] An even more important
aspect of these studies is that they have called attention to the possible cooperation between host factors and chemotherapeutic agents in the elimination
of invading bacteria. Synergistic bactericidal effects of penicillin and leuco-
cyte derived factors[61] or polymorphonuclear leukocytes[62] have also been described.

We have encountered a case of these types of phenomena in some strains of
Streptococcus faecium. Treatment with a number of beta lactams caused primarily
an inhibition of growth and loss of viability with a moderate rate. However,
addition of lysozyme to the growth medium caused a great acceleration in the
loss of viability and provoked lysis, provided that the bacteria have been also
treated with penicillins (Fig. 8). The rate of loss of viability and lysis was
proportional to the concentration of lysozyme. An observation of potential
clinical importance is also shown in the Figure. Streptococci treated with high
concentrations of penicillin are completely resistant to the bactericidal effect
of these antibiotics ("zonal" effect). Bacteria treated with a combination of
such high concentrations of penicillin (100 x MIC) plus lysozyme nevertheless
still lysed and lost viability although higher concentration of lysozyme was
needed to achieve a rapid rate.

A plausible biochemical basis of these sensitization effects may be the
phenomenon of penicillin-induced surface-polymer secretion. Treatment with penicillin or other cell wall inhibitors (but not with inhibitors of protein, RNA
or DNA synthesis) induces the rapid and massive release of a number of bacterial
surface components; the list of which by now includes such diverse compounds as
the Forssman antigen,[10] polyglycerophosphate-type lipoteichoic acids[54] and
murein precursors,[36] capsular material (Horne and Tomasz, unpublished),

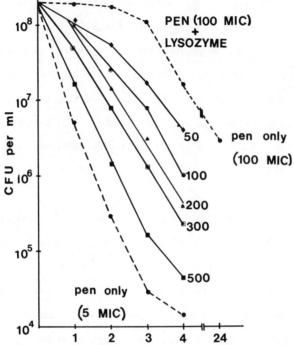

Fig. 8. Sensitization of <u>Streptococcus</u> <u>Faecium</u> to exogenous lysozyme by treatment with penicillin. Cultures of Str. Faecium strain
495 were grown in Todd Hewitt broth and treated with different concentrations of lysozyme (concentrations indicated by numbers) plus
penicillin (100 x MIC). The effect of penicillin treatment alone
(at 5 x and 100 x MIC) are shown by the dashed lines.

polysaccharides,[58] lipids[55] and membrane proteins (Hakenbeck and Tomasz, un-

published). The release of these surface components does not seem to represent

an irreversible stage of cellular disintegration (lysis) since lysis-defective

and lysis-prone bacteria both release these substances; release is not affected

by osmotic stabilizers but it may be suppressed by inhibition of metabolic ac-

tivity and the process can be reversed by the timely removal of the antibiotic.[52]

Also, under the appropriate conditions, release of material is restricted to

cell surface components. Several of the released substances have powerful bio-

logical activities such as triggering of the alternative pathway of comple-

ments,[63] autolysin inhibitors, antiphagocytic components (capsule) and putative

factors involved with bacterial adhesion.[64] The loss of such surface components during antibiotic treatment in vivo may indeed influence the inter-action of some bacterial pathogens with host factors and cells. Thus, relative-ly subtle surface alterations that may be repaired by the bacteria during in vitro cultivation, may become fatal vulnerabilities if host factors are also present in the environment. Thus, the widely accepted notion that beta lactams may act by essentially the same antimicrobial mechanism in vitro and in vivo[65] may not be completely true for all bacteria. The interaction of chemothera-peutic agents and host factors is likely to become an exciting and important area of experimentation in the future.

SUMMARY

This brief overview of various aspects of beta lactam action demonstrates the immense complexity and variability in the antibacterial effects of these anti-biotics. The biochemical activities of the beta lactam-sensitive target pro-teins are not fully understood. It seems that selective inhibition of these PBPs may cause distinct antimicrobial effects. The mechanism of the pharmaco-logically most useful, irreversible effects is also unclear. Analysis of the process of bacterial lysis in pneumococci has resulted in the proposition that in some bacteria inhibition of the primary biochemical targets (PBP) may be a necessary, but not sufficient, condition to cause bacterial death and lysis. The irreversible effects may be caused by the uncontrolled (suicidal) activity of the pneumococcal murein hydrolase, the normal regulation of which is upset in the penicillin-treated bacterium. In this model, the direct physiological con-sequence of the inhibition of PBPs may be a reversible inhibition of growth, i.e., the type of response exhibited by autolysin-defective mutants of pneumo-cocci or Str. sanguis. It may be worthwhile pointing out that the mechanism of a reversible growth inhibition by penicillins is far from obvious. It is con-ceivable that inhibition of cellular growth, i.e., cessation of all major poly-mer syntheses, by inhibitors of cell wall synthesis would occur via an as yet unrecognized control mechanism, in a manner analogous to the operation of the R_c control system during aminoacid starvation of bacteria. However, in some other species of bacteria (e.g., group A streptococci) and in the case of some beta lactams (e.g., mecillinam acting on $\underline{E}$. $\underline{coli}$) autolysin activity may not be part of the antimicrobial mechanism.

Recent investigations have produced more questions than answers concerning the mode of action of beta lactams, and several issues that were formerly thought to be settled have resurfaced in new, interesting contexts. Nevertheless, there is little doubt that the powerful and selective inhibitory activity of beta lactams is directed at the metabolism of bacterial cell wall. Perhaps, the best evidence for this is still provided by the old observation that in an appropriate environment (high osmolality and presence of membrane protective agents) several species of bacteria can escape the lethal consequences of penicillin treatment by converting to wall-deficient forms.[66] Bacteria may grow and multiply in these special environments as L-forms or spheroplasts indicating that in these cases all the inhibitory effects of penicillins (including reversible inhibition of growth) are by-passed once bacterial survival has become independent of the replication of cell wall. A particularly interesting case is that of a Proteus L-form capable of rapid proliferation in the presence of penicillin.[28] Addition of certain other beta lactams (notably mecillinam or cefoxitin) together with penicillin to the growth medium caused inhibition of growth again implying that multiple inhibitory targets exist in these cells.[67]

A full characterization of the biochemical targets of beta lactams and the elucidation of the "pathway" leading from inhibited targets to inhibited bacterial cell, would require a better understanding of the biochemical details of cell wall synthesis; its role in the organization of non-murein components of the cell envelope; the mechanism of control of autolysins and the mechanisms by which wall synthesis is coordinated with the division of the bacterial cell. With the emergence of novel types of beta lactam resistant bacteria, our ability to rapidly develop effective new antibacterial agents will depend on a better understanding of the mechanism of beta lactam action, which, in turn, will depend on the production of more basic knowledge concerning the chemistry of the bacterial cell surface.

ACKNOWLEDGMENTS

Investigations described in this paper have been supported by grants from the National Science Foundation (PCM 7812770), National Institutes of Health (AI 09423 and AI 12932) and from the Smith-Kline and French Laboratories. C. de Freitas is the recipient of a career development award from the National Research Council of Brazil.

REFERENCES

1. Nierlich, D. (1978) Ann. Rev. Microbiol. 32, 393-407.
2. Inouye, M. (1971) J. Bacteriol. 106, 539-542.
3. Cohen, S.S. and Barnes, M.D. (1955) J. Bacteriol. 69, 59-65.
4. Dougherty, T.J. and Saukkonen, J.J. (1978) Abstract No. 252, Interscience Conf. Antimicrob. Agents Chemotherap.
5. Horne, D., and Tomasz, A. (1977) Antimicrob. Agents Chemother. 11, 888-896.
6. Tomasz, A., Albino, A. and Zanati, E. (1970) Nature 227, 138-140.
7. Goodell, E.W., Lopez, R. and Tomasz, A. (1976) Proc. Natl. Acad. Sci. U.S.A 73, 3293-3297.
8. Lopez, R. et al. (1976) Antimicrob. Agents Chemother. 10, 697-706.
9. Spratt, B.G. (1977) In D. Schlessinger [ed.] Microbiology 1977. American Society for Microbiology, Washington, D.C., p. 182-194.
10. Tomasz, A. and Waks, S. (1975) Proc. Natl. Acad. Sci. U.S.A. 72, 4162-4166.
11. Suzuki, H. et al. (1978) Proc. Natl. Acad. Sci. U.S.A. 75, 664-668.
12. Matsuhashi, M. et al. (1977) Proc. Natl. Acad. Sci. U.S.A. 74, 2976-2979.
13. Matsuhashi, M. et al. (1978) Proc. Natl. Acad. Sci. U.S.A. 75, 2681-2685.
14. Spratt, B.G. (1975) Proc. Natl. Acad. Sci. U.S.A. 72, 2999-3003.
15. Greenwood, D. and O'Grady, F. (1973) J. Infect. Dis. 128, 791-794.
16. Tamaki, S. et al. (1977) Proc. Natl. Acad. Sci. U.S.A. 74, 5472-5476.
17. Spratt, B.G. (1977) Eur. J. Biochem. 72, 341-352.
18. Greenwood, D. and O'Grady, F. (1973) J. Clin. Pathol. 26, 1-6.
19. Lund, F. and Tybring, L. (1972) Nature [New Biol.] 236, 135-137.
20. Matsuhashi, S. et al. (1974) J. Bacteriol. 117, 578-587.
21. Aono, R. et al. (1979) J. Bacteriol. 137, 839-845.
22. Grunberg, E. et al. (1976) Antimicrob. Agents Chemotherap. 9, 589-594.
23. Park, J.T. and Burman, L. (1973) Biochem. Biophys. Res. Commun. 51, 863-868.
24. Braun, V. (1975) Biochim. Biophys. Acta 415, 335-377.
25. Spratt, B.G. (1976) J. Bacteriol. 131, 293-305.
26. Tipper, D.J. and Strominger, J.L. (1968) J. Biol. Chem. 243, 3169-3179.
27. Ghuysen, J.M. (1977) In D. Schlessinger [ed.] Microbiology 1977. American Society for Microbiology, Washington, D.C., p. 195-208.

222

28. Martin, H.H. (1964) J. Gen. Microbiol. 36, 441-450.
29. Blumberg, P.M. and Strominger, J.L. (1974) Bacteriol. Rev. 38, 291-335.
30. Tipper, D.J. and Strominger, J.L. (1965) Proc. Natl. Acad. Sci. U.S.A. 54, 1133-1141.
31. Wise, E.M., Jr. and Park, J.T. (1965) Proc. Natl. Acad. Sci. U.S.A. 54, 75-81.
32. Hamilton, T.E. and Lawrence, P.J. (1975) J. Biol. Chem. 250, 6578-6585.
33. Ayusawa, D. et al. (1975) J. Bacteriol. 124, 459-469.
34. Rogers, H.J. and Forsberg, C.W. (1971) J. Bacteriol. 108, 1235-1243.
35. Mirelman, D. et al. (1972) Proc. Natl. Acad. Sci. U.S.A. 69, 3355-3359.
36. Ward, J.B. (1974) Biochem. J. 141, 227-241.
37. Kitano, K. and Tomasz, A. (1979) Abstract A(H) 17 Annual Meeting of Amer. Soc. Microbiol.
38. Schwarz, U. et al. (1969) J. Mol. Biol. 41, 419-429.
39. Tomasz, A. (1974) Ann. N.Y. Acad. Sci. 235, 439-447.
40. Mosser, J.L. and Tomasz, A. (1970) J. Biol. Chem. 245, 287-298.
41. Tomasz, A. and Westphal, M. (1971) Proc. Natl. Acad. Sci. U.S.A. 68, 2627-2630.
42. Sabath, L.D. et al. (1977) Lancet 1, 443-447.
43. Best, G.K. et al. (1974) Antimicrob. Agents Chemother. 6, 825-830.
44. Mayhall, C.G. et al. (1976) Antimicrob. Agents Chemother. 10, 707-712.
45. Weidel, W. and Pelzer, H. (1964) Advances in Enzymology 26, 193-232.
46. Rogers, H.J. (1970) Nature 213, 31-33.
47. Rogers, H.J. (1970) Bacteriol. Rev. 34, 194-214.
48. Shockman, G.D. et al. (1974) Ann. N.Y. Acad. Sci. 235, 161-197.
49. Holtje, J.V. and Tomasz, A. (1975) Proc. Natl. Acad. Sci. U.S.A. 72, 1690-1694.
50. Cleveland, R.F. et al. (1975) Biochem. Biophys. Res. Commun. 67, 1128-1135.
51. Cleveland, R.F. et al. (1976) J. Bacteriol. 126, 192-197.
52. Waks, S. and Tomasz, A. (1978) Antimicrob. Agents Chemother. 13, 293-301.
53. Hakenbeck, et al. (1978) Antimicrob. Agents Chemother. 13, 302-311.
54. Horne, D. and Tomasz, A. (1979) J. Bacteriol. 137, 1180-1184.
55. Horne, D. et al. (1977) J. Bacteriol. 132, 704-717.
56. Tomasz, A. and Holtje, J.V. (1977) In D. Schlessinger [ed.] Microbiology 1977. American Society for Microbiology, Washington, D.C., p. 209-215.
57. Tomasz, A. et al. (1975) J. Supramol. Biol. 3, 1-16.
58. Warren, G.H. and Gray, J. (1967) Canad. J. Microbiol. 321-328.
59. Friedman, H. and Warren, G.H. (1974) Proc. Soc. Exp. Biol. Med. 146, 707-711.
60. Friedman, H. and Warren, G.H. (1976) Proc. Soc. Exp. Biol. Med. 153, 301-304.
61. Lahav, M. and Ginsburg, I. (1977) Inflammation, 2, 165-170.
62. Molari, A. et al. (1978) Abstr. 18th Interscience Conf. Antimicrob. Ag. Chemotherap., p. 203.
63. Winkelstein, J.A. and Tomasz, A. (1977) J. Immunol. 118, 451-454.
64. Beachey, E.M. and Ofek, I. (1976) J. Exp. Med. 143, 759-771.
65. Eagle, H. et al. (1952) J. Lab. Clin. Med. 122, 122-132.
66. Lederberg, J. (1975) J. Bacteriol. 73, 144.
67. Martin, H.H. and Gmeiner, J. (1979) Eur. J. Biochem. 95, 487-495.

DISCUSSION

ONDETTI: Are you postulating that PBP 1 is not really a cell wall
synthesizing enzyme, but a protein that has as a function to trigger the autolytic mechanism?

TOMASZ: No.

ONDETTI: Good. Could you elaborate on that?

TOMASZ: I am postulating a pathway leading from the PBP 1 function, whatever
that is, to the triggering of the autolytic enzyme(s). That does not mean that
PBP 1 itself is an inhibitor of the autolysin. Inhibition of a murein
synthetizing enzyme (e.g., the transpeptidase) would have metabolic consequences
for instance, precursors would accumulate. One of those may be what I have
referred to as the "signal", which then causes dissociation of inhibitor from
enzyme, and that, in turn would initiate the suicidal autolytic activity. You
probably are aware of the work of Suzuki et al., who isolated double mutants[1]
of PBP 1b and 1a. The mutants were defective in PBP 1b and temperature
sensitive in PBP 1a. These cells would lyse when shifted to the higher temperature.

ONDETTI: Apparently the 1b, is a more critical penicillin binding protein
than 1a. The PBP 1a will become more critical, however, if the amount of PBP
1b is decreased. I mean, if the relative amounts of those components changed
then components that were not critical before, become more critical for the
survival of the cell.

TOMASZ: Yes.

CHU: Have you tried a penicillin analog, which is not active, to see
whether or not it binds to PBP 1? For example, 6-APA or some other ester types,
which are not active analogs, do they bind to PBP 1?

TOMASZ: We have not yet done experiments of this sort.

CHU: You mentioned that the inhibition of the enzyme by penicillin is
reversible. But normally one considers penicillins and cephalosporins a kind
of irreversible inhibitors of the enzyme. Can you clarify this point?

TOMASZ: Even if the inhibition of the enzyme is irreversible, you still
have to explain why the bacteria do not regenerate the enzyme, after the
removal of the inhibitor. The case of group A Streptococcus may illustrate
this point. Penicillin treatment of this bacterium causes rapid loss of
viability, but there is no evidence of structural damage in the cells. This
may be an organism in which penicillins irreversibly and quantitatively inactivate all the lethal targets or enzyme molecules. Yet, this is still not enough
to explain, why the cell is dead. You would have to make the extra assumption

e.g., that penicillin may also inhibit protein synthesis in these bacteria. In other words, you have to consider two kinds of reversibility in a bacterium. One is the reversibility of the primary reaction with the target protein and the other is the recovery of enzyme through *de novo* synthesis.

CHU: One thing has always interested me but I do not know the answer is that if the cell bursts and the proteins are released into the host; how does the host eliminate those proteins? Because I am worrying about the immune response.

TOMASZ: I do not know what the fate of such bacterial proteins is. There are interesting extra complexities that one must consider when the bacterium is exposed to penicillin inside an infected host rather than in culture medium. There are immune factors present and the fact that penicillin-treated bacteria loose surface components (a fact I did not have a chance to document here) may be of consequence for their survival in the infected host. There is a great deal of evidence, which indicate that one can actually sensitize bacteria to host factors by antibiotic treatment. For instance, tolerant bacteria which are not killed in the test tube by penicillin, may loose viability by the combined action of penicillin and immune cells. In some other cases we find sensitization to soluble host factors.

REFERENCES

1. Suzuki, H., Nishimura, Y. and Hirota, Y. (1978) Proc. Natl. Acad. Sci. USA 75, 664.

NUCLEAR ANALOGS OF β-LACTAM ANTIBIOTICS:
TOTAL SYNTHESIS AND PROPOSED MECHANISM OF ACTION

KENNETH G. HOLDEN, JOHN G. GLEASON, WILLIAM F. HUFFMAN, AND CARL D. PERCHONOCK
Research & Development Division, Smith Kline & French Laboratories,
Philadelphia, PA 19101

The combination of broad antibacterial spectrum, high potency, and remarkably low mammalian toxicity displayed by β-lactam antibiotics has made them
the therapy of choice against most bacterial infections. All of the penicillins
and cephalosporins currently in use by the medical profession are derived from
fermentation products by partial chemical synthesis. During the process of
discovering and developing these drugs, many thousands of derivatives of the
general structural types 1 and 2 were prepared and tested against a variety of
gram-positive and gram-negative bacteria. Until recently, however, analogous
compounds with more profound structural modifications, particularly new ring
systems, were virtually unexplored. This did not stem from a lack of interest
in such derivatives, but rather resulted from their relative inaccessibility.
The preparation of each new derivative required either extensive degradation and
resynthesis starting from the natural products or a multistep total synthesis.
Moreover, the stereochemical requirements and lability of the β-lactam ring in
such bicyclic structures presented special synthetic difficulties. We have
recently developed a versatile synthetic route to a variety of β-lactam antibiotic nuclear analogs, some of which have antibacterial activity comparable to
naturally derived penicillins and cephalosporins.

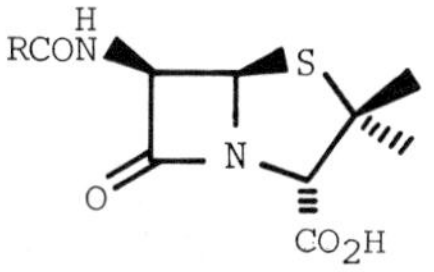

$$1 \qquad\qquad\qquad 2$$

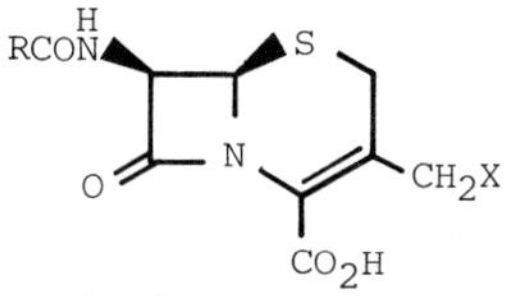

When we began our studies on the total synthesis of β-lactam antibiotic
nuclear analogs in the early 1970's, there were two major sources of information to guide us in selecting target structures. One was the proposed mechanism of action of penicillins and cephalosporins; the other was structure-
activity relationships developed from modified derivatives of these antibiotics.

In 1965 Tipper and Strominger[1] proposed a mechanism of action for penicillin that gained wide acceptance and, with modification and additions, remains so today. Based on earlier observations which showed penicillin to be a highly specific inhibitor of bacterial cell wall synthesis and new information about the detailed chemical structure and biosynthesis of cell wall components, they proposed that penicillin (1) mimics the D-alanyl-D-alanine terminus (3) of a cell wall glycopeptide. A transpetidase enzyme utilizes this substance in completing the final step in cell wall biosynthesis: cross-linking of glyco-peptide chains. In the absence of cross-linking, the fragile underlying cyto-plasmic membrane is susceptible to osmotic shock, and cell lysis results. At the molecular level, penicillin was postulated to inactivate the transpeptidase irreversibly by acylation of the enzyme active site.

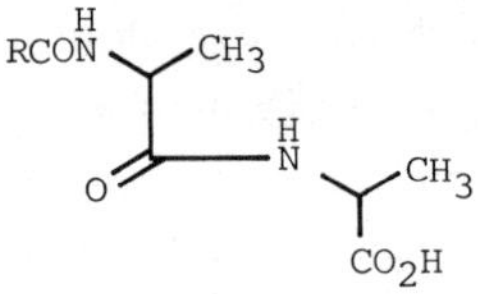

That the β-lactam carbonyl is indeed reactive and could function in this manner is well known. The source of this reactivity was originally postulated by Woodward[2] who recognized that inhibition of amide resonance by ring strain could account for this. The amount of ring strain is considerably increased by fusion of a second ring to the β-lactam. Thus, x-ray analysis[3] shows that, in penicillins and cephalosporins with potent antibacterial activity, the β-lactam nitrogen is significantly distorted from the plane defined by the three other atoms to which it is joined. On the other hand, monocyclic β-lactams and Δ^2-cephalosporins*, which are essentially inactive as antibacterial agents, have nearly planar structures. The distortion measured by x-ray diffraction is

*For the nuclear analogs discussed in this paper, the numbering system is analogous to the penicillins for 4:5 ring systems and to cephalosporins for 4:6 systems. The term "iso" penicillin or cephalosporin has been used to designate ring systems in which the hetero atom has been moved one position around the ring to the 2-position.

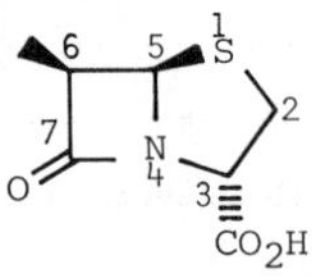

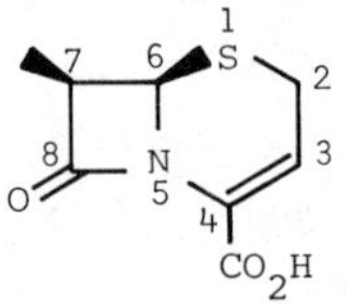

also reflected in an increased stretching frequency for the β-lactam carbonyl band in the infrared and an increased rate of reaction with nucleophiles.[4,5]

From structure-activity relationships among modified penicillins and cephalosporins,[6] it was clear that the integrity of both rings of these bicyclic structures was essential for activity. In the case of 4:6-ring systems, it appeared that a Δ^3 double bond was also required, since Δ^2-cephalosporins[7] and saturated nuclear analogs[8,9] are inactive. Furthermore, a cis relationship between the bridgehead hydrogen and the adjacent hydrogen bearing the side chain amide nitrogen was required. A carboxylic acid residue at C-3(4) and an acylated amine at C-6(7) were also apparently essential.[6]

Based on the proposed mechanism of action and known structure-activity relationships, it appeared that compounds represented by structure 5 might reasonably be expected to be recognized by the transpetidase enzyme and possess sufficient reactivity to inactivate it through acylation at the active site. In considering how one might construct molecules of this type, it is clear that an intermediate such as 4 possesses a number of desirable structural features. The β-lactam ring and acylamino function with cis stereochemistry are established early in the synthetic route, while the ester group and the unsubstituted β-lactam nitrogen represent functionalities which might allow fusion of a second ring. Since the β-lactam ring is relatively unstrained and unreactive until ring fusion is accomplished, postponing this step until late in the synthetic scheme should minimize involvement of the β-lactam in undesirable side reactions.

The synthesis of 4 was accomplished as follows.[10,11] Azidoacetic acid was activated as its mixed anhydride and reacted with the imine formed in situ from methyl glyoxylate and 2,4-dimethoxybenzylamine. The resulting β-lactam 6 possessed the desired cis stereochemistry; none of the trans isomer was detected.[12] Removal of the 2,4-dimethoxybenzyl group was accomplished by an oxidative procedure to give 7 and 2,4-dimethoxybenzaldehyde which could be recycled to the amine if desired. Reduction of the azide function followed by acylation with, for example, phenoxyacetyl chloride gave 4 (R = PhOCH$_2$, R' = Me).

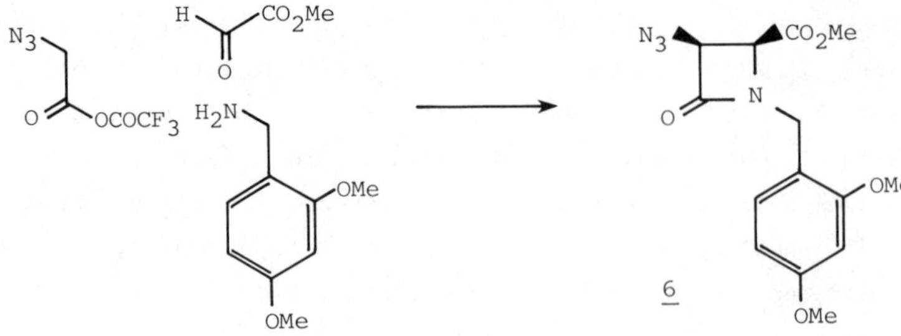

6

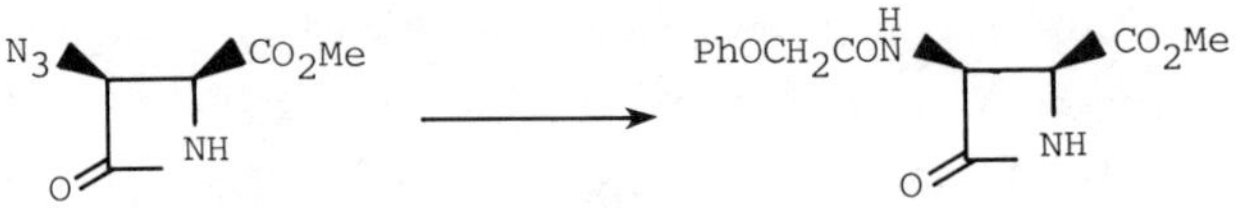

7   4

With the key monocyclic intermediate 4 in hand, its conversion to nuclear analogs of penicillin was next investigated. Selective reduction of the methyl ester followed by conversion of the resulting alcohol to an amine afforded 8. The imine resulting from reaction of 8 with benzyl glyoxylate was cyclized with acetyl chloride to give 9a as a mixture of carboxylate epimers. Quantitative cleavage of the benzyl ester was effected by catalytic hydrogenation to give 9b. This penicillin nuclear analog proved to be so reactive that the β-lactam was readily hydrolyzed in aqueous solution ($t_{1/2}$ = 2 hr; 37°C, pH 7.0).[10] Despite its instability under biological test conditions, 9b did exhibit antibacterial activity against a few gram-positive and gram-negative organisms. Growth inhibition of Bacillus subtilis, Staphylococcus aureus, and Shigella paradysenteriae was observed at concentrations of 10, 100 and 400 µg/ml, respectively.

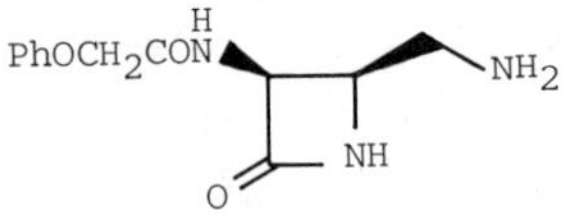

8

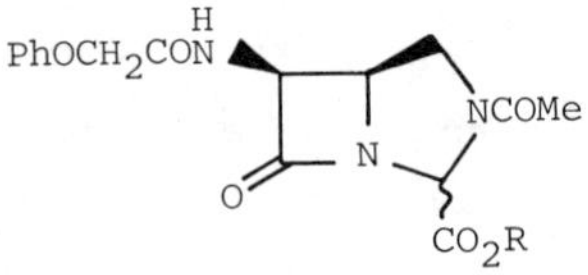

9a, R=CH$_2$Ph
 b, R=H

The antibacterial activity displayed by 9b seemed to validate our hypothesis that structures of the type 5 would be recognized by the transpeptidase and have sufficient reactivity as acylating agents to inactivate it. However, in this case the reactivity of the system was so great that hydrolysis by water occurred rapidly enough to effectively reduce its antibacterial potency. To decrease ring strain and hence reactivity, we next investigated the synthesis of the corresponding penicillin nuclear analog in which the nitrogen in the fused ring of 9b is replaced by a larger sulfur atom. Intermediate 7 was converted to 10 in a series of steps[13] analogous to the preparation of 8. Acid-catalyzed addition of benzyl glyoxylate to the β-lactam nitrogen followed by reaction of the resulting carbinolamide with thionyl chloride and in situ displacement with potassium thioacetate gave 11a as a mixture of carboxylate epimers. Hydrolysis under mildly basic aqueous conditions gave largely 11b along with the desired penicillin nuclear analog 12a. Although 11b could be readily isolated and purified, a different approach was necessary in order to obtain a pure sample of the relatively unstable nuclear analog 12. Treatment of 11b with excess cyclohexylamine in methylene chloride cleanly gave the desired product as its cyclohexylamine salt (12b). Surprisingly, both the

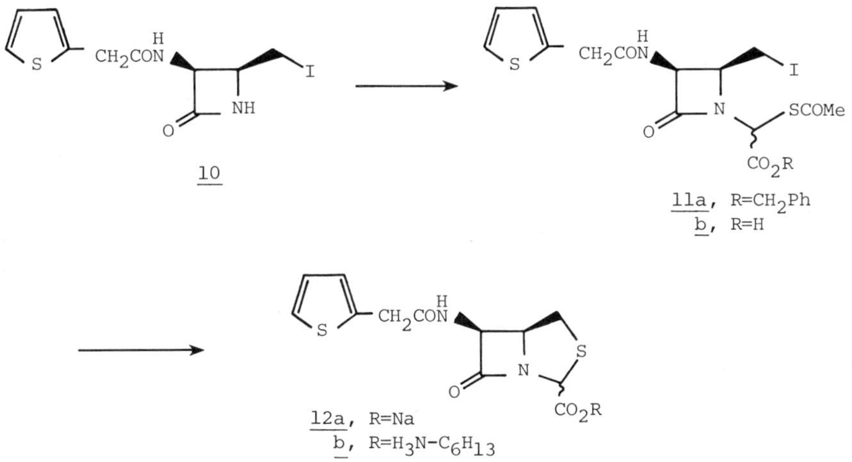

10

11a, R=CH₂Ph
 b, R=H

12a, R=Na
 b, R=H₃N-C₆H₁₃

monocyclic precursor 11b and the isopenicillin 12b showed considerable antibacterial activity against a representative group of organisms (Table 1). Compared to the penicillin and cephalosporin with the same thienyl side chain, the synthetic compounds 11b and 12b were approximately equipotent against gram-negative organisms. However against gram-positive organisms (Staph. and

Strep.) the penicillin and cephalosporin were clearly superior. When one
takes into account that the synthetic compounds are both racemic and a mixture
of carboxylate epimers, a single stereoisomer of 11b or 12b might be expected to
exhibit in vitro activity at lower concentrations than those shown in Table 1.

The unexpected antibacterial activity of the monocyclic precursor 11b de-
serves further comment. Since monocyclic β-lactams are not strained enough to
act as acylating agents, a different explanation for the observed antibacterial
action was sought. In situ hydrolysis of the thioacetyl group of 11b
(possibly enzymatic) followed by spontaneous cyclization to yield the active
species (12b) was an attractive possibility. To test this hypothesis we prepared a number of analogs (13) in which X and Y were varied.[14] The antibacterial activity of this series of compounds correlates very well with
the expected rates of hydrolysis and cyclization. Thus, thiobenzoate 13b was
less active than thioacetate 13a while those derivatives (13c-e) which could
not yield a thiol were inactive. In the series 13a, f-m only those derivatives capable of cyclizing by virtue of a good leaving group were active. A
notable exception is homologous iodide 13m. The cyclization product of 13m
was prepared and found to be inactive, presumably because of insufficient ring
strain (see below).

13

	X = CH$_2$I				Y = SCOMe	
	Y	Relative Potency*			X	Relative Potency
a	SCOMe	A		a	CH$_2$I	A
b	SCOPh	A-		f	CH$_2$Br	A
c	OCOMe	I		g	CH$_2$Cl	A
d	H	I		h	CH$_2$OTs	A-
				i	CH$_2$OAc	I
				j	CH$_2$OH	I
e	N—N (S—S—Me)	I		k	CH$_2$SR	I
				l	CO$_2$Me	I
				m	CH$_2$CH$_2$I	I

* A = good activity, A- = weak activity,
  I = inactive at 200 μg/ml.

Turning our attention to nuclear analogs of cephalosporins, we next investigated the synthesis of isocephalosporins (16) in which the sulfur atom has been
moved one position around the ring.[11] Intermediate 10 was converted to the

TABLE 1

MINIMUM INHIBITORY CONCENTRATIONS (MIC) EXPRESSED IN μg/ml

Compound	Staph. aureus SK&F 23390	Strep. faecalis HH 34358	E. coli SK&F 12140	E. coli HH 33779	Kleb. pneumoniae SK&F 1200	Serratia marcescens ATCC 13880	Proteus morgani 179	Enterobacter aerogenes ATCC 13048
11b[a]	3.1	50	6.3	12.5	3.1	50	50	12.5
12[a]	6.3	50	25	25	25	200	>200	25
Thienyl Penicillin[b]	0.2	1.6	12.5	12.5	25	50	>200	25
Cephalothin	0.1	6.3	3.1	3.1	1.6	>200	>200	6.3

[a] racemic. [b] R.R. Chauvette, et al. (1962) J. Amer. Chem. Soc., 84, 3401.

TABLE 2

MINIMUM INHIBITORY CONCENTRATIONS (MIC) EXPRESSED IN μg/ml

Compound[a]	Staph. aureus SK&F 23390	Strep. faecalis HH 34358	E. coli SK&F 12140	Kleb. pneumoniae SK&F 1200	Salmonella paratyphi ATCC 12176	Serratia marcescens ATCC 13880	Enterobacter aerogens ATCC 13048	Enterobacter cloacae HH 31254
16b (racemic)[b]	12.5	>200	12.5	6.3	3.1	200	25	25
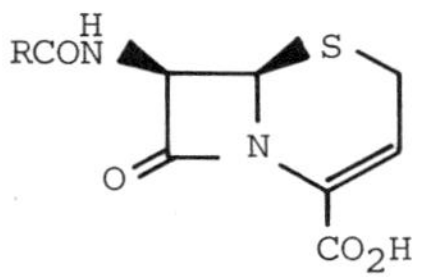 (structure)	1.6	100	25	3.1	3.1	>200	>200	>200

[a] R = 2-thienylmethyl. [b] One isomer of 16b would be expected to have twice the activity of the racemic mixture.

corresponding thiol (14) by displacement with the sodium salt of trityl
mercaptan followed by cleavage of the trityl group with silver nitrate.
Alkylation of 14 with benzhydryl bromopyruvate afforded the bicyclic carbinolamide 15 which was dehydrated to 16a and deblocked to give the free acid (16b)
of the desired isocephalosporin.

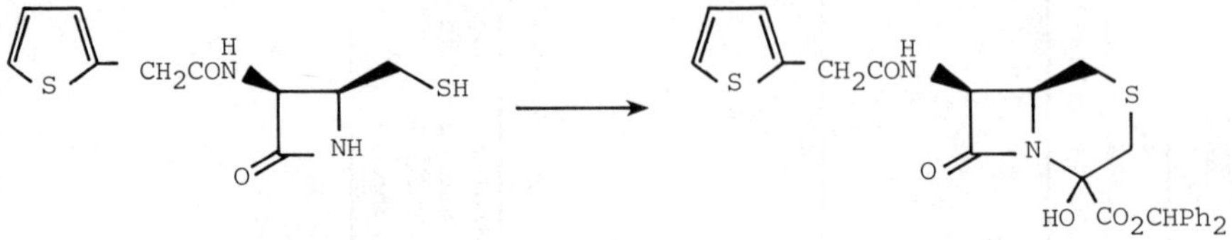

14

15

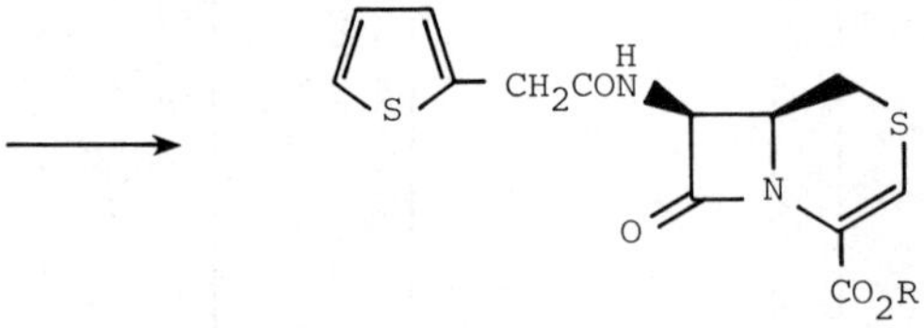

16a, R=CHPh$_2$
 b, R=H

The antibacterial activity of 16b is compared to the corresponding cephalosporin in Table 2. The naturally derived compound shows considerably better
gram-positive activity; but, against gram-negative organisms, the totally
synthetic isocephalosporin (16b) is generally superior.

A functionalized C-3 methyl group, as is present in naturally occurring
cephalosporins, generally leads to compounds possessing enhanced antibacterial
activity.[15] Therefore the synthesis of corresponding derivatives in the
synthetic isocephalosporin series was undertaken. Using a route analogous to
that described above, thiol 17 was prepared from 4. Addition of tert-butyl
3-bromo-2-oxobutyrate gave a mixture of two diastereomeric carbinolamides 18.
Dehydration of one of the diastereomers afforded 19a, which was deblocked to
acid 19b. Free radical bromination of 19a gave the 3-bromomethyl derivative
19c, which was reacted with potassium acetate to afford, after removal of the
t-butyl ester, the 3-acetoxymethyl compound 19d. Contrary to the natural

cephalosporin series, the C-3 substituted isocephalosporins proved to be less potent antibacterial agents than the unsubstituted compound (16b).

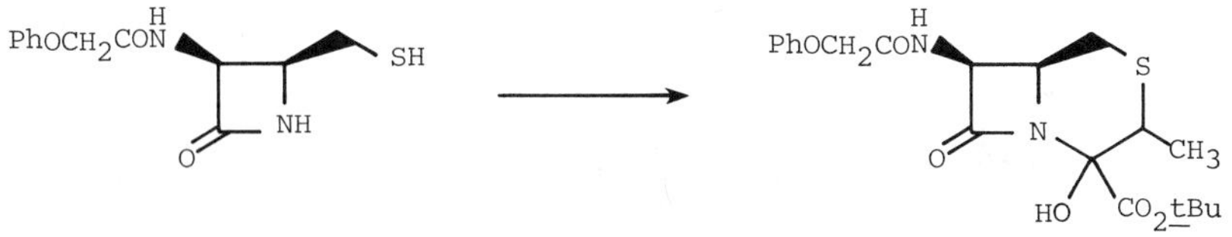

17

18

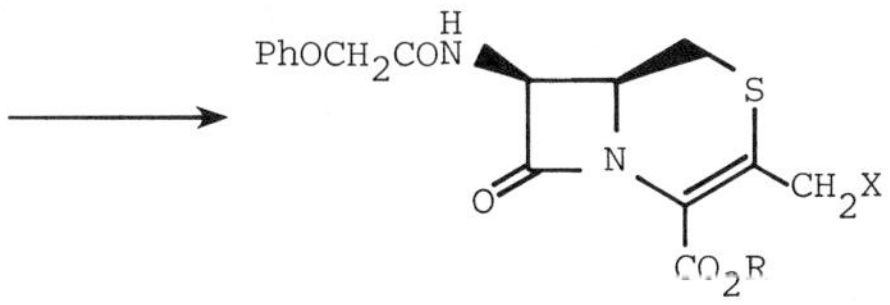

19a, R = t-Bu, X = H
  b, R = H, X = H
  c, R = t-Bu, X = Br
  d, R = H, X = OAc

A somewhat different approach was used to synthesize the benzofused nuclear analogs 22[16] and 25.[17] In the initial β-lactam ring formation step, a benzaldehyde derivative was substituted for glyoxylate. Again, only the desired cis isomers 20 and 23 were formed. In the case of 20, the use of phthaloylglycyl chloride in place of the mixed anhydride of azidoacetic acid led to 20b in greatly improved yield. Both 20a and 20b could be converted to ylide 21 in a series of steps. Hydrolysis of the acetal produced the desired cyclized product 22a directly. Intermediate 23 was likewise converted to the analogous 3-hetero derivative 25a via 24 in a series of steps paralleling the synthesis of the isoazapenicillin nuclear analog (9). Acids 22b and 25b proved to be inactive against a spectrum of gram-positive and gram-negative organisms at concentrations as high as 1000 μg/ml. An exception was B. subtilis which was sensitive to 22b at 25 μg/ml. Since carbocyclic nuclear analogs of cephalosporin lacking the fused benzo ring[18-20] retain good antibacterial activity, the finding of little or no activity for 22b suggests that additional steric bulk or other factors resulting from benzo fusion at positions 1 and 2 are detrimental to binding at the killing site. That reactivity of the β-lactam is not the explanation for the lack of activity of 22b was demonstrated by measuring its rate of reaction with hydroxylamine. Compared to several biologically active desacetoxycephalosporins, 22b reacted approximately 20 times faster.

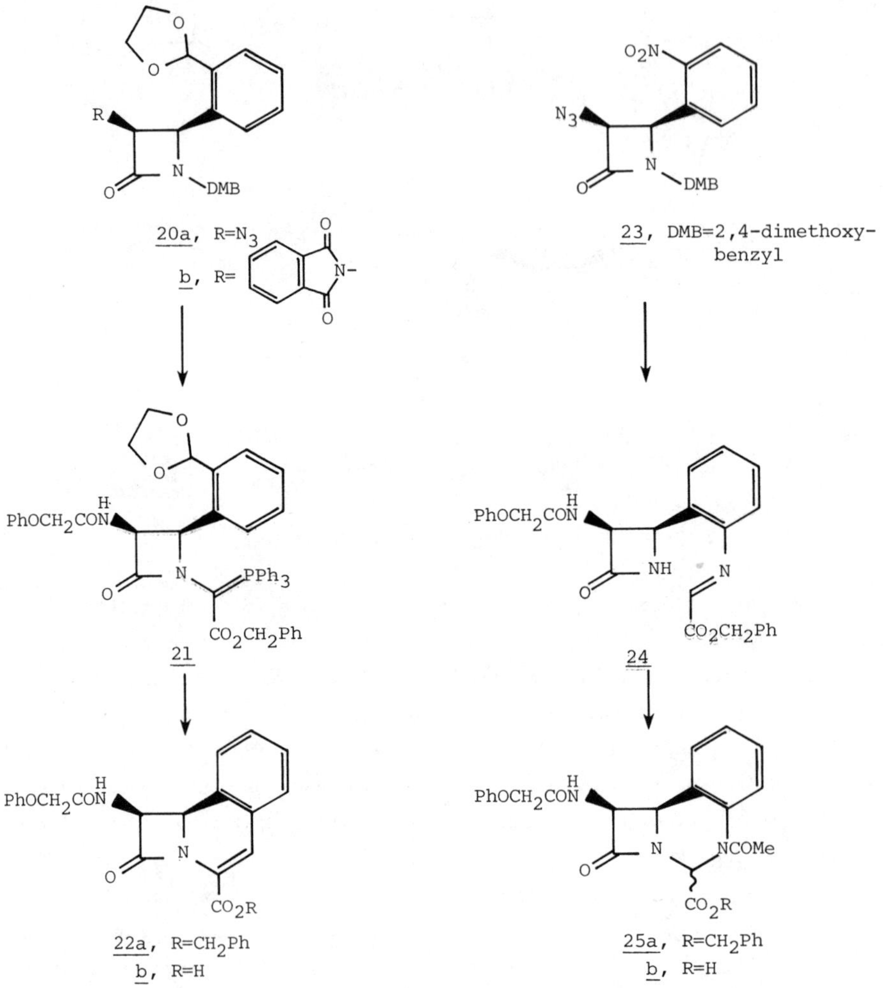
R
O
N
DMB
O
20a, R=N3
b, R=
N-
O_2N
N_3
23, DMB=2,4-dimethoxy-benzyl
PhOCH2CON
H
PPh3
CO2CH2Ph
21
NH
24
NCOMe
CO2R
22a, R=CH2Ph
b, R=H
25a, R=CH2Ph
b, R=H

Since benzo fusion proved detrimental in the case of 22b, 3-hetero structures analogous to 25b which lack benzo fusion were investigated.[21] Hydrolysis of the ester function of monocyclic intermediate 4 followed by coupling with various hydrazines in the presence of dicyclohexylcarbodimide gave hydrazides 26. Cyclization with benzyl glyoxylate followed by hydrogenolysis of the

benzyl ester gave nuclear analogs 27-30 as mixtures of carboxylate epimers.
In the case of 27, the epimers were separated and tested for antibacterial
activity. Both showed modest activity against Staph. aureus (MIC = 200 µg/ml).
Compound 28 showed somewhat improved activity (MIC = 25 µg/ml) while 29 and 30
were inactive against B. subtilis at 500 µg/ml.

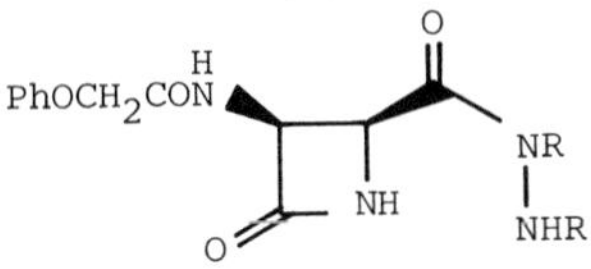

26a, R + R' = $CH_2CH_2CH_2CH_2$
b, R + R' = $CH_2CH_2CH_2$
c, R + R' = CH_2CH_2CO
d, R = H, R' = CO_2CH_3

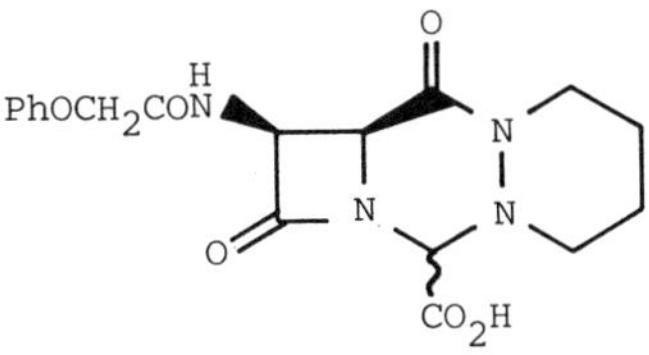

27

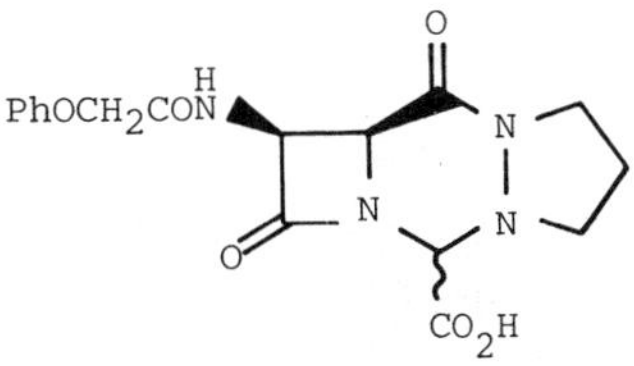

28

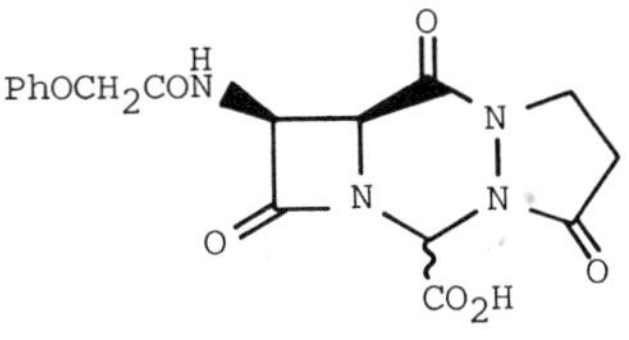

29

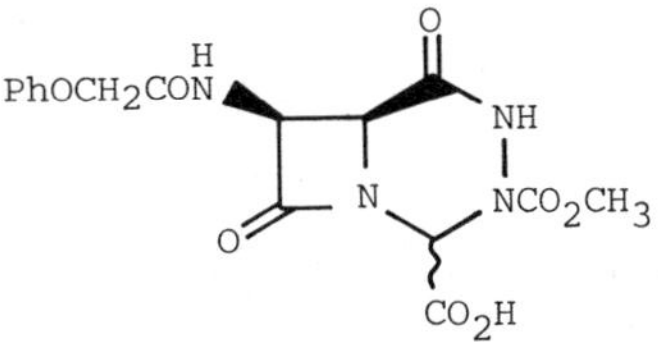

30

Since the carbonyl function at position 1 and additional heteroatom at
position 2 in structures 27-30 were additional complications in assessing the
effect of ring size on antibacterial activity, we prepared ring-expanded
analogs of isoazapenicillin 9 (32)[22] and isopenicillin 11 (33)[22] as well as

the oxa analog (34).[23]   Photolytic Arndt-Eistest homologation of 6 followed by
reduction gave alcohol 31 which served as a common intermediate for 32-34.

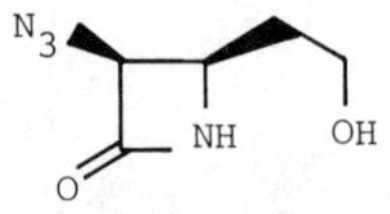

31

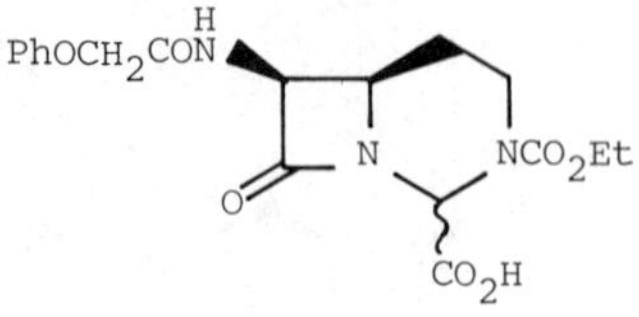

32

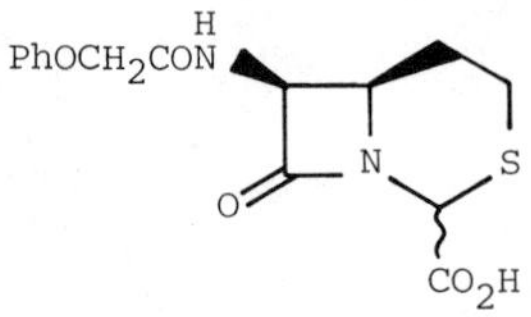

33

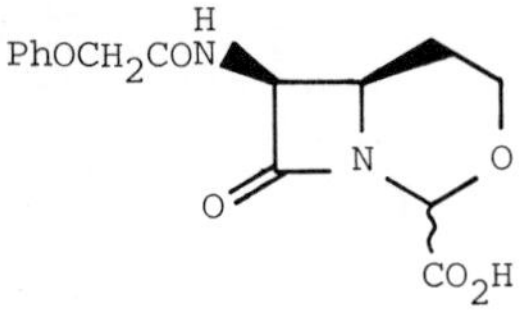

34

All of the 3-heterocephalosporin derivatives (32-34) lacked appreciable
antibacterial activity (MIC >500 µg/ml vs. B. subtilis). This finding is not
unanticipated since a number of other saturated 4:6 bicyclic β-lactams prepared by other research groups[7-9, 24-26] were also found to be inactive,
presumably because of the absence of significant ring strain. In light of
these results it was clear that additional steric or electronic activation of
the β-lactam would be required to obtain antibacterial activity in ring systems
of this type.

With this goal in mind we undertook the synthesis[27] of a C-2 functionalized
derivative of 34. Intermediate 6 was converted to 35a by selective reduction
of the ester function to an alcohol followed by reoxidation. Condensation with
nitromethane followed by dehydration and reduction gave 35b which was converted
directly to dimethoxyacetal 35c by a modified Nef reaction. Oxidative cleavage
of the 2,4-dimethoxybenzyl group followed by thermal condensation with benzyl
glyoxylate produced carbinolamide 36 as separable mixture of diastereomers.
Cyclization of one of the diastereomers gave 37 whose structure was tentatively
assigned on the basis of nmr coupling constants and mechanistic considerations.
The other diastereomer gave an inseparable mixture of cyclic acetals 38 which
were epimeric at C-2. Reduction of the azide function of 37 and 38 followed by

acylation with phenoxyacetyl chloride or O-formylmadelic acid and hydrogenolysis of the benzyl ester gave 39 and 40. The antibacterial activities
of acids 39a, 40a and 39b are compared with the analogous naturally derived
cephalosporins in Table 3. Stereoisomers 39a and 39b exhibited diminished
gram-positive activity but were somewhat superior to the analogous cephalosporins against gram-negative bacteria. Moreover, low doses of 39b protected
rats against a lethal infection of E. coli. The oral (P.O.) dose required for
protection was significantly lower than the corresponding cephalosporin.
Surprisingly, the corresponding α-carboxylic acids (40a) were not active at
400 µg/ml. Acids 40b (not in table) were much less active than 39b when
compared vs. B. subtilis at 100 and 500 µg/ml.

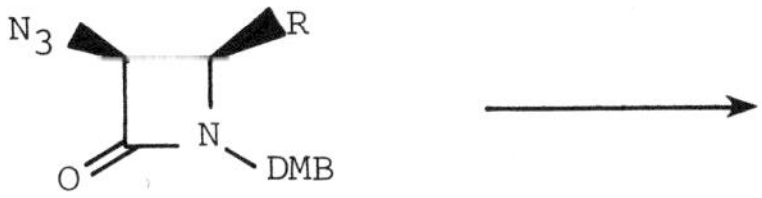

35a, R = CHO
b, R = CH$_2$CH$_2$NO$_2$
c, R = CH$_2$CH(OMe)$_2$

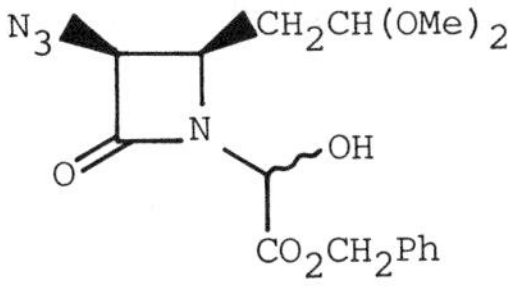

36

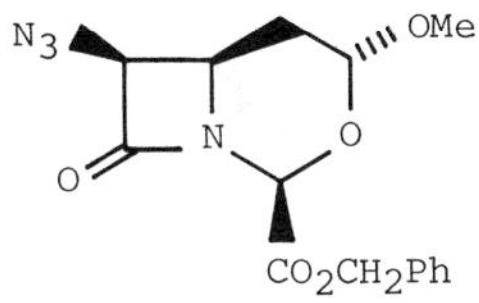

37

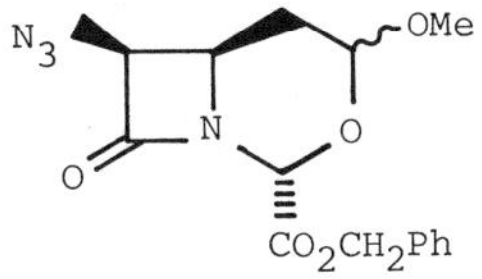

38

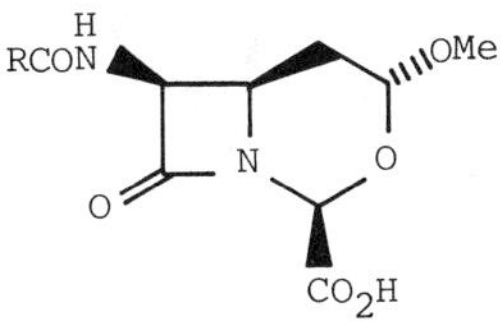

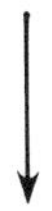

39a, R = PhOCH$_2$
b, R = PhCH(OCHO)

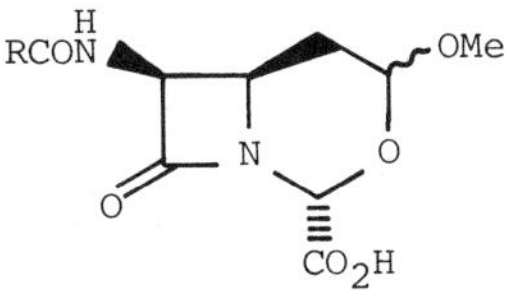

40a, R = PhOCH$_2$
b, R = PhCH(OCHO)

TABLE 3

MINIMUM INHIBITORY CONCENTRATIONS (µg/ml)

STRUCTURE	Staph. aureus HH 127	Strep. faecalis HH 34358	E. coli SK&F 12140	Kleb. pneumoniae SK&F 1200	Proteus morgani 179	Salmonella paratyphi ATCC 12178	Serratia marcescens ATCC 13880	Enterobacter cloacoe HH 31254	IN VIVO: ED$_{50}$ [a] E. coli SK&F 12140 S.C.	IN VIVO: ED$_{50}$ [a] E. coli SK&F 12140 P.O.
39a [b]	50	>200	100	50	200	50	>200	200		
40a (PhOCH$_2$CONH–cephem, 3‑CH$_3$, 4‑CO$_2$H)	>400	>400	>400	>400	>400	>400	>400	>400		
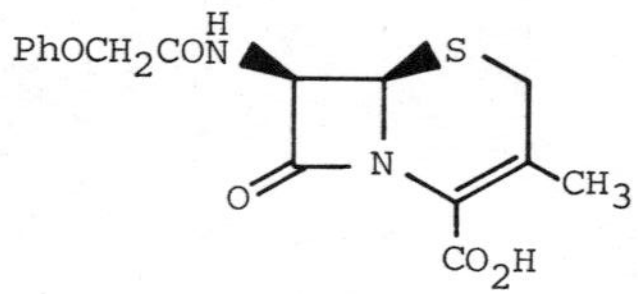	0.8	200	>400	>400	>400	>400	>400	>400		
39b [b] (PhCH(OH)CONH–cephem, 3‑CH$_2$OCOMe, 4‑CO$_2$H)	100	>200	6.3	6.3	25	3.1	25	6.3	15.5	25
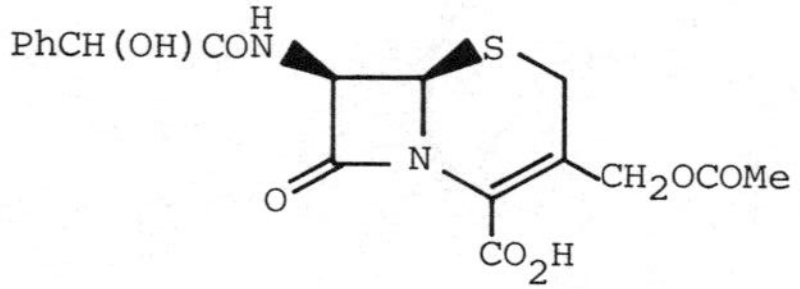	16	25	3.1	1.6	200	1.6	200	3.1	6.2	100

a) Protective dose (mg/kg) against a lethal infection of E. coli bacterium in rats.

b) One isomer of 39a and 39b would be expected to have twice the activity of the racemic mixture.

The observation of potent antibacterial activity for 4:6 bicyclic β-lactams lacking unsaturation in the six-membered ring was quite unexpected and would appear to be of considerable theoretical importance. As previously noted, none of the related saturated 4:6 bicyclic β-lactams possess significant anti-bacterial activity; even an isomeric 2-oxa-3-ethoxy structure did not exhibit useful activity.[28] Beside the lack of precedent for antibacterial activity in saturated systems of this type, the assigned configuration of the carboxylic acid in both biologically active isomers 39a and 39b is opposite to that of the naturally occurring penicillins. To provide further information about strain and to determine unambiguously the stereochemistry of this novel ring system, an x-ray crystallographic study of 37 was undertaken. The results of this analysis are summarized and compared with other β-lactams in Table 4. The molecular geometry is illustrated in Figure 1.

TABLE 4

STRUCTURAL CHARACTERISTICS OF 3-OXACEPHALOSPORIN AND REPRESENTATIVE β-LACTAM ANTIBIOTICS[a]

Compound	Sum of Bond Angles about Nitrogen (deg)	Distance of N Atom from Plane of Three Substituents (Å)	β-Lactam Bond (N-CO) Length (Å)
37	350.5	.24	1.360
Cephaloridine	350.7	.24	1.382
Cephalosporin-C	345	.32	1.385
Penicillin V	337	.40	1.46
Δ^2-Cephem	359.3	.06	1.355

[a] All data other than that for 37 abstracted from Sweet, R.M. (1972) in "Cephalosporins and Penicillins; Chemistry and Biology" Flynn, E.H., Ed., Academic Press, N.Y., Chapter 7.

In the crystal state, the six membered ring exists in a chair conformation with the carboxyl group in an equatorial conformation and the methoxy group axial, as predicted above. The β-lactam nitrogen is not planar, but is 0.24Å above the plane defined by the β-lactam carbonyl, C-4 and the bridgehead carbon. This deformation, which significantly increases the reactivity of the β-lactam, presumably results from fusion of the second ring. The magnitude of the deformation is similar to that observed for active cephalosporins and is significantly greater than the inactive Δ^2-cephalosporin isomers.[13] The observed spatial orientation of the carboxylic acid group is very similar to

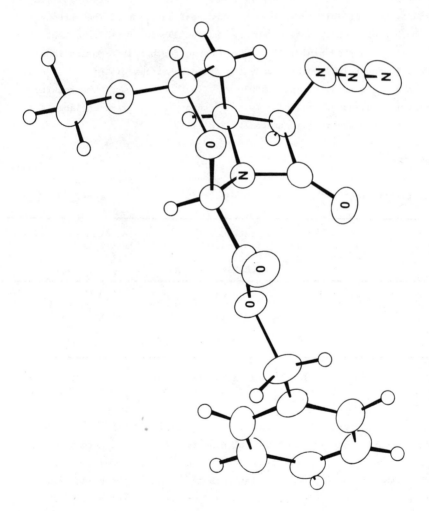

Figure 1. The x-ray structure of 3-oxacephalosporin 37.

that seen in the active Δ^3-cephalosporins.[3] This would suggest that the relationship between the carboxyl group and the β-lactam bond, and not the relative configuration of the carboxyl, may be important for enzyme recognition and antibacterial activity.

The lack of antibacterial activity of the desmethoxy analog (34) suggests that the methoxyl group contributes significantly to biological activity. In the crystal state, the methoxy group does not appear to be sterically crowded, and it is therefore unlikely that the observed effect is purely of steric origin. However, from the available data, it is not possible to ascertain if the methoxyl group merely serves to increase the strain and hence the reactivity of the β-lactam, or if further fragmentation to a reactive species following enzymatic cleavage of the β-lactam is important in imparting the observed potent antibacterial activity.

The concept of further fragmentation to reactive species can be illustrated with cephalosporins (41a) where the group X has been shown to be expelled during β-lactam cleavage.[29] There is also an apparent correlation between antibacterial activity and the ability of X to act as a leaving group.[5, 30, 31] This trend appears more pronounced in the cephamycins (41b) since 41b (X = H)[32] is virtually inactive compared to 41b (X = OAc)[33] while 41a (X = H) retains considerable activity compared to 41a (X = OAc).

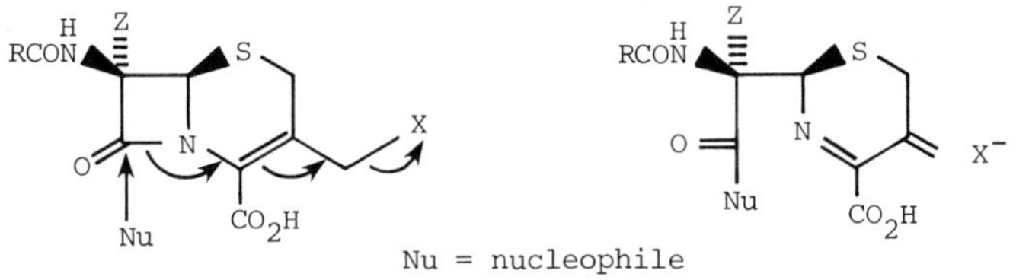

Nu = nucleophile

41a, Z = H
b, Z = OMe

42

When X is itself an antibacterial agent increased antibacterial activity has been observed.[34-36] Whether or not 42, by virtue of its reactive conjugated imine functionality, might also further react when generated in the active site of the target enzyme is not known.

For both penicillins and cephalosporins two additional modes of fragmentation in which sulfur participates are possible. For example, penicillin (43)
can react with a nucleophile (Nu) at the β-lactam carbonyl to produce 44.
Structure 44 contains imine and sulfhydryl groups, both potential enzyme
inactivators. Alternatively, abstraction of the amide proton by a base (B)
results in penicillenic acid (45). This highly reactive substance has been
implicated in penicillin allergy by virtue of its ability to bind covalently
to serum proteins.[37]   It has been observed that rearrangement to penicillenic
acid is markedly accelerated by imidazole,[38] a moiety which might be present in
an enzyme active site in the form of a histadine residue.

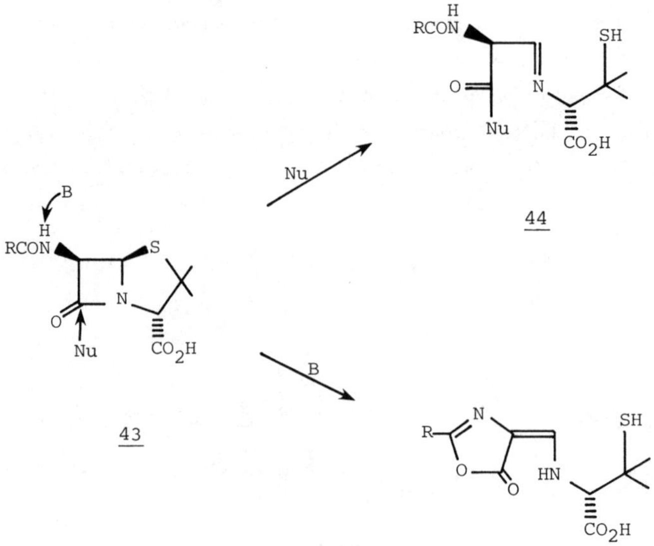

Whether or not species such as 42, 44 and 45 are actually generated in the
active sites of enzymes crucial to bacterial survival and contribute to the
antibacterial activity of penicillins and cephalosporins is not known. However, speculation along these lines led us to choose certain of the nuclear
analogs described above as targets for synthesis and may aid in the explana-

tion of some of our unexpected findings. For example, isopenicillin (11) and related structures can be envisaged to fragment to 46 as shown below. Similarly, 3-oxacephalosporin 39 could yield 47.

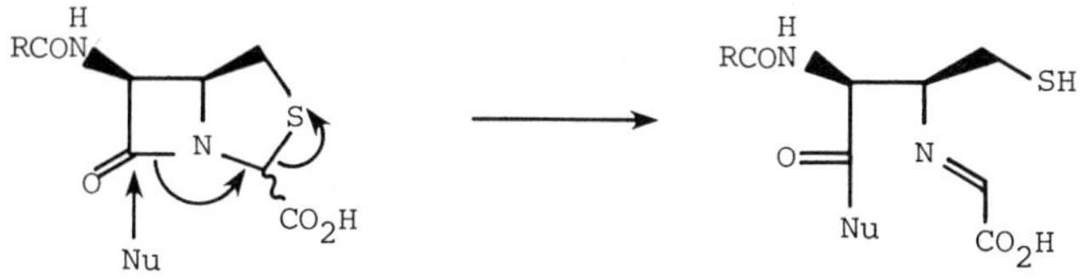

11

46

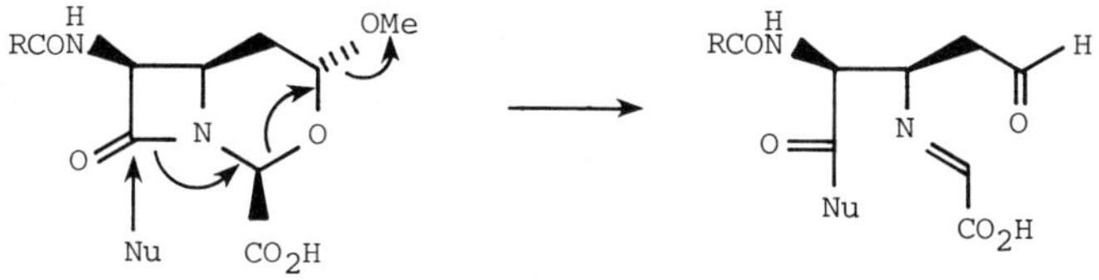

39

47

Since we began our nuclear analog program in the early 1970's, a number of research groups have made important contributions to our understanding of the mechanism of action of β-lactam antibiotics and of the structural requirements for good antibacterial activity. Several other groups have been active in the field of nuclear analog total synthesis.[39,40] During this same time period, two new types of β-lactam antibiotics were isolated from fermentation broths. One of these, clavulanic acid (48), has antibacterial activity, but is most useful as an irreversible inhibitor of bacterial β-lactamase enzymes.[41] The other structural type, represented by thienamycin (49),[42] contains a highly strained and reactive β-lactam system. Thienamycin displays unusually potent antibacterial activity against a broad spectrum of gram-positive and gram-negative microorganisms. Of particular interest is its activity against normally resistant Pseudomonas spp. and its ability to withstand hydrolysis by β-lactamases. The unique structural features of 48 and 49, particularly the complete lack of an amide side chain in 48 and the substitution of a hydroxyethyl group with a trans configuration in 49, required that we revise our previous concepts about the structural requirements for antibacterial activity of bicyclic β-lactams. In a series of steps we were able to prepare the isopenicillin precursors 50[43] and 51[22] corresponding to clavulanic acid and thienamycin. However, although they were expected to undergo in situ cyclization to the isopenicillin nucleus, neither showed antibacterial activity at 500 μg/ml. The failure of 51 to show significant activity is consistent with the reported low potency of the corresponding hydroxyethyl penams and cephams.[44] On the other hand, the penicillin derivative with no functionality at C-6[45] retains weak but signifi-cant activity, and the analogous sulfoxide is reported[46] to be a potent irreversible inhibitor of β-lactamases.

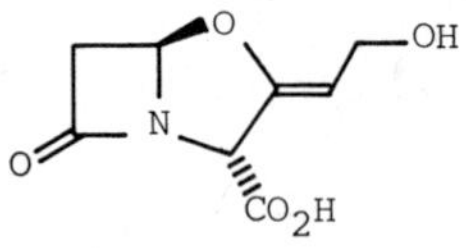

48

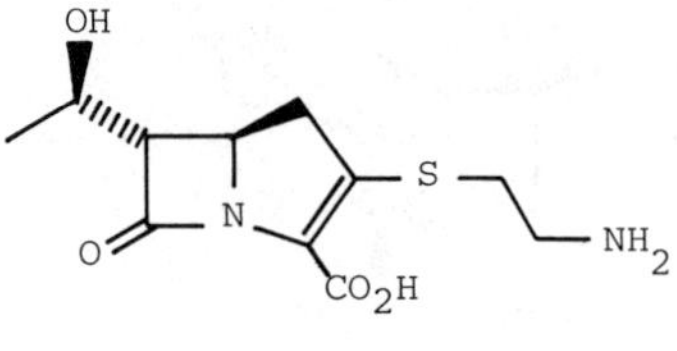

49

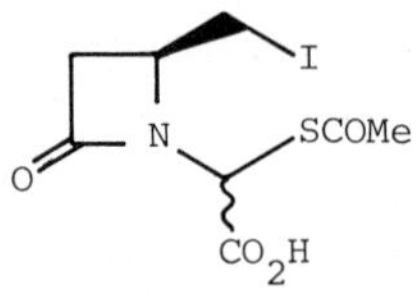

50

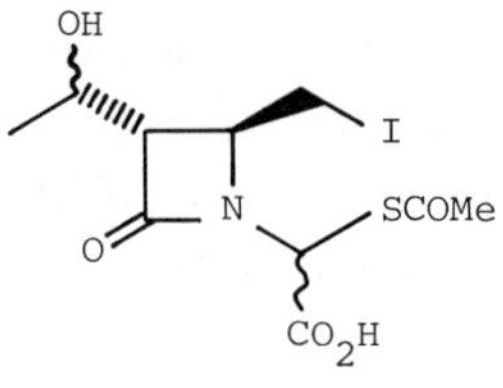

51

More recent mechanism of action studies on β-lactam antibiotics now make it clear that the original proposal by Tipper and Strominger[1] is an oversimplifi-cation. Multiple binding sites for penicillin and related β-lactam anti-biotics have been detected in the membranes of all bacteria that have been

examined and several penicillin-sensitive enzymes that apparently correspond
to some of the binding sites have been identified.[47, 48] The observation that
the concentration of a given β-lactam antibiotic required to compete with
radiolabeled penicillin for irreversible binding sites parallels the concentration required for growth inhibition implies that the binding sites are
synonymous with killing sites.[49] Six distinct penicillin binding proteins
have been identified in the inner membrane of E. coli.[50, 51] On electrophoresis in gels containing sodium dodecylsulfate, they separate according to
molecular weight and have been numbered in order of decreasing size (91,000 →
40,000 daltons). The two smallest proteins, 5 and 6, have been shown to be
equivalent to D-alanine carboxypeptidase which also appears as a doublet under
these conditions of electrophoresis. Although sensitive to penicillin, this
enzyme is not believed to be a normal killing site for most β-lactam antibiotics. Protein 4 is also an unlikely candidate because mutants have been
reported that lack this protein but grow normally[52]. Protein 3 is believed to
be involved in septum formation and cell division.[50, 51] Selective inhibition
of this protein causes the normally rod-shaped cells to become filamentous.
Protein 2 has been shown to be necessary for maintenance of cell shape.[53] Mutants which lack this protein, or normal bacteria treated with an agent that
selectively inhibits it, grow as osmotically stable spherical cells.[50]
Finally, protein 1, which sometimes appears as a doublet (1A and 1B), has been
identified as the peptidoglycan transpeptidase originally described by Tipper
and Strominger[1] as the killing site for penicillin. Selective inhibition of
this enzyme preferentially inhibits cell elongation and causes cell lysis.[50,51]

Although most β-lactam antibiotics bind covalently to some or all of the
same 6 proteins, there are decided differences among them in terms of their
relative affinities. For example, cefoxitin fails to bind to protein 2 while
cephacetrile binds very slowly to proteins 5 and 6. Cephaloridine binds most
avidly to protein 1, the transpeptidase, and inhibits cell elongation and
causes lysis at its minimum inhibitory concentration (MIC). On the other hand,
cephalexin binds preferentially to protein 3 and causes inhibition of cell
division and filament formation at its MIC.[50, 51] CP-35,587, a novel penicillin in which the 3-carboxylic acid has been replaced by a tetrazole, has
the same effect and was found not to be an inhibitor of peptidoglycan transpeptidase.[54]

Mecillinam, a penicillin derivative having an amidine in place of an amide
at C-6, was observed to display an unusual antibacterial spectrum when compared
to ampicillin and benzylpenicillin and to cause the formation of osmotically

stable spherical cells.[55] This antibiotic was subsequently found to bind only to protein 2.[53]

The generality of the findings with E. coli appears to extend to other gram-negative bacteria including Pseudomonas aeruginosa.[56] The observation of multiple binding and killing sites, and the relative specificity of some β-lactams for one or more of these sites makes the exact mechanism of action of a given compound difficult to assess without detailed studies. Although we have observed unexpected results with some of our nuclear analogs in terms of potency and antibacterial spectrum, it is not possible to assign specific mechanisms of action without much more refined experiments. Superimposed on the ability of various β-lactams to irreversibly inactivate specific enzymes required for bacterial cell wall synthesis are questions regarding their stability to spontaneous or enzymatic (β-lactamase)[57] inactivation by hydrolysis as well as their ability to penetrate to the site of action.[58-60] Penetration is of particular concern in the case of gram-negative organisms which are protected by an outer membrane composed largely of lipopolysaccharides.

In summary, total synthesis has provided a number of new bicyclic β-lactams, some of which have antibacterial activity comparable with clinically useful penicillins and cephalosporins. The structural requirements for antibacterial activity and the mechanism of action of these agents are not completely defined. However, a reactive (strained) β-lactam that can function as an acylating agent seems to be required, and enzymes involved in bacterial cell wall synthesis are probably the major target.

REFERENCES

1. Tipper, D.J. and Strominger, J.L. (1965) Proc. Natl. Acad. Sci. U.S.A., 54, 1133.
2. Woodward, R.B. (1949) in "The Chemistry of Penicillin," Clarke, H.T., Johnson, J.R. and Robinson, R., Ed., Princeton University Press, Princeton, N.J., p 440.
3. Sweet, R.M. and Dahl, L.F. (1970) J. Amer. Chem. Soc., 92, 5489.
4. Morin, R.B., Jackson, B.G., Mueller, R.A., Lavagnino, E.R., Scanlon, W.B. and Andrews, S.L. (1969) J. Amer. Chem. Soc., 91, 1401.
5. Indelicato, J.M., Norvilas, T.T., Pfeiffer, R.R., Wheeler, W.J. and Wilham, W.L. (1974) J. Med. Chem., 17, 523.
6. Hoover, J.R.E. and Stedman, R.J. (1970) in "Medicinal Chemistry" 3rd ed., Burger A. Ed., Wiley-Interscience, N.Y., p 371.
7. Van Heynigen, E. and Ahern, L.K. (1968) J. Med. Chem., 11, 933 (1968).
8. Brunwin, D.M., Lowe, G. and Parker, J. (1971) J. Chem. Soc. C, 3756.
9. Brunwin, D.M. and Lowe, G. (1973) J. Chem. Soc. Perkin I, 1321.
10. Huffman, W.F., Holden, K.G., Buckley, T.F., Gleason, J.G., and Wu, L. (1977) J. Amer. Chem. Soc., 99, 2352.
11. Bryan, D.B., Hall, R.F., Holden, K.G., Huffman, W.F. and Gleason, J.G. (1977) J. Amer. Chem. Soc., 99, 2353.

12. Moore, H.W., Hernandez, L. and Chambers, R. (1978) J. Amer. Chem. Soc., 100, 2245.

13. Huffman, W.F., Hall, R.F., Grant, J.A. and Holden, K.G. (1978) J. Med. Chem., 21, 413.

14. Huffman, W.F., Hall, R.F., Perchonock, C.D., Bryan, D.B. and Gleason, J.G., unpublished results.

15. Gorman, M. and Ryan, C.W. (1972) in "Cephalosporins and Penicillins; Chemistry and Biology", Flynn, E.H., Ed., Academic Press, N.Y., Chapter 12.

16. Finkelstein, J., Holden, K.G. and Perchonock, C.D. (1978) Tetrahedron Lett., 1629.

17. Huffman, W.F., unpublished results.

18. Guthikonda, R.N., Cama, L.D. and Christensen, B.G. (1974) J. Amer. Chem. Soc., 96, 7584.

19. Firestone, R.A., Fahey, J.L., Maciejewicz, N.S., Patel, G.S. and Christensen, B.G. (1977). J. Med. Chem., 20, 551.

20. Doyle, T.M., Conway, T.T., Lim, G. and Luh, B.-Y. (1979) Can. J. Chem., 57, 227.

21. Finkelstein, J., Holden, K.G., Sneed, R. and Perchonock, C.D. (1977) Tetrahedron Lett., 1855.

22. Huffman, W.F. and Hall, R.F., unpublished results.

23. Gleason, J.G. and Siler, P., unpublished results.

24. Lowe, G. (1975) Chem. Ind., 459.

25. Woodward, R.B. (1970) Pharm. J., 205, 562.

26. Kukolja, S. (1972) J. Amer. Chem. Soc., 94, 7590.

27. Gleason, J.G., Buckley, T.F., Holden, K.G. and Siler, P. (1979) J. Amer. Chem. Soc., in press.

28. Doyle, T.W., Belleau, B., Luh, B.-Y., Ferrari, C.F. and Cunningham, M.P. (1977) Can. J. Chem., 55, 468.

29. O'Callaghan, C.H., Kirby, S.M., Morris, A., Waller, R.E. and Duncombe, R.E. (1972) J. Bacteriol. 110, 988.

30. Topp, W.C. and Christensen, B.G. (1974) J. Med. Chem., 17, 342.

31. Boyd, D.B., Hermann, R.B., Presti, D.E. and Marsh, M.M. (1975) J. Med. Chem., 18, 408.

32. Jen, T., Frazee, J. and Hoover, J.R.E. (1973) J. Org. Chem., 38, 2857.

33. Cama, L.D., Leanza, W.J., Beattie, T.R., and Christensen, B.G. (1972) J. Am. Chem. Soc., 94, 1408.

34. Russell, A.D. and Fountain, R.H. (1971) J. Bacteriol., 106, 65.

35. O'Callaghan, C.H., Sykes, R.B. and Staniforth, S.E. (1976) Antimicrob. Agents Chemother., 10, 245.

36. Greenwood, D. and O'Grady, F. (1976) Antimicrob. Agents Chemother., 10, 249.

37. Levine, B.B. (1961) Arch. Biochem. Biophys., 93, 50 (1961).

38. Bundgaard, H. (1971) Tetrahedron Lett., 4613.

39. Christensen, B.G. and Ratcliffe, R.W. (1976) in "Annual Reports in Medicinal Chemistry", Clarke, F.H., Ed., Academic Press, N.Y., Vol. 11, Chapter 28.

40. Cama, L.D. and Christensen, B.G. (1978) in "Annual Reports in Medicinal Chemistry", Clarke, F.H., Ed., Academic Press, N.Y., Vol. 13, Chapter 16.

41. Reading, C. and Cole, M. (1977) Antimicrob. Agents Chemother., 11, 852.

42. Alkers-Schonberg, G., Arison, B.H., Hensens, O.D., Hirshfield, J., Hoogsteen, K., Kaczka, E.A., Rhodes, R.E., Kahan, J.S., Kahan, F.M., Ratcliffe, R.W., Walton, E., Ruswinkle, L.J., Morin, R.B., and Christensen, B.G. (1978) J. Amer. Chem. Soc., 100, 6491 and references cited therein.

43. Huffman, W.F. and Grant, J.A., unpublished results.

44. DiNinno, F., Beattie, T.R. and Christensen, B.G. (1977) J. Org. Chem., 42, 2960.

45. Evrard, E., Claesen, M. and Vanderhaeghe, H. (1964) Nature, 201, 1124.

248

248

46. English, A.R., Retsema, J.A., Girard, A.E., Lynch, J.E. and Barth, W.E. (1978) Antimicrob. Agents and Chemother., 14, 414.
47. Blumberg, P.M. and Strominger, J.L. (1974) Bacteriol. Rev., 38, 291.
48. Frere, J-M. (1977) Biochem. Pharmacol., 26, 2203.
49. Park, J.T., Edwards, J.R. and Wise, E.M. (1974) Ann. N.Y. Acad. Sci., 235, 300.
50. Spratt, B.G. (1975) Proc. Natl. Acad. Sci. U.S.A., 72, 2999.
51. Spratt, B.G. (1977) Eur. J. Biochem., 72, 341.
52. Matsuhashi, M., Takagaki, Y., Maruyama, I.N., Tamaki, S., Nishimura, Y., Suzuki, H., Ogino, U. and Hirota, Y. (1977) Natl. Acad. Sci. U.S.A., 74, 2976.
53. Spratt, B.G. and Pardee, A.B. (1975) Nature, 254, 516.
54. Presslitz, J.E. (1978) Antimicrob. Agents Chemother., 14, 144.
55. Lund, F. and Tybring, L. (1971) Natur New Biol., 236, 135.
56. Noguchi, H., Matsuhashi, M., Takaoka, M. and Mitsuhashi, S. (1978) Antimicrob. Agents Chemother., 14, 617.
57. Sykes, R.B. and Matthew, M. (1976) J. Antimicrob. Chemother., 2, 115.
58. Costerton, J.W. and Cheng K.-J. (1975), J. Antimicrob. Chemother., 1, 363.
59. Zimmermann, W. and Rosselet, A. (1977) Antimicrob. Agents Chemother., 12, 368.
60. Sawai, T., Matsuba, K. and Yamagishi, S. (1977) J. Antibiot., 30, 1134.

DISCUSSION

CHU: In your isopenicillin series, you have an intermediate, which can give you the oxygen analogs. Do you have a reason why you did not go into the oxygen series?

HOLDEN: The oxapenicillin, in which the heteroatom is simply replaced, is very unstable[1]. We have actually tried to make the corresponding iso-oxapenicillin without any success, and we think that is becuase it is just too unstable.

CHU: In your O-methoxy series, the configuration of the carboxyl group is reversed, compared to the most active penicillin analogs. Do you have an explanation for this?

HOLDEN: Yes, I can comment on that. If you examine the X-ray structure, the carboxyl group is equitorial and lies close to the plane of the 6-membered ring. In the case of the cephalosporins, which have a Δ^3-double bond, the carboxyl lies in a similar environment because the bond is trigonal. Although the carboxyl of penicillins lies below the plane of the ring, the spacial relationship of this group relative to the β-lactam carbonyl is not very different from the cephalosporins and our active 3-oxacephem isomer. On the other hand, the inactive 3-oxacephem has an axial carboxyl which places it in a decidedly different relative position. In other words, the carboxyl group in our active analog is oriented in such a way that it probably resembles cephalosporins and penicillins closely enough to be recognized by the bacterial enzymes.

HABER: In the isocephem series, where you functionalized the 3-position, have you placed what traditionally are better groups out there to see enhanced activity?

HOLDEN: We have put a few traditionally better groups in the 3-position, but the results were disappointing.

HABER: Would you care to speculate, why the functionalized isocephem was less active than the unfunctionalized one?

HOLDEN: I do not have a good explanation for it. One would think it could eliminate in the same way as occurs in cephalosporins. Whether the sulfur being on the double bond would have an adverse effect on this process and hence on the activity I cannot really say.

DONALD B. BOYD (Lilly Research Laboratories, Eli Lilly and Co., Indianapolis, IN; invited comments): Using hand-held molecular models, it was evident to earlier investigators that a structural analogy existed between penicillins and what seemed to be possible transition state (TS) structures for the scission of the peptide bond in the D-Ala-D-Ala substrate of the peptidoglycan-regulating enzymes. Tipper and Strominger hypothesized a TS structure in general terms of having a nonplanar amide C-N bond so that the bond is weakened. Recently, some preliminary but detailed structural information on the TS's of a dipeptide became available from molecular orbital calculations[2]. In these calculations, glycylglycine was used as a simplified model of D-Ala-D-Ala, and OH$^-$ was used as a nucleophile to approach the peptide carbonyl carbon on either the α or β face. Produced were two transition intermediates with tetrahedral hybridization at the amide nitrogen (Figure 1). Least-squares fitting of the

Figure 1.

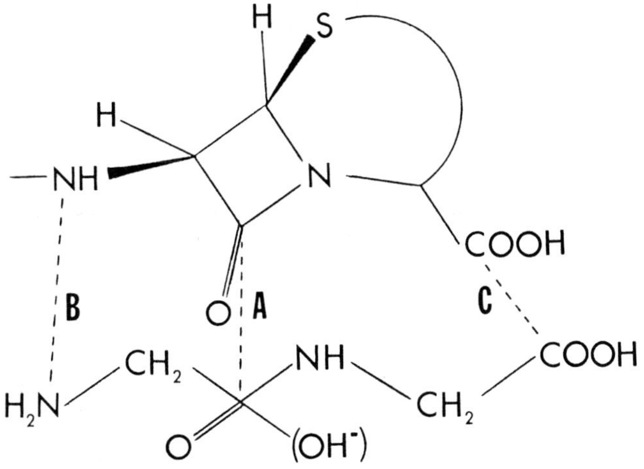

three-dimensional structures of the dipeptide models and some penicillins and cephalosporins was done on the basis of minimizing the distances A, B, and C.

Although further refinement of the dipeptide geometries would be desirable, the findings so far corroborate the idea that the β-lactam antibiotics can, in fact, be acting as TS analogues. Thus, the antibiotics are able to inhibit bacterial cell-wall enzymes by structurally mimicking one of the early geometries in the presumed reaction path for cleavage of the C-terminal D-Ala of the natural substrate. Since the antibiotic structures display a range of dimensions between some of the key atoms, the functionalities in the active sites may be able to adjust position upon binding to the inhibitors or substrate. The flexibility of the peptide substrate and the ability of the antibiotics to conformationally match the parent dipeptide not too poorly make understandable the fact that other large molecules besides the enzymes (such as vancomycin) can have an affinity for either.

Some recent theoretical work has been reported[3] for clavulanic acid. The five-membered ring was found to prefer a single conformation with 3α-COOH roughly axial, which is one of the two conformations that a thiazolidine ring of penicillins may adopt. It was speculated that clavulanic acid may competitively inhibit β-lactamases because it exists as a single conformer, whereas penicillins would exist as a mixture of axial and equatorial conformers with the latter being more stable. Further investigation would be valuable in determining the importance of the conformational properties of clavulanic acid relative to the reactivity properties of the acyl-enzyme intermediates* that it can form[5].

REFERENCES

1. Cama, L.D., and Christensen, B.G. (1978) Tetrahedron Lett. 4233.
2. Boyd, D.B., (1979) J. Med. Chem. 22, 533.
3. Rao, V.S.R., Joshi, N.V., and Virudachalam, R. (1978) Curr. Sci. India 47, 933.
4. Fisher, J.F. (1979) this volume.
5. Fisher, J., Charnas, R.L. and Knowles, J.R. (1978) Biochemistry 17, 2180.

---

*The topic of Dr. Fisher's presentation[4].

β-LACTAMASE INHIBITION AND INACTIVATION *VIA* ACYL-ENZYME INTERMEDIATES

JED F. FISHER[*]
Department of Chemistry, Harvard University, 12 Oxford Street, Cambridge,
Massachusetts 02138

SUMMARY

    Bacterial resistance to β-lactam antibiotics most often arises from the
acquisition by the bacterium of the β-lactamase enzyme.[1,2] We have been interested in the mechanistic aspects of this enzyme, and in particular whether an
understanding of its mechanism[3] might explain the ability of some of the newer
classes of β-lactams to inhibit this enzyme. From this understanding the
structural features responsible for such inhibition may be identified, perhaps
allowing the more rational design of a β-lactam that combines immunity to β-
lactamase action with the retention of antibiotic activity.

    To illuminate the pathway by which the *E. coli* RTEM-1 β-lactamase catalyzes
the hydrolysis of β-lactam substrates, the hydrolysis of a 7α-methoxy-cephalo-
sporin, cefoxitin, has been studied. Cefoxitin is hydrolyzed sufficiently
slowly to permit direct observation of the formation, and then the rate-
limiting decomposition of an intermediate during the course of each turnover.
The existence of this intermediate has been corroborated by chemical and
spectroscopic means, that have allowed its identification as an acyl-enzyme
species.[4] This is the first clear indication that β-lactamase catalysis passes
through an acyl-enzyme intermediate. Not only does this raise the possibility
of acyl-enzyme formation as an initial event in the enzymatic hydrolysis of
other substrates, but it also clarifies the interpretation of the mechanism of
the known substrate inactivators of the enzyme.[5] The available evidence,
married to the notion of an acyl-enzyme, suggests that inactivation involves the
formation from the acyl-enzyme, of a chromophoric species possessing a double
bond between C-5 and C-6 in which both rings have been opened. This sequence
of acylation followed by fragmentation may account for β-lactamase inactivation
by clavulanic acid,[6-11] 6β-bromopenicillanic acid[12,13] and by the penicillin
sulfones.[10,14,15] Should this hypothesis be sustained, the structural criteria
for inactivators of the β-lactamase may be enumerated. The β-lactam
inactivator must possess a hydrogen on C-6, and an adequate leaving group on

---

[*]Present address: Department of Chemistry, University of Minnesota,
Minneapolis, Minnesota 55455

C-5, to permit facile fragmentation. Further, the β-lactam must be one that forms a relatively long-lived acyl-enzyme, to provide maximal opportunity for fragmentation to compete with de-acylation. As an illustration of the predictive success of these principles, we have extended the ideas of English *et al*.[14] and of Cartwright and Coulson[10] regarding penicillin sulfone inactivators, to the synthesis of (*inter alia*) quinicillin sulfone.[15] This molecule incorporates the features mentioned above, and is one of the most efficient inactivators of the RTEM β-lactamase.

The experiments described are fully reported in the proceedings of two very recent meetings: "Enzyme Inhibitors as Drugs" (ref. 15) and "50 Years After Fleming" (ref. 5).

REFERENCES

1. Abraham, E.P. (1977), J. Antibiotics, 30, S1-S26.
2. Fisher, J. and Knowles, J.R. (1978), Ann. Rep. Med. Chem., 13, 239-248.
3. Cama, L.D. and Christensen, B.G. (1978), Ann. Rep. Med. Chem., 13, 149-158.
4. Fisher, J., Belasco, J.G., Khosla, S. and Knowles, J.R. (1979), manuscript in preparation.
5. Fisher, J., Belasco, J.G., Charnas, R.L. and Knowles, J.R. (1979), Phil. Trans. Roy. Soc. London, in press.
6. Charnas, R.L., Fisher, J. and Knowles, J.R. (1978), Biochemistry, 17, 2185-2189.
7. Fisher, J., Charnas, R.L. and Knowles, J.R. (1978), Biochemistry, 17, 2180-2184.
8. Charnas, R.L., Fisher, J. and Knowles, J.R. (1978) in Enzyme-Activated Irreversible Inhibitors, Seiler, N., Jung, M., and Koch-Weser, J., Eds. Elsevier-North-Holland Press, Amsterdam, pp. 315-322.
9. Labia, R. and Peduzzi, J. (1978), Biochim. Biophys. Acta, 526, 572-579.
10. Cartwright, S.J. and Coulson, A.F.W. (1979), Nature (London), 278, 360-361.
11. Reading, C. and Hepburn, P. (1979), Biochem. J., 179, 67-76.
12. Pratt, R.F. and Loosemore, M.J. (1978), Proc. Natl. Acad. Sci. U.S.A., 75, 4145-4149.
13. Knott-Hunziker, V., Orlek, B.S., Sammes, P.G. and Waley, S.G. (1979), Biochem. J., 177, 365-367.
14. English, A.R., Retsema, J.A., Girard, A.E., Lynch, J.E. and Barth, W.E. (1978), Antimicrob. Agents Chemother., 14, 414-419.
15. Fisher, J. and Knowles, J.R. (1979) in Enzyme Inhibitors as Drugs, Sandler, M., Ed., Macmillan Press, Ltd., London, in press.

DISCUSSION

QUESTION from the audience: You presented a possible mechanism for β-lactamase inactivation by the olivanic acid carbapenems, of acyl-enzyme formation followed by deprotonation at C-6 and consequent elimination of the sulfate to form an α,β-unsaturated carbonyl system. Does this imply that an olivanic acid derivative that has only an hydroxyethyl sidechain would be no good as an inhibitor?

FISHER: Not necessarily. The experimental data suggests that a very good *competitive* inhibitor (which the Pfizer compound, CP 45,899, is) would also act synergistically with other β-lactam antibiotics and would, therefore, be efficacious *in vivo*. So, as far as these non-sulfated carbapenems are concerned, they may well show synergy *in vivo*, as a consequence of competitive inhibition rather than irreversible inactivation of the enzyme.

HABER: The mechanism that you show for the inactivation by clavulanic acid of the β-lactamase, shows protonation of the allylic double bond during the elimination across the C_5-C_6 bond. Some people have suggested that one could write an equally good mechanism having protonation of the allylic alcohol, leading to an α,β-unsaturated ketone, which provides another mechanism for perhaps a double inactivation of the enzyme. Do you have any evidence in favor of the mechanism you propose, over this alternative one?

FISHER: I think what you are saying is that the allylic hydroxyl would then be essential to the inactivation mechanism, right?

HABER: Yes, I would think that for clavulanate, *per se,* it might be involved. I know that the synthetic group at Beecham have made a number of analogs, but until the bound system is actually isolated, one may not be able to tell.

FISHER: Well, this mechanism was certainly a valid possibility, that we were aware of when we began our work on clavulanic acid. As a result, we asked the group at Beecham if they could kindly supply us with 9-deoxyclavulanic acid, which has had the allylic hydroxyl removed by catalytic hydrogenation. When we looked at this compound, we found that it duplicated clavulanic acid in its behaviour, in every respect that we could quantify. This implies that the allylic hydroxyl of clavulanic acid is completely irrelevant as far as the inactivation of the β-lactamase is concerned.

JUNG: Your mechanism for the β-lactamase inactivation implies a basic residue in the active-site responsible for the abstraction of the α-hydrogen atom on C-6. Would you care to speculate if that residue plays any role in the acylation or deacylation of the enzyme reacting with a normal substrate?

FISHER: We had considered this as a possibility ourselves, and in particular we wished to determine whether or not solvent deuterium is incorporated
into C-6 of the product released during normal substrate hydrolysis. The
answer to this is a resounding no. The conclusion that you are left with is
that this is either a unique feature of the active site that appears only with
these inactivators, or that it is a reflection of the chemical instability of
the acyl-enzymes formed by these inactivators.

JUNG: May I make a suggestion. A couple of years ago, Prof. B. Belleau
(Dept. of Chemistry, McGill University, Montreal) suggested during a conference
at the Centennial Meeting of the American Chemical Society (New York, April
1976) that the normal deacylation occurs as follows: a basic group of the
enzyme abstracts the hydrogen form the amide on C-6, this triggers azalactone
formation with concomitant elimination of the acylated enzyme residue. Since
the hydrogen atom at C-6 is in this vicinity, is it possible that the same
basic group given no other choice, can remove this hydrogen atom?

FISHER: Yes, that is an interesting possibility. An area of this whole
field that chemists, including ourselves, I am sorry to say, have been
negligent in is in looking at the chemical structures of the products produced
during these reactions. One of the complications that is encountered in doing
this is the fact that not only are many of the β-lactams intrinsically unstable, but the products resulting from β-lactam cleavage are even more so.
Nevertheless, there is certainly room for this sort of mechanistic investigation to proceed. The presence of a 6-amide substituent is not necessary to
the efficient enzymatic hydrolysis of a β-lactam, however; the C-6 unsubstituted penem shown below, is hydrolyzed at a rate fully 36% of benzylpenicillin
using the RTEM-1 β-lactamase as a catalyst.

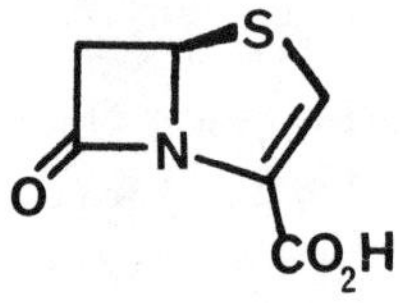

KALMAN: Is there any analogy between the fragmentation of clavulanic acid,
when it is bound to the β-lactamase, and the fragmentation of penicillins
bound to the penicillin binding target proteins?

FISHER: Clavulanate is particularly exemplary of the chemical instability
that follows β-lactam cleavage; the chemists at Beecham have detected upward

of a half a dozen products arising from chemical solvolysis of clavulanate. Although this is not meant to imply that penicillins and cephalosporins yield only a single product from their solvolysis[1]. What is interesting, though, is that the release of the penicillin product(s) from the penicillin binding proteins does not correspond to a simple deacylation of an acyl-enzyme, even though an acyl-enzyme is initially formed[2,3]. This raises the possibility that the inactivation of the β-lactamase by specific inactivators, and the inactivation of the penicillin binding proteins by penicillins and cephalosporins, may have some common mechanistic features.

REFERENCES

1. Ross, G. and O'Callaghan, C. (1975) Methods Enzymol. 43, 69-85.
2. Kozarich, J. and Strominger, J. (1978) J. Biol. Chem. 253, 1272-1278.
3. Adriaens, P., Meesschaert, B., Frère, J.-M., Vanderhaeghe, H., Degelaen, J., Ghuysen, J.-M. and Eyssen, H. (1978) J. Biol. Chem. 253, 3660-3665.

IV
Molecular Design

Published 1979 by Elsevier North Holland, Inc.
Kalman, ed. Drug Action and Design: Mechanism-Based Enzyme Inhibitors

AFFINITY LABELING OF SERINE PROTEASES WITH AN ACTIVE SITE DIRECTED IRREVERSIBLE
INHIBITOR

MICHAEL CORY[+], DAVID H. BING[++] AND JUDITH M. ANDREWS[++]
[+]Organic Chemistry Department, Burroughs Wellcome Co., 3030 Cornwallis Rd.,
Research Triangle Park, NC 27709; [++] Center for Blood Research, 800 Huntington
Avenue., Boston, MA 02115

INTRODUCTION

Serine proteases comprise a class of enzymes characterized by a serine
residue at the catalytic site.[1] Serine proteases are involved in a wide
variety of biologic functions including digestion, blood coagulation, complement activation, reproduction and fibrinolysis. The specificity exhibited
by enzymes of this class varies greatly; from general proteases like trypsin[2]
and chymotrypsin[3] with very broad substrate specificity to the complement
proteins which will hydrolyze only one or two protein substrates.[4,5]

The specificity exhibited by these enzymes can be divided into two
general types. The first type of specificity is determined by the C-terminal
amino acid residue of the peptide bond to be cleaved. Therefore, while both
trypsin and chymotrypsin hydrolyze many of the same protein substrates,
trypsin hydrolyzes a peptide bond C-terminal to a lysyl or arginyl residue[2]
and chymotrypsin cleaves a peptide bond C-terminal to an aromatic amino acid.[3]
In the case of the tryptic enzymes the presence of an aspartate residue in the
binding site accounts for the specificity for positively charged amino acids.[3]

The second type of specificity exhibited by serine proteases is more
poorly understood. For example, plasmin, thrombin and C1s̄, a subcomponent of
the first component of complement are all tryptic proteases with specificity
for a peptide bond with a C-terminal lysyl or arginyl residue.[6-8] However,
while plasmin will hydrolyze a wide variety of protein substrates,[7] thrombin
will hydrolyze only a few,[6,9] and C1s̄ is known to hydrolyze only the second
and fourth components of complement.[4] The chemical basis for the exquisite
specificity of these enzymes is not known.

Active site directed irreversible inhibitors (affinity labeling reagents)
such as diisopropylfluorophosphate (DIFP) and phenylmethanesulfonylfluoride
have been used extensively to investigate the reactive groups in the active
site (A of Figure 1) of enzymes.[10] These reagents react with residues
within the catalytic site of the enzyme and have been designated by Baker as
"endo" affinity labeling reagents.[11] Baker and his coworkers have charac-

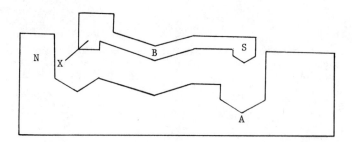

Figure 1.

terized a second type of affinity labeling reagent, the "exo" reagent.[11]
The exo affinity labeling reagent binds to residues outside the catalytic
site and consists of three distinct regions of activity.[11,12] The first
region of activity is a group (S of Figure 1) which will interact with the
enzyme active site; the second (B of Figure 1) consists of a bridging or
spacer group; and the third is a chemically reactive group (X of Figure 1)
located near an enzyme surface nucleophilic group.

The approach to the design of such an "exo" reagent was first described
by Baker.[12] First, a systematic exploration of the active site binding is
carried out. This is followed by a search for a bulky substituent which will
be accommodated by the enzyme surface. Finally, a reactive group such as a
chloroketone or fluorosulfonyl is attached to the distal end of the bridge.
This reactive group can then form a covalent bond with a functional group on
the enzyme surface which is not explicitly required for catalytic activity.
It was Baker's hypothesis[12] that the bridging group gives the "exo" reagent
a degree of specificity not obtainable with an "endo" reagent.

In a series of papers, Baker and his coworkers described compounds which
inhibited bovine trypsin and guinea pig complement at micromolar concentrations.[13] The aim of this work was to synthesize compounds which were
highly active, specific inhibitors of various serine proteases. One of the
compounds developed in this work has proved particularly useful in the study
of the human plasma serine proteases, thrombin, plasmin and C1s.[14,15]

MATERIALS AND METHODS

Enzymes. Bovine trypsin (3X crystallized) was obtained as the salt-free
lyophilized powder from Worthington Biochemicals, Freehold, NJ. It was 63 to

65% active as determined by NPGB titration[10] and assuming $E_{280}^{1\%} = 15.6$[16] and
molecular weight of $23,991$[1]. $\overline{\text{C1s}}$, the esterase subcomponent of C1, was
purified from Cohn fraction I as described by Bing et al.[17] It has 84.6%
of the theoretically possible enzymatic activity based on the V_{max} and k_{cat}
with respect to N-Z-L-Tyr-ONp.[18] Human α thrombin 97 to 98.3% α, 94.2 to
84.9% active by NPGB titration and 2.6 to 2.2 U.S. (NIH) clotting units/μg of
protein were generously provided by Dr. John W. Fenton, II, Division of
Laboratories and Research, New York Dept. of Health, Albany, NY. Preparation
of thrombin has been described.[19] Plasmin (29.3% active by NPGB titration)
was made by streptokinase activation of plasminogen isolated from outdated
plasma by affinity chromatography on lysine-Sepharose[20], and purified further
by gel filtration on ACA 34 ultragel (LKB) in 0.1 M KPO_4 buffer, pH 7.4. The
plasminogen was stored as a 50% $(NH_4)_2SO_4$ slurry at 4° until used. The
slurry was centrifuged at 10,000 rpm at 4° and dissolved to 1 to 2 mg/ml in
100 mM Tris-acetate-500 mM NaCl-20 mM lysine-10 mM EDTA, pH 8.1. It was
activated with streptokinase purified by affinity chromatography on Cibracron
Blue Sepharose from streptokinase (generously provided by Kabi Co.) at a
molar ration of 100:1 for 15 min at 37°. The molecular weight of streptokinase was taken as 45,000 and plasminogen as 83,800.[21] An $E_{280}^{1\%}$ of 17.1
was used for plasminogen and 9.49 for streptokinase. The streptokinase
activated plasminogen was used immediately without further treatment. It was
about 90% converted to heavy and light chain as judged by electrophoresis of
reduced (0.5% mercaptoethanol 30 min, 37°) and S-pyridylated (1% 4-vinyl-
pyridine, 30 min, 37°) in 5% polyacrylamide gels in the presence of 0.1% SDS
at pH 7.1 according to the method of Weber and Osborn.[22]

Labeling Reagents and Other Compounds

The reagent m-[o-(2-chloro-5-fluorosulfonylphenylureido)phenoxybutoxy]-
benzamidine, I, and its analog o-(2-chloro-5-fluorosulfonylphenylureido)-
methoxybenzene, III, were synthesized as previously described.[13,14]
Tritiation of m-(o-aminophenoxybutoxy)-benzamidine was accomplished by
catalytic exchange of 100 mg with 10 Ci of tritium gas (New England Nuclear,
Boston, MA) and the isotopically labeled reagent [^{3}H]-I was prepared with a
specific activity of 0.43 to 0.12 Ci/mole by the condensation of nitrophenyl)-
N-(2-chloro-5-fluorosulfonylphenyl)carbamate.[13] The reagent [^{14}C]DIFP was
obtained with a specific activity of 100 Ci/mole from New England Nuclear.
All compounds used in synthesis were purchased as reagent grade. Buffered
solution were made with deionized, distilled water and salts meeting ACS

specifications. All organic chemicals were obtained from Aldrich Chemical except for N-Z-L-Tyr-ONp and NPGB which were obtained from ICN Chemicals.

Examination of Inactivation Kinetics

The time course of inactivation was analyzed in the following manner: one to one-half milliliter samples of enzyme (6 to 10 μM) were prepared in 60 mM NaCl/5 mM Tris-acetate at pH 8.1. Plasmin was prepared in the Tris-NaCl-lysine-EDTA buffer discussed above. A stock solution of 100 μM trypsin in 1 mM HCl was diluted into 0.1 M Tris-HCl buffer pH 6.0 or 7.0 containing 1 mM $CaCl_2$. These were mixed with 50 μl of 990 μM I or III in methanol or solvent alone for controls, then were incubated at 24°, and 50 μl samples were withdrawn at 2 to 5 minute intervals. The amount of enzyme activity of $C1\bar{s}$ and thrombin was determined with N-Z-L-Tyr-ONp by measuring the absorbancy of p-nitrophenol released at 410 nm with a Gilford 240 spectrophotometer. Trypsin activity was assayed spectrophotometrically with N-Ts-L-Arg-OMe at 257nm.[23]

The log percent of the activity remaining at each sample time gives the pseudo-first-order constant (k_{1st}) for inactivation. In other experiments, the initial velocity (v_o) of inactivation was determined by the method of Mares-Guia and Shaw,[24] as modified by Childs and Bardslay[25]. The preceding protocol was followed except that the concentration of the reagent I in methanol was varied from 103 to 162 μM (Figure 2). These data were analyzed on the basis of the reaction scheme in which the enzyme (E) initially reacts with the inhibitor reactant (I) to form a reversible enzyme-inhibitor complex (EI) and subsequently an irreversible complex (EI'), as a consequence of forming a covalent bond (Eq. 1).

$$E + I \underset{k_{-1}}{\overset{k_1}{\rightleftharpoons}} EI \overset{k_2}{\longrightarrow} EI' \tag{1}$$

Assuming steady state conditions where d(EI/dt) = 0 and $k_1 >> k_{-1}$, then one finds the loss of enzyme activity per unit time (-d(E)/dt) approximates the velocity [v = d(EI')/dt = k_2(EI)] in the initial stages of the reaction [$v=v_o$, (E)=(E_o), (I)=(I_o)]. This may be expressed by a simple rectangular function (Eq. 2).

$$v_o = \frac{-d[E_o]}{dt} \cong \frac{k_2[E][I]}{K_L + [I]} \tag{2}$$

which contains the affinity labeling constant $K_L = (k_{-1} + k_2)k_1$, analogous to

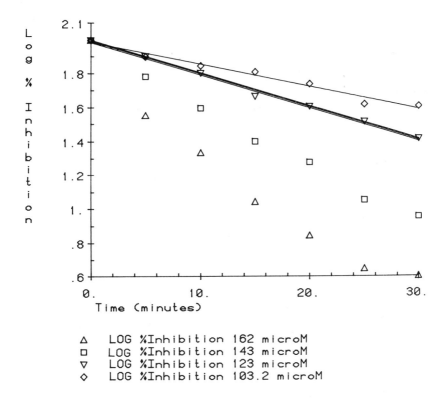

Figure 2. Inhibition of plasmin by I.

the Michaelis-Menten constant of simple enzyme-substrate kinetics.[26] The
plot of the reciprocal velocity (1/v) against the reciprocal reagent concentration 1/[I] consequently has an intercept of $1/(k_2[E_o])$ and a slope of
$K_L/(k_2[E_o])$. The slope/intercept is K_L, whereas the reciprocal of the
intercept divided by the enzyme concentration $[E_o]$ give k_2.
Calculations of kinetic constants and their statistical errors were performed
with the NIH PROPHET computer system.[27] All plots had r values of 0.95 or
better. The standard deviation of regression was ± 0.003 with the confidence
level at the 0.001 to 0.005 level.

Examination of Labeling Products

Enzyme samples reacted with isotopically labeled reagents were dissolved directly in 10 ml of Biofluor (New England Nuclear) scintillation fluid. Radioactivity was measured with a Searle Mark III scintillation counter, and isotope specific activities were determined for a minimum of three samples.

The distribution of labeled trypsin thrombin, plasmin and $C\bar{1}s$ products was examined in 0.1% SDS-0.1 M $NaPO_4$ pH 7.4 - in 5%, 10% or 15% PAA gels according to Weber and Osborn,[22] except that 20 μl of N,N,N',N'-tetraethylene-diamine were used to catalyze gel polymerization and 6 M urea was included in all gels. Gel calibrations were based on mobility of standards of known molecular weight in the appropriate % PAA gel. Protein components were assessed by means of staining with Coomassie blue (Schwartz-Mann).[22] Radioactivity distributions were determined by sectioning gels with a Savant Autogel Divider, where the pulverized gel slices were suspended directly in Biofluor scintillation fluid (New England Nuclear) for counting (Figure 3).

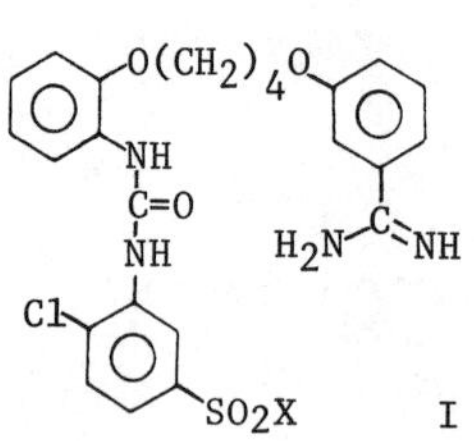

I   X = F
II X = OH

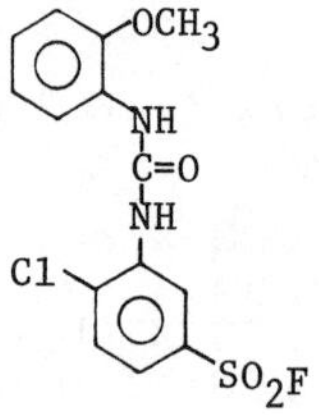

III

RESULTS

Benzamidines are well established competitive inhibitors of plasmin, thrombin and $C\bar{1}s$ [18]. The extended side chain of the affinity labeling reagent I considerably enhances the binding of the compound over simple benzamidines. Alkaline hydrolysis of compound I converts the sulfonylfluoride to a sulfonic acid, compound II. This yields a competititve inhibitor of enzyme activity in plasmin, thrombin, $C\bar{1}s$ and trypsin with an inhibition constant, K_i, at least two orders of magnitude lower than benzamidine.

Sulfonylfluorides are known to react with the active site, or DIFP sensitive serine.[28] This serine has enhanced reactivity over other serines

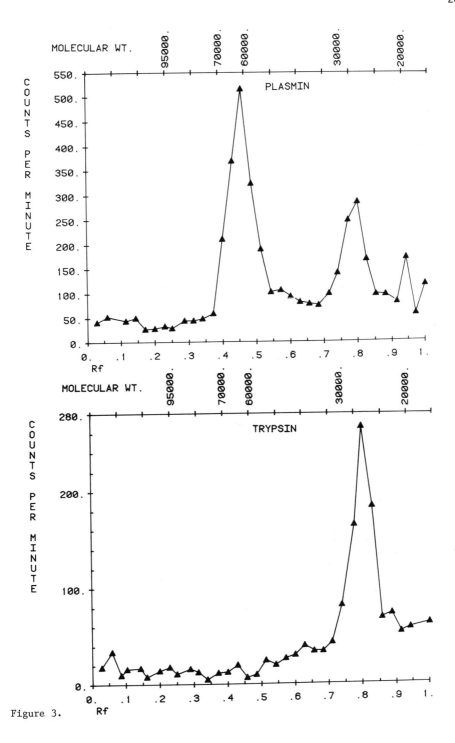

Figure 3.

because of its position in the catalytic center. Cardinaud and Baker[29] found evidence that sulfonylfluoride of an extended chain compound, such as I, could react with residues other than the serine in the catalytic mechanism. The bulky extended chain of compound I should place the reactive fluoride group well outside the active center and prohibit reaction with the catalytic serine. In a low energy conformation of compound I, the distance between the reactive fluoride atom and the amidino carbon was calculated to be 1.7 nm (Figure 4). By comparison, the carbonyl carbon of the tryptic enzyme substrate p-nitrophenylguanidinobenzoate is approximately 0.65 nm from the cationic guanidine carbon atom. The distance between the anionic binding site of trypsin and functionally reactive serine is approximately 0.7 nm.[14]

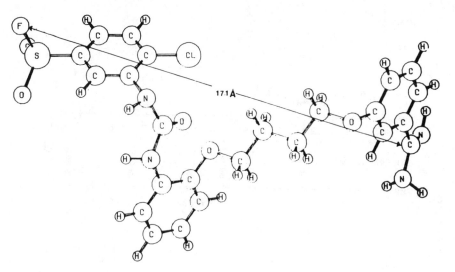

Figure 4.

The criteria for demonstrating affinity labeling have been set forth in detail by Baker[12], Singer[30] and Shaw[31]. In this study, four independent methods were used to establish affinity labeling of the serine proteases with compound I. First, a 2-7 fold molar excess of I caused a relatively rapid pseudo first order inactivation of each of the enzymes. See Table 1. This inactivation is consistent with the kinetics predicted for affinity labeling reagents. In experiments in which the reagent concentration was varied, the rate of initial inactivation followed the double reciprocal relationship characteristic of simple enzyme-substrate kinetics. Second, the presence of the alkaline hydrolyzed form of the reagent II protected the enzymes from labeling with I and diisopropylfluorophosphate. This indicates that compound I binds at the active site. Third, I is stoichiometrically incorporated into each of the enzymes where present in a slight molar excess. See Table 2. However, stoichiometric uptake did not occur if the enzymes were previously inactivated with diisopropylfluorophosphate. Fourth, a slight molar excess of compound III, which contains the chemically reactive sulfonylfluoride, but not the butoxybenzamidine moiety of I, did not react with the enzymes to a significant extent.

TABLE 1.

KINETIC CONSTANTS FOR INHIBITION OF PLASMA PROTEASES BY COMPOUND I

	K $\sec^{-1}10^{-4}$	I μM	K_L^d μM	k_2^e $\sec^{-1}10^{-3}$	K_i^f	k_2 $\sec^{-1}10^{-3}$
Thrombin[a]	30.9	49.3	115.0	3.82	3.65	2.89
C1s[b]	1.5	233	87.3	3.06	4.6	3.62
Plasmin	26.9	54.1	71.8	0.691	N.D.	N.D.
Trypsin[c]	46.4	9.9	N.D.[g]	N.D.	N.D.	N.D.

[a] Ref. 15
[b] Ref. 14
[c] Bing et al. (1977) in Chemistry and Biology of Thrombin, Lundblad, R.,
Fenton, J.W. II, and Mann, K.G. eds., Ann Arbor Science Press, pp. 159-177.
[d] K_L affinity labeling constant, see equation 1.
[e] determined as $k_2 = [E_0] = V_{max}$
[f] determined for hydrolyzed compound II $k_2 = K_i(v_0/[I_0][E_0])$
[g] N.D., not determined.

TABLE 2

INCORPORATION OF $[^3H]$-I INTO SERINE PROTEASES

	$[E]$ μM	$[^3H]$-I μM	mole label/mole enzyme	enzyme protected
α-Thrombin	76	382	1.05	0.00[b]
C1s	3	39.9	1.08	0.37[c]
Plasmin	13.8	129	0.99[a]	N.D.
Trypsin	17.3	129	0.65[a]	N.D.

[a] based on NPGB titration of untreated enzyme
[b] stoichiometrically inactivated with $[^{14}C]$DIFP 0.73 mole label/mole α thrombin
[c] inactivated 60 min with 1 mM DIFP at 23°

Together, these experiments demonstrate that compound I reacts with the active site of the enzyme with kinetics appropriate for an enzyme-substrate reaction; the reaction of the chemically reactive sulfonylfluorides requires binding of I at the active site; and one mole of I reacts with one mole of enzyme. Thus, compound I fulfills the criteria for an affinity labeling reagent of bovine trypsin and the human plasma proteases plasmin, thrombin and $\overline{Cls}$, and offers a tool for further investigation of the specificity of these enzymes.

REFERENCES

1. Walsh, K.A. (1975) in Proteases and Biological Control, Reich, E., Rifkin, D.B. and Shaw, E., eds., Cold Spring Harbor Laboratory, Cold Spring Harbor, N.Y.,p. 1.
2. Johnson, D. and Travis, J. (1976) Anal. Biochem. 72, 573.
3. Blow, D.M. (1971) in The Enzymes, Vol. III. Boyer, P.D. ed., Academic Press, New York, N.Y. p. 185.
4. Muller-Eherhard, H.J. (1970) in Progress in Immunology, Amos, C.B., ed., Academic Press, New York, N.Y. p. 568.
5. Cooper, N.R., and Ziccardi, R.J. (1978) Immunol. 119, 1664.
6. Takayi, T. and Doolittle, R.F. (1974) Biochemistry, 13, 750.
7. Robbins, K.C. and Summaria, L. (1970) Methods Enzymol. 19, 184.
8. Walsh, K.A. (1970) Methods Enzymol. 19, 41.
9. Cohen, I., Bohak, Z., de Vries, A. and Katchalski, W. (1969) Eur. J. Biochem. 10, 388.
10. Shaw, E. (1975) in Proteases and Biological Control, Reich, E., Rifkin, D.B. and Shaw E., eds. Cold Spring Harbor Laboratory, Cold Spring Harbor, N.Y. p. 455.
11. Baker, B.R. (1964) J. Pharm. Sci. 53, 347.
12. Baker, B.R. (1967) Design of Active Site Directed Irreversible Enzyme Inhibitors, Wiley, New York, N.Y.
13. Baker, B.R. and Cory, M. (1971) J. Med. Chem. 14, 805 and references therein.
14. Bing, D.H., Laura, R., Andrews, J.M. and Cory, M. (1978) Biochemistry, 17, 5713.
15. Bing, D.H., Cory, M. and Fenton, J.W. II (1977) J. Biol. Chem. 252, 8027.
16. Worthington Enzyme Manual (1972) Worthington Biochemical Corp., Freehold, N.J. p. 125.
17. Bing, D.H., Andrews, J.M. and Cole, E. manuscript in preparation.
18. Bing, D.H. (1969) Biochemistry 8, 4503.
19. Fenton, J.W., Fasco, M.J., Stackrow, A.B., Aronson, D.L., Young, A.M., Finlayson, J.S. (1977) J. Biol. Chem. 252, 3587.
20. Deutsch, G.D. and Mertz, E.T. (1970) Science, 170, 1095.
21. Castellino, F.J., Sodetz, J.M., Brockway, W.J. and Siefring, G.E. Jr., (1976) Methods Enzymol. 45, 1244.
22. Weber, K. and Osborn, H. (1975) in The Proteins Neurath, H. and Hill, R.L. eds., 3rd ed. Academic Press, New York, N.Y. p. 180.
23. Schoellman, G. and Shaw, E. (1962) Biochemistry, 2, 252.
24. Mares-Guia, M. and Shaw, E. (1967) J. Biol. Chem. 242, 5782.
25. Childs, R.E. and Bardsley, W.G. (1975) J. Theor. Biol. 53, 381.
26. Morris, J.G. (1975) in a Biologist's Physical Chemistry, Addison-Wesley, Reading, MA. p. 283.
27. Fed. Proc. (1973) 32, 1744.

28. Fahrney, D.E. and Gold, A.M. (1963) J. Amer. Chem. Soc. 85, 997.
29. Cardinaud, R. and Baker, B.R. (1971) J. Med. Chem. 14, 119.
30. Singer, S.J. (1967) Adv. Protein Chem. 22, 1.
31. Shaw, E. (1970) in The Enzymes, Vol. I, Boyer, P.D. ed., Academic Press, New York, N.Y. p. 99.

DISCUSSION

LAWSON: Do you have any idea which serine, if any, is modified with that reagent? Do you actually know, whether it is a serine that is modified?

CORY: No. We do not know that it is a serine for sure, other than the fact that there was some preliminary work a decade ago in Prof. B.R. Baker's lab with a chymotrypsin reagent, which showed that the sulfonyl fluoride did react with a serine. It could be threonine and, unfortunately, these particular proteases have a lot of serines and threonines in them. So there are a number, four likely ones, that it could reach.

LAWSON: One thing I could suggest trying would be that if in the case of chymotrypsin it happens to be serine-195, and you treat it with base you ought to produce anhydrochymotrypsin, which would be identical to that produced by other means unambiguously and if it were, let us say another serine, then going through the same procedure it would probably give you active enzyme.

CORY: Since we know that it labels both chains in enzymes such as thrombin and C1s, we know that at least some of the label is not going to serine-195.

LAWSON: To what extent is that going to the other chain in a nonspecific way? How much is going to the A chain with your nonspecific sulfonyl fluoride reagent? Could you, for example, tie up the active site in some other way and still get it going on the A chain or is it really specifically binding in the pocket and react with the A chain?

CORY: It is hard to show that we could tie up the active site in any way that would not also prevent the benzamidine from binding. So, admittedly, the diisopropylfluorophosphate modification may prevent the benzamidine from binding within the pocket.

CHOWDHRY: I am curious, if you have tried any cleavable reagents, where your bridge is in fact cleavable; that may answer the question that was just raised. In other words, you first bind the benzamidine in the active site, let it react, then cleave the bridge, get the reversibly bound fragment out and that should give your activity back.

CORY: That is a very good idea. But we have not done that. The approach which we will be using is to try to isolate the actual amino acid that has the label on it.

QUESTION from the audience: It is difficult to assume that only one residue is labeled, because with a fairly reactive reagent, like the one you have, considering the microheterogeneity, one would expect to label several residues within a certain radius. Have you done any amino acid hydrolysis?

CORY: No. That would be the next step, to do the amino acid hydrolysis and find out where the reagent goes. It is admittedly not a very specific reagent in the sense that it labels all of the proteases tested to date.

EDITOR's comments: Regarding the previous question, high reactivity and selective modification may go hand in hand. Horse liver alcohol dehydrogenase is inactivated in the presence of NADPH by 4-(p-bromoacetamidophenyl)butyramide 4 orders of magnitude faster than by bromoacetamide, apparently *via* active site directed exoalkylation[1] of a single methionine residue, without any detectable reaction with cysteines.[2] In the absence of the coenzyme, the reagent inactivates the enzyme 4-fold slower with concomitant alkylation of 6 cysteine residues, but no methionine becomes modified. It was proposed[2] that in the presence of NADPH, the carbonyl oxygen of the butyramide moiety of the reagent is liganded to the active site zinc ion allowing the alkylating C-atom to reach the sulfur of Met-306 some 14 $\overset{\circ}{A}$ away from the zinc.

REFERENCES

1. Baker, B.R., (1967) Design of Active Site Directed Irreversible Enzyme Inhibitors, Wiley, New York.
2. Chen, W.-S. and Plapp, B.V. (1978) Biochemistry, 17, 4916.

THE DESIGN OF ACTIVE-SITE-DIRECTED REVERSIBLE INHIBITORS OF EXOPEPTIDASES

MIGUEL A. ONDETTI, DAVID W. CUSHMAN, EMILY F. SABO AND HONG S. CHEUNG
The Squibb Institute for Medical Research, Princeton, New Jersey   08540

ANGIOTENSIN-CONVERTING ENZYME INHIBITORS

Angiotensin-converting enzyme is an exopeptidase that cleaves dipeptide units from the C-terminal end of a peptide chain, and has been designated in the systematic nomenclature as peptidyldipeptide carboxy hydrolase[1] (EC 3.4.15.1). Its two most important natural substrates are the decapeptide angiotensin I and the nonapeptide bradykinin. Angiotensin I is converted by the action of this enzyme into the very potent hypertensive octapeptide angiotensin II, and the hypotensive nonapeptide bradykinin is degraded to inactive hepta- and pentapeptide fragments (Figure 1). Because of the latter reaction angiotensin-converting enzyme is also known under the trivial name of kininase II.[2] The net result of

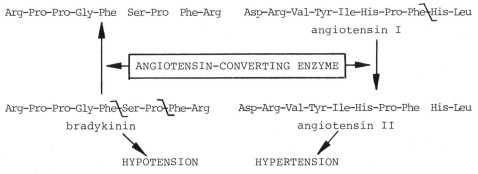

Figure 1: Action of angiotensin-converting enzyme (kininase II) on its two natural substrates: angiotensin I and bradykinin.

the action of angiotensin-converting enzyme on these two substrates is the elevation of blood pressure, either by generation of a hypertensive agent or by destruction of a hypotensive agent. This is the reason why inhibitors of this enzyme exert a pronounced antihypertensive effect and are becoming very important additions to the therapy of human hypertension.[3,4,5]

Angiotensin-converting enzyme is capable of hydrolyzing a large variety of peptidic substrates, provided they have a free C-terminal carboxylic group. It does not have the restricted specificity of the well-known pancreatic carboxypeptidases A and B, but it will not hydrolyze substrates with C-terminal acidic amino acids like aspartic and glutamic acid, and substrates with a penultimate proline residue. Skeggs and collaborators,[6] the discoverers of this converting enzyme, had already pointed out its sensitivity towards inhibition by EDTA, and many subsequent investigations have confirmed that most metal chelators are powerful inhibitors.[7] Utilizing homogeneous rabbit lung angiotensin-converting enzyme, Das and Soffer[8] have shown that it contains approximately one gram-atom of zinc per mole of protein.

Skeggs et al., had also uncovered another very characteristic feature of this enzyme, the requirement of chloride or other monoanions for the display of optimal activity. This chloride ion requirement has been qualified as absolute (no measurable hydrolysis in the absence of chloride ions) in the case of the synthetic substrate hippuryl-glycyl-glycine.[9] With other substrates, the chloride concentration required for optimal activity varies; with angiotensin I it is approximately ten-times greater than with bradykinin.[10]

Angiotensin-converting enzyme resembles the well-known pancreatic carboxypeptidases A and B in its exopeptidase nature and zinc content. Bünning et al.,[11] have recently identified at the active site of angiotensin-converting enzyme the following catalytically important amino acid residues: glutamic (or aspartic) acid, tyrosine, arginine and lysine. The first three are also known to play an important catalytic role in carboxypeptidase A.[12] All of these observations would indicate that both enzymes have similar mechanisms of action.

The first important inhibitors of angiotensin-converting enzyme were peptides isolated from the venom of the South American snake Bothrops jararaca. Ten peptides were isolated and characterized from the crude extracts of this venom.[13,14] Eventually, seven of them were synthesized, and their availability has played a significant role in the clarification of the biochemical, physiological and pathological role of this enzyme. The two most important inhibitors from this group are the pentapeptide BPP_{5a} (bradykinin potentiating peptide 5_a, also designated by the Squibb Institute code number SQ 20,475), and the nonapeptide SQ 20,881 (BPP_{9a}).

SQ 20,475 BPP_{5a} <Glu-Lys-Trp-Ala-Pro

SQ 20,881 BPP_{9a} <Glu-Trp-Pro-Arg-Pro-Gln-Ile-Pro-Pro

The studies of Cushman et al.,[15] indicated that with the isolated rabbit lung converting enzyme the pentapeptide BPP_{5a} was more potent (K_i: 0.06 μM) than the nonapeptide SQ 20,881 (K_i: 0.56 μM). However, the pentapeptide lost all its inhibitory properties upon ten to fifteen minutes preincubation with the enzyme, while the nonapeptide inhibitory activity was completely stable under those conditions. Thin layer chromatography indicated that the pentapeptide was cleaved by the converting enzyme with the release of the dipeptide Ala-Pro. Unlike angiotensin I, the pentapeptide is cleaved more slowly in the presence of chloride ion.

This peculiar behavior with respect to chloride ion concentration was later analyzed in more detail utilizing three synthetic substrates with the C-terminal dipeptide sequences of angiotensin I, bradykinin and the pentapeptide inhibitor BPP_{5a}. The results are summarized in Table 1. A broad range of chloride ion

Table 1

COMPARISON OF SYNTHETIC SUBSTRATES OF ANGIOTENSIN-CONVERTING ENZYME

Enzymatic Property	Substrate		
	Hip-His-Leu	Hip-Phe-Arg	Hip-Ala-Pro
Effect of Cl^-			
Conc. for optimal activity (mM)	300	20	0
Activity change (%) (0 mM to 300 mM Cl^-)	+4800	+300	-400
K_m (μM)			
Optimal conditions	2200^a	420^b	630^c
pH 8.3 and 300 mM Cl^-	2200	330	30
k_{cat} (s^{-1})			
Optimal conditions	260	1015	2400
pH 8.3 and 300 mM Cl^-	260	725	115
k_{cat}/K_m ($\mu M^{-1}s^{-1}$)			
Optimal conditions	0.1	2.4	3.8
pH 8.3 and 300 mM Cl^-	0.1	2.2	3.8

a: pH 8.3, 300 mM NaCl; b: pH 8.3, 20 mM NaCl; c: pH 7.8, no NaCl

concentration requirements for optimal activity was observed. Hippuryl-His-Leu hydrolysis is strongly activated by chloride ion, while an inhibitory effect is actually observed in the case of hippuryl-Ala-Pro. The substrate efficiency of these tripeptides increase in opposite direction to that of their chloride ion requirement, and in the case of hippuryl-His-Leu and hippuryl-Phe-Arg it parallels that observed with their longer counterparts, angiotensin I and bradykinin. Since these three synthetic substrates differ only in their C-terminal dipeptide, it is reasonable to assume that the interaction of these amino acid residues with the enzyme plays a key role in the catalytic process, because it must be responsible for the large differences in k_{cat}/K_m ratios and in chloride ion requirements.

At high chloride ion concentrations hippuryl-Ala-Pro binds strongly to the enzyme (K_m = 3 x 10^{-5} M) but has a low turn-over number, while in the absence of chloride this binding energy is "expended" to accelerate hydrolysis, giving a high K_m (6.3 x 10^{-4} M) and a high turn-over number. This increased binding and low catalytic efficiency at high chloride ion concentrations would explain why peptides containing an Ala-Pro C-terminal sequence will behave as inhibitors vis-a-vis substrates with His-Leu or Phe-Arg C-terminal sequences, such as angiotensin I and bradykinin.

The chloride ion might induce a conformation of the enzyme complementary to that of the C-terminal dipeptide product of the enzymatic reaction. Since this complementarity cannot be realized upon binding of the substrate until this is "distorted" to resemble the product, this complementarity might constitute the main driving force of the hydrolytic reaction. Since the dipeptide product will fit this complementary enzyme without any major energy expenditure, the result will be strong binding, and, therefore, inhibitory activity. The fact that angiotensin-converting enzyme is strongly inhibited by dipeptides has been pointed out by a number of investigators.[8,16,17,18]

The major significance of the C-terminal dipeptide binding in the interaction of substrates with angiotensin-converting enzyme, made this enzyme a very attractive example to explore the concept of "biproduct" analog inhibitors developed by Byers and Wolfenden.[19] These authors had pointed out that benzylsuccinic acid was a potent inhibitor of carboxypeptidase A because it combined in one molecule the mode of binding of the two products of the enzymatic reaction (Figure 2). In applying this concept to the angiotensin I-converting enzyme[20,21] we elected to mimic the C-terminal dipeptide sequence Ala-Pro of the venom inhibitor BPP$_{5a}$ because it lead to tighter binding in the presence of chloride ion, as it was later confirmed with the model hippuryl substrates described above. The compound targeted for synthesis had, besides the binding features of L-alanyl-L-proline sequence, a carboxyl function which would contribute some of the modes of binding of the other product of the enzymatic reaction. The compound thus obtained D-2-methylsuccinyl-L-proline (Figure 2) was a potent and specific inhibitor of angiotensin I-converting enzyme with a K_i value of 2.5 µM. The study of a number of structural modifications of this molecule indicated that the optimal activity was obtained with those compounds

in which the methyl substituent of the succinyl moiety and the proline moiety
were isosteric with an L-alanyl-L-proline dipeptide, indicating that the mode
of binding of these inhibitors was similar to that of the C-terminal dipeptides
of the substrates. We had also assumed that the free carboxyl of the succinyl
moiety was bound to the enzyme surface by becoming a ligand of the zinc ion
present at the active site,[20,21] as schematized in the hypothetical model of
Figure 5. It has been recently concluded that on the basis of the X-ray evidence for the binding of benzylsuccinic acid with thermolysin, the β-carboxyl
of benzylsuccinic acid is probably bound to the zinc ion in carboxypeptidas A[22]
through one of its oxygen atoms.

CARBOXYPEPTIDASE A   ANGIOTENSIN-CONVERTING ENZYME

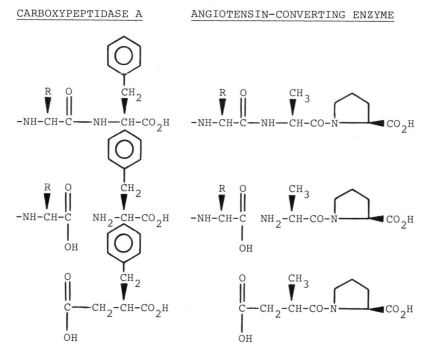

Figure 2. "Biproduct" analogs of carboxypeptidase A and angiotensin-converting
enzyme.

A large number of structural modifications of D-2-methylsuccinyl-L-proline
were then undertaken to uncover functions that would provide stronger ligands
for the zinc atom, thereby increasing the total binding of the inhibitor molecule. Of the many functionalities tested, the hydroxycarbamoyl,[23] the phosphonyl[24] and the sulfhydryl[21] were found to provide a more efficient

interaction with the zinc ion, since they lead to considerably more potent
inhibitors than their carboxyl counterparts. This was particularly the case
for the sulfhydryl derivatives which lead to a thousand-fold enhancement in inhibitory activity (Table 2). The fact that sulfur is a better ligand than

Table 2

MODIFICATION OF ZINC-BINDING FUNCTIONALITY IN ANGIOTENSIN-
CONVERTING ENZYME INHIBITORS

No.	Structure	I_{50} µM
1.	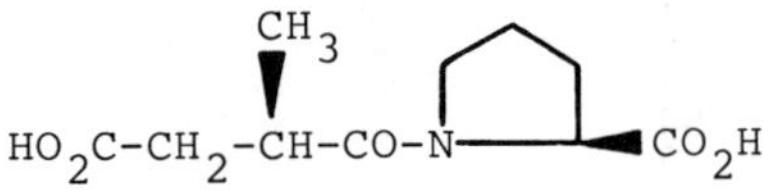 CH$_3$ HO$_2$C-CH$_2$-CH-CO-N—⟨⟩—CO$_2$H	22
2.	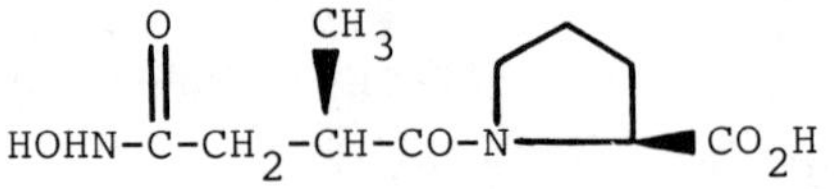 O CH$_3$ ‖ HOHN-C-CH$_2$-CH-CO-N—⟨⟩—CO$_2$H	0.6
3.	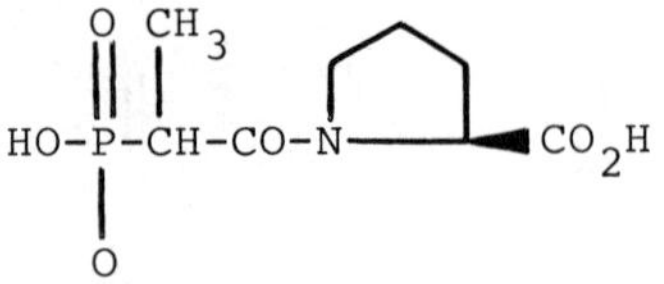 O CH$_3$ ‖ ‖ HO-P-CH-CO-N—⟨⟩—CO$_2$H ‖ O	31
4.	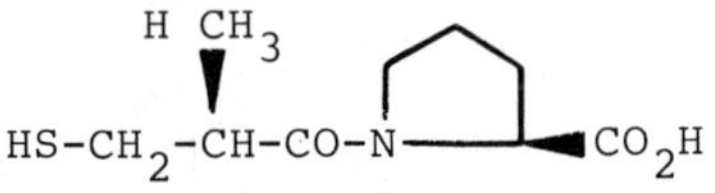 H CH$_3$ HS-CH$_2$-CH-CO-N—⟨⟩—CO$_2$H (SQ 14,225)	0.02

oxygen for zinc,[25] supports the assumption that in these functionalities the
oxygen or sulfur atom is bound to the metal at the first sphere of coordination
(Figure 4) and not through the intermediacy of a water molecule (Figure 3).
Cleland[26] has postulated that substrates of carboxypeptidase A bind to the
enzyme surface with the oxygen of the scissile amide bond coordinated to the
zinc through a water molecule as in Figure 3, while Breslow and Wernick[27] propose that this mode of binding only occurs with esters, and that in amide substrates the carbonyl oxygen displaces the water molecule to bind in the first
sphere of coordination. The structure-activity relationships with angiotensin-

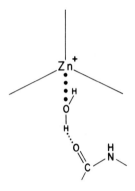

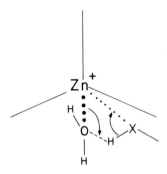

Figure 3. Binding of the scissile amide bond to the zinc atom at the active-site.

Figure 4. Binding of the zinc-binding function of angiotensin-converting enzyme inhibitors to the active-site zinc ion with displacement of coordinated water.

converting enzyme inhibitors indicate that in order to obtain significant inhibitory activity the zinc binding moiety of the inhibitors should carry an oxygen or sulfur atom with a potentially ionizable hydrogen to counteract the residual positive charge present on the zinc atom of the enzyme active site. It is assumed that, as is the case in carboxypeptidase A and B,[12,28] one of the enzyme ligands of zinc is a carboxylate so that the net residual charge on zinc is +1.

Even though the sulfur-zinc interaction plays a very important role in the binding of an inhibitor such as SQ 14,225 to the converting enzyme, this interaction is by no means the only critical one.[21] As it can be seen in Table 3, deletion of any of the functional groups in SQ 14,225 or alteraction of its stereochemistry can lead to a substantial decrease in inhibitory activity, from a ten-fold for the elimination of the alpha methyl side chain in the mercapto propanoyl moiety to a 10,000-fold for the elimination of the proline carboxyl.

These relative activities are not necessarily a direct measure of the contribution of each particular functional group to the binding of the whole molecule, since every alteration will also modify the general physico-chemical properties of the molecule (e.g., hydrophobicity) in a manner that is difficult to quantitate.

278

TABLE 3

STRUCTURE-ACTIVITY RELATIONSHIPS IN MERCAPTOALKANOYL AMINO ACID
INHIBITORS

No.	Structure	I_{50} μM
1.	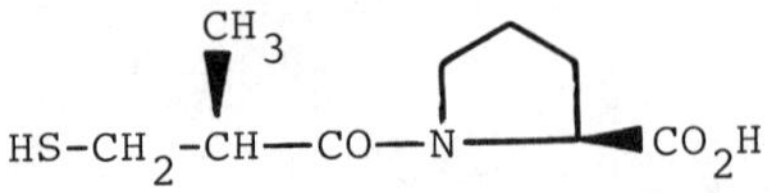 CH_3 HS-CH$_2$-CH—CO—N⟨ring⟩CO$_2$H	0.02
2.	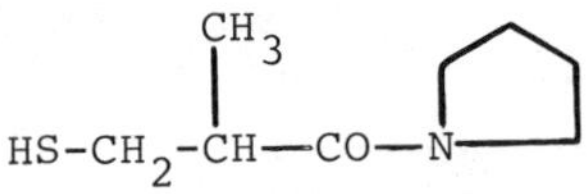 CH_3 HS-CH$_2$-CH—CO—N⟨ring⟩	250
3.	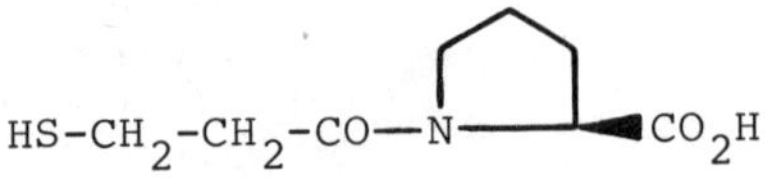 HS-CH$_2$-CH$_2$-CO—N⟨ring⟩CO$_2$H	0.2
4.	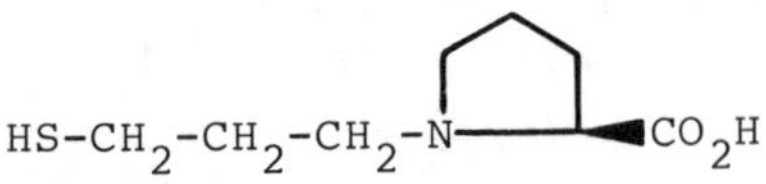 HS-CH$_2$-CH$_2$-CH$_2$-N⟨ring⟩CO$_2$H	240
5.	HS-CH$_2$-CH$_2$-CO—NH—CH$_2$-CO$_2$H	2.4
6.	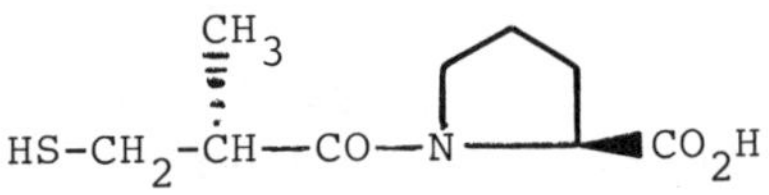 CH_3 HS-CH$_2$-CH—CO—N⟨ring⟩CO$_2$H	2.4

In any case, it is evident that these inhibitors are capable of establishing
a number of binding interactions with the active site of the angiotensin-
converting enzyme, as it is schematically described in the hypothetical model
of the active site of this enzyme shown in Figure 5.

By analogy with carboxypeptidase A we postulate that the carboxylic group of
substrates and inhibitors bind at a cationic center on the enzyme surface, most
likely provided by an arginine residue. However, the distance between the C-
terminal carboxyl binding site and the zinc atom should be longer in

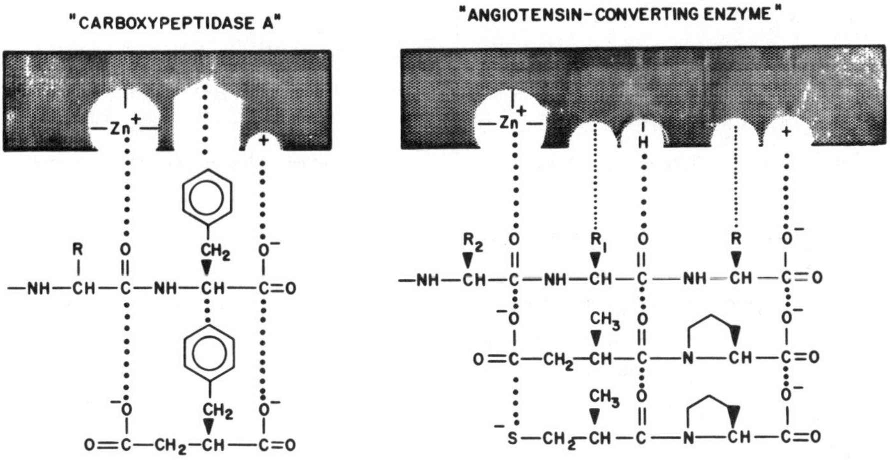

Figure 5. Mode of binding of substrates and inhibitors to the active sites of carboxypeptidase A and angiotensin-converting enzyme.

angiotensin-converting enzyme than in the carboxypeptidase A by approximately one amino acid residue, since it is the penultimate peptide linkage the one that will be cleaved in the case of the converting enzyme. The last amide linkage of the peptide chain is probably a very important recognition point in the substrate structure since it is the most characteristic feature of the di-peptide product of the enzymatic reaction. It is likely that the interaction between this amide linkage and the enzyme surface takes place through a hydro-gen bond to the oxygen atom of the amide carbonyl. As in the case of all mammalian peptidases the side chains of the two C-terminal amino acid residues of angiotensin-converting enzyme substrates must be of the L-configuration, and in the case of the inhibitors the corresponding side chains must be placed so that the structure becomes isosteric with an L-L dipeptide as is clearly the case for SQ 14,225. It is difficult to describe accurately the nature of the binding sites for the side chains of the two C-terminal amino acids. On the basis of the structure-activity relationships with substrates and inhibitors it appears that these binding sites are predominantly hydrophobic in nature.

The active site of angiotensin I-converting enzyme provides the opportunity for a multiplicity of binding interactions that can be utilized advantageously in the design of multibinding active-site-directed reversible inhibitors. The development of SQ 14,225 (captopril) is a clear and successful example of this approach, that could also be applied to other metalloproteases.

INHIBITORS OF CARBOXYPEPTIDASES A AND B

The architecture of the active-site of carboxypeptidases A and B is well known as a result of extensive enzymological studies by a number of investigators and the clarification of the tridimensional structure by X-ray crystallography.[12,20,28] There is, therefore, nothing hypothetical in regard to the active-site models of these enzymes. Figure 6 describes schematically the features that are known to be present at these sites: (1) a cationic center for the binding of the C-terminal carboxyl group of substrates; (2) a purely hydrophobic pocket for the binding of the side chain of the C-terminal amino acid in the case of carboxypeptidase A, and an anionic and partially hydrophobic pocket for the binding of the basic C-terminal amino acids in the case of carboxypeptidase B; (3) a zinc atom to polarize the carbonyl of the scissile amide bond.

Benzylsuccinic acid, the biproduct analog inhibitor developed by Byers and Wolfenden[19] binds to the active site of carboxypeptidase A by triple interaction with the cationic center, the hydrophobic pocket and the zinc atom. Since benzylsuccinic acid is also a fairly potent inhibitor of carboxypeptidase B,[29] it is tempting to speculate that it binds to this enzyme in a reverse direction, allowing for only partial penetration of the benzyl group in the anionic hydrophobic pocket and thereby avoiding the unfavorable interaction of the hydrophobic phenyl ring with the anionic charge. Succinic acid derivatives with a basic amino or guanidino side chain have been recently synthesized and shown to be potent and specific inhibitors of carboxypeptidase B.[30]

If the zinc binding functionality of benzylsuccinic acid; namely, the β-carboxyl group, is replaced with a functional group that has strong affinity for the zinc atom and practically none for the cationic center, the ambiguity of binding of benzylsuccinic acid could be eliminated. The inhibitors thus obtained[31] would show higher potency because of the more efficient zinc-ligand interaction and greater specificity than the dicarboxylic acids. Two compounds were synthesized following these guidelines; 2-mercaptomethyl-3-phenyl-propionic acid (SQ 14,603) and 2-mercaptomethyl-5-guanido pentanoic acid (SQ 24,798). In Table 4 their activities as inhibitors of angiotensin-converting enzyme and carboxypeptidases A and B are compared with those of SQ 14,225. The extreme potency and specificity of these inhibitors is quite apparent.

The design of multibinding active-site-directed reversible inhibitors rests

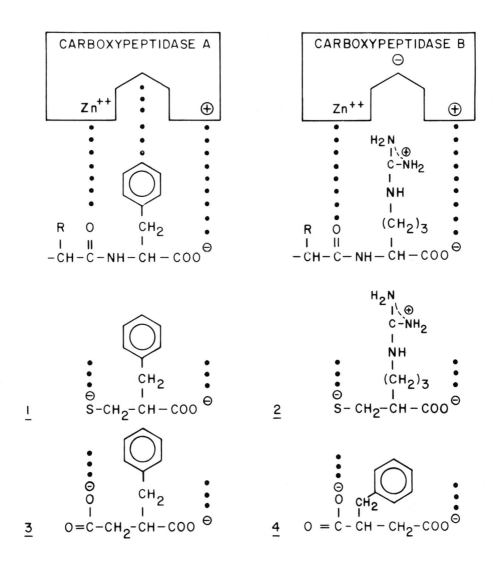

Figure 6. Schematic representation of substrates and proposed mode of binding of inhibitors to the active sites of carboxypeptidase A and B. 1, SQ 14,603; 2, SQ 24,798; 3, benzylsuccinic acid; 4, benzylsuccinic acid shown binding to carboxypeptidase B in the reverse direction with a partial interaction of its aromatic ring with the anionic-hydrophobic pocket. [Reprinted with permission from M. A. Ondetti et al., Biochemistry, 18, 1427 (1979). Copyright by the American Chemical Society.]

TABLE 4

SPECIFICITY OF TIGHT-BINDING COMPETITIVE INHIBITORS OF CARBOXY-PEPTIDASES A AND B AND ANGIOTENSIN-CONVERTING ENZYME[a]

Inhibitor	K_i (nM)		
	Carboxy-peptidase A	Carboxy-peptidase B	Angiotensin-Converting Enzyme
$CH_2C_6H_5$ $HSCH_2\overset{\|}{C}HCO_2H$ (SQ 14,603)	11	163,000	58,000
$NHC(=NH)NH_2$ $(CH_2)_3$ $HSCH_2\overset{\|}{C}HCO_2H$ (SQ 24,798)	11,600	0.42	288,000
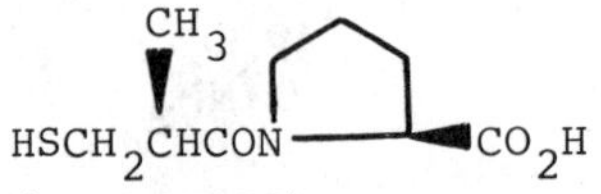 CH_3 $HSCH_2CHCON-\!\!\!\!\triangleleft\!\!\!\!-CO_2H$ (SQ 14,225)	623,000	>250,000	1.7

a) Reprinted with permission from M. A. Ondetti et al., Biochemistry, 18, 1427 (1979), copyright by the American Chemical Society.

on the hypothetical or actual knowledge of the enzyme active site, and the potential binding interactions that can be established between the enzyme and the substrate and products of the enzymatic reaction. If somewhere along the reaction coordinate further interactions come into play to stabilize transition states, a knowledge or a working hypothesis of the molecular nature of these interactions will be extremely helpful for the purpose of inhibitor development. Finally, as it has been shown in the case of the metallo exopeptidases discussed above, the design of inhibitory molecules should not aim only at duplicating these binding interactions, but to increase their efficiency so that a more favorable competition with substrates can be achieved.

REFERENCES

1. Soffer, R. L. (1976) Ann. Rev. Biochem., 45, 73. Cf. also Ganten, D. (1978) Klin. Woch, 56 (suppl. 1) 187.
2. Erdös, E. G. (1977) Fed. Proc., 36, 1760.

3. Case, D. B., Wallace, J. M., Keim, H. J., Weber, M. A. Drayer, J. I. M., White, R. P., Sealey, J. E., Laragh, J. H. (1976) Am. J. Med. 61, 790.
4. Brunner, H. R., Gavras, H., Waeber, B., Kershaw, G. R., Turini, G. A., Vukovich, R. A., McKinstry, D. N., Gavras, I. (1979) Ann. Int. Med. 90, 19.
5. Case, D. B., Atlas, S. A., Laragh, J. H., Sealey, J. E., Sullivan, P. A., McKinstry, D. N. (1978) Progress Cardiovasc. Dis., 21, 195.
6. Skeggs, L. T., Kahn, J. R. and Shumway, N. P. (1956) J. Exp. Med., 103, 295.
7. Cushman, D. W. and Cheung, H. S. (1971) Biochem. Pharmacol., 20, 1637.
8. Das, M. and Soffer, R. L. (1975) J. Biol. Chem. 250, 6762.
9. Dorer, F. E., Kahn, J. R., Lentz, K. E., Levine, M. and Skeggs, L. S. (1976) Biochem. Biophys. Acta, 429, 220.
10. Dorer, F. E., Kahn, J. R., Lentz, K. E., Levine, M. and Skeggs, L. S. (1974), Circ, Res., 34, 824.
11. Bünning, P., Holmquest, B., Riordan, J. F. (1978) Biochem. Biophys. Res. Commun., 83, 1442.
12. Quiocho, F. A. and Lipscomb, W. N. (1971) Adv. Prot. Chem., 25, 1.
13. Ferreira, S. H., Bartelt, D. C. and Greene, L. J. (1970) Biochemistry, 9, 7583.
14. Ondetti, M. A., Williams, N. J., Sabo, E. F., Pluscec, J., Weaver, E. R. and Kocy, O. (1971) Biochemistry, 10, 4033.
15. Cheung H. S. and Cushman, D. W. (1973) Biochem. Biophys. Acta, 293, 451.
16. Yang, H. Y. T., Erdös, E. G. and Levin, Y. (1971) J. Pharmacol. Exp. Ther., 177, 291.
17. Sanders, G. E., West, D. W. and Huggins, C. G. (1971) Biochem. Biophys. Acta, 242, 662.
18. Cushman, D. W., Ondetti, M. A. and Cheung, H. S. (1978) Fed. Proc., 37, 657.
19. Byers, L. D. and Wolfenden, R. (1973) Biochemistry, 12, 2070.
20. Ondetti, M. A., Rubin, B. and Cushman, D. W. (1977) Science, 196, 441.
21. Cushman, D. W., Cheung, H. S., Sabo, E. F. and Ondetti, M. A. (1977) Biochemistry, 16, 5484.
22. Bolognesi, M. C. and Matthews, B. W. (1979) J. Biol. Chem., 254, 634.
23. Ondetti, M. A., Sabo, E. F., Losee, K. A., Cheung, H. S., Cushman, D. W. and Rubin, B. (1977) in Peptides Proceed. 5th Am. Peptide Symposium, M. Goodman and J. Meinehofer Eds., John Wiley & Sons, New York, p. 576.
24. Petrillo, Jr., E. W., Ondetti, M. A., Cushman, D. W., Weaver, E. R. and Heikes, J. E. (1978) 176th ACS National Meeting, Abstract Medi, 27.
25. Vallee, B. and Coleman, J. E. (1964) Compr. Biochem., pp. 165-210.
26. Cleland, W. W. (1977) Adv. Enzymol., 45, 273.
27. Breslow, R. and Wernick, D. L. (1977) Proc. Natl. Acad. Sci. U.S.A., 74, 1303.
28. Schmid, M. F. and Herriott, J. R. (1976) J. Mol. Biol., 103, 197.
29. Zisapel, N. and Sokolowski, M. (1974) Biochem. Biophys. Res. Commun., 58, 951.
30. McKay, T. J. and Plummer, Jr., T. H. (1978) Biochemistry, 17, 401.
31. Ondetti, M. A., Condon, M. E., Reid, J., Sabo, E. F., Cheung, H. S. and Cushman, D. W. (1979) Biochemistry, 18, 1427.

DISCUSSION

LAWSON: ... with carboxypeptidase A and B, in the case of the isomeric
benzylsuccinic acids, one enantimer might bind better to one and one to the
other.

ONDETTI: Yes, that is correct. In the case of carboxypeptidase B
Sokolowski[1], who did a study with benzylsuccinic acid did not use the specific
isomers, which were synthesized by Byers and Wolfenden[2], he used the D,L-form.
So I cannot comment on that. But I could comment on what to me was always a
little bit surprising, that in the results of Byers and Wolfenden with carboxypeptidase A, there is less than a tenfold difference between the inhibition
caused by the D and the L isomer. And I think that one would have expected a
considerably larger difference. The fact that you see such a small difference,
might be attributable to the fact that the opposite, that we call (unfortunately, there is a certain ambiguity in terms) the "wrong" isomer still combines
with the enzyme. Not as efficiently, but in the reverse form. The ambiguity
that I mentioned is that it just happens that the form of benzylsuccinic acid
that is isosteric with L-phenylalanine happens to be in the Fisher-Rosanow
notation the D-benzylsuccinic acid, which Byers and Wolfenden originally
called "L" (in quotation marks). Those who quote them call this isomer L
(without the quotation marks), but it is the D-benzylsuccinic acid. But in
any case, the difference between the inhibitor activity of the D and the L is
comparatively small and I think the reason for this small difference might be
the possible existence of an alternative binding mode for the "wrong" isomer.*

P. BARTLETT: The species, which is bound to the enzyme is the thiolate and
the species, which is presumably the predominant one in solution is the thiol.
Thus, the inhibition constant should reflect the ionization equilibrium between
the thiol and the thiolate and your true equilibrium constant may in fact be
in the picomolar range. Have you considered taking advantage of this
additional binding interaction by using thiocarboxylate, as the coordinating
group? In this case you would have an ionized thiolate at neutral pH.

ONDETTI: We have considered it, but those studies have not yet been
completed.

---

*Editor's note: It is interesting that the D,L-mixtures of guanidinoethyl-
mercaptosuccinic acid and aminopropylmercaptosuccinic acid are about equipotent with D,L-benzylsuccinic acid as inhibitors of carboxypeptidase B, but
essentially inactive against carboxypeptidase A,[3] indicating that in this
case neither isomer is capable of interacting with carboxypeptidase A, in
contrast to the case of the benzylsuccinic acid isomers discussed above.

P. BARTLETT: Do you see a pH dependence on the inhibition?

ONDETTI: We have not looked into that.

YOUNG: Do you have any feeling as to the nature of the nucleophile in the hydrolysis reaction catalyzed by the angiotensin converting enzyme? Is it an enzymic residue, which attacks or just water?

ONDETTI: I cannot really comment on that, except by saying that the mechanism is probably similar to that of carboxypeptidase A, which still not everybody completely agrees upon. It has been proposed[4] that in the case of esters, it is through the formation of a mixed anhydride and in the case of a peptide substrate it might be through general base catalysis.

YOUNG: Do you think that there is an assistance by partial protonation of the amide nitrogen by the enzyme?

ONDETTI: You mean, in the catalytic mechanism?

YOUNG: Right.

ONDETTI: It is possible that protonation plays a role in some of the inhibition that we and other people have observed with the dipeptides. In some cases the inhibition caused by the dipeptides reflects a combination of the binding interaction of the amino acids plus the ionization constant of the N-terminal amino group. So, protonation may play a role here, but there is not much known about the details of the actual peptide bond cleavage step by this enzyme to say how protonation may be involved there.

JONES: Is my assumption correct, that your choice of proline was determined by your model studies on the three hippuryl tripeptides?

ONDETTI: It really stems from our studies of the inhibitors isolated from snake venom[5]. The studies of the hippuryl tripeptides were done somewhat later. It was clear from the study of the venom peptides that proline led to the most active inhibitors in the presence of chloride.

EDITOR's comments: It may be of interest trying to draw some conclusions from Dr. Ondetti's elegant studies, which may apply to the general design of *specific* chelating inhibitors of metallo-enzymes.

(1) It is evident that high potencies approximating those of covalently interacting inhibitors can be achieved;

(2) A structural feature for recognition (be it substrate, product or transition state like) is essential not only for the required specificity, but also for the high overall affinity;

(3) The chelating type of inhibitor is relatively more sensitive to structural modifications, since even small changes in the orientation of the chelating moiety may result in drastic destabilization of the complex. This is a

consequence of the multidentate nature of the complementary structure, which rigidly defines the location of the immobilized protein-bound metal ion[6], in contrast to the more flexible and mobile side chains of the cationic arginine and lysine residues, which are able to tolerate larger changes in distances and orientation. As is demonstrated, however, a favorable structural geometry can yield uniquely superior inhibitory activities for many specific chelating agents, both in terms of potency and specificity (see Table 4).

Some of the results of our recent studies[7] of orotidylate (OMP) decarboxylase inhibitors also support these conclusions. A plausible mechanism of the pyridoxal-P independent OMP decarboxylase catalyzed reaction, which we have considered, may be divided into two distinct steps: (1) formation of an enzyme-activated covalent intermediate (2) decarboxylation; as outlined below:

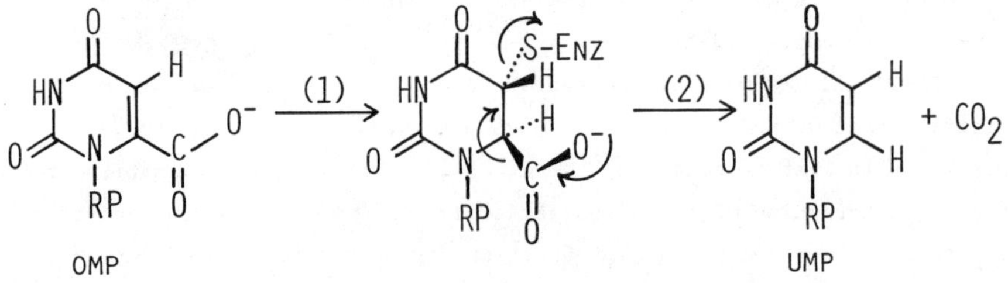

In step (1) a charge neutralization of the carboxylate is likely to be involved in substrate recognition and binding, and is *essential* for effective nucleophilic attack at C-5. In step (2) a relocalization of the negative charge on the carboxylate is a *prerequisite* for decarboxylation accompanied by reformation of the 5,6-double bond and the expulsion of the enzymic nucleophile *via* the reversed Michael route. It was tempting to speculate that the cationic site of the enzyme crucial for the initial interaction with the carboxylate group of the substrate may be a positively charged Zn-ion* bound to the protein:

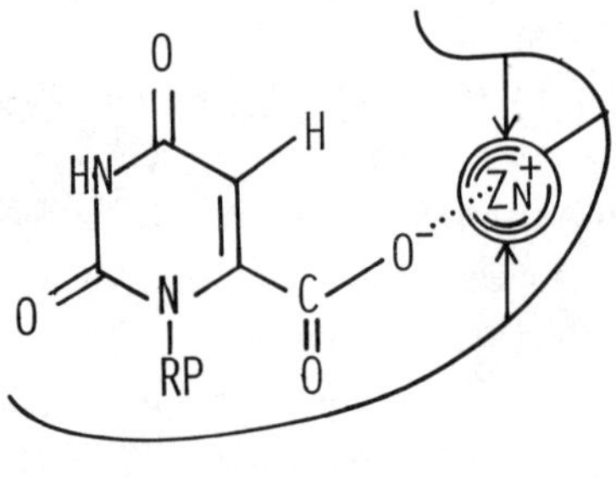

---

* There is only indirect evidence at the present for the existence of enzyme-bound Zn.

During formation of the intermediate in step (1) the saturation of the 5,6-double bond changes the hybridization of C-6 from sp^2 to sp^3, forcing the carboxylate group out of the plane of the pyrimidine ring and consequently also out of the coordination sphere of the Zn-ion. The reversal of the ligand exchange reaction which is likely to accompany the initial substrate binding would serve to restore full coordination around the zinc.

Based on the above mechanistic working hypothesis, the carboxamide (6-$CONH_2$-UMP) and the thiocarboxamide (6-$CSNH_2$-UMP) derivatives of OMP were designed as molecular probes to test the nature of the carboxylate binding-site of the enzyme:

6-$CONH_2$-UMP   6-$CSNH_2$-UMP

They were evaluated as inhibitors of yeast OMP decarboxylase. Preliminary experiments yielded I_{50}-values of 10^{-3} M and $2-3 \times 10^{-8}$ M for 6-$CONH_2$-UMP and 6-$CSNH_2$-UMP, respectively. Thus, the simple replacement of the O-atom of the carbonyl group with sulfur resulted in a > 30,000-fold increase in potency. The apparent K_i of 6-$CSNH_2$-UMP was estimated to be < 10^{-10} M. These results are consistent with the postulated heavy metal complexation mechanism. Further work is required however, to demonstrate conclusively the functional participation of protein-bound zinc in the enzymic decarboxylation of OMP and explore the utility of this approach for the rational design of selective enzyme inhibitors.

REFERENCES

1. Zisapel, N., and Sokolowski, M. (1974) Biochem. Biophys. Res. Commun. 58, 951.
2. Byers, L.D. and Wolfenden, R. (1973) Biochemistry, 12, 2070.
3. McKay, J.J. and Plummer, T.H., Jr. (1978) Biochemistry, 17, 401.
4. Breslow, R. and Wermick, D.L. (1977) Proc. Natl. Acad. Sci. U.S.A. 74, 1303.
5. Ondetti, M.A., Williams, N.J., Sabo, E.F., Pluscec, J., Weaver, E.R. and Kocy, O. (1971) Biochemistry, 10, 4033.
6. Vallee, B.L. and Williams, R.J.P. (1968) Proc. Natl. Acad. Sci. U.S.A. 59, 498.
7. Kalman, T.I. and Landesman, P.W., to be published.

USE OF ELECTROSTATIC FINGERPRINTS TO DETERMINE THE RECEPTOR
SITE CONFORMATION OF ENKEPHALINS

ROBERT P. SHERIDAN, SUSAN L. BRANTLEY, AND LELAND C. ALLEN
Department of Chemistry, Princeton University, Princeton, N. J. 08544, USA

INTRODUCTION

There has been considerable research recently on the use of molecular electrostatic potentials as a method to correlate structure and activity of drugs
and biomolecules.[1] The electrostatic potential at some point near a molecule
is defined as the work necessary to bring an infinitesimal positive point
charge from infinity to that point. The potential is a function of the electronic distribution and the position of nuclei in the molecule and is computed
from molecular wavefunctions.[2] We and others[3,4] have shown that the potential
field around a molecule is relatively insensitive to perturbing effects of
nearby molecules.

The electrostatic energy dominates the medium-to long-range interaction
between closed shell molecules with permanent multipoles and electrostatic
potential field calculations on small molecules have been used to successfully
predict the site of hydrogen bonding, protonation, and electrophilic attack.[2]
By extension it is assumed that electrostatic fields of drug molecules can be
related to binding at the corresponding receptors. Such a relationship is not
unreasonable since much of any drug-receptor interaction is likely to be
through hydrogen bonding, whose strength and geometry is very well predicted by
electrostatic potential. The pattern of equipotential energy contours in three
dimensional space around a drug molecule has been called the 'interaction
pharmacophore'[5] in contrast to less informative pharmacophores based on the
position of functional groups, steric arrangement of atoms, or other purely
structural features. It is expected that drug molecules with similar activities will have similar interaction pharmacophores, i.e., the electrostatic
potential contour maps around pharmacophorically significant parts of the molecules would resemble each other in shape and magnitude. Ab initio and semiempirical electrostatic potentials have been calculated for a number of
pharmacological compounds, including cholinergic and muscarinic compounds[5,6]
adrenergics[7], neuroleptics[8], opiates[1,9,10], carcinogens[11], indolealkylamines[12],
teratogens[13], etc. Some useful correlations have been drawn between the
potential fields and chemical and biological activities.

While the electrostatic potential is a well-defined physical property, its use requires further assumptions about molecular conformation and charge state since details of the receptor are not available:

(1) Ideally one would like to know the receptor-bound conformation of a drug molecule. Usually, what is done is simply to use crystallographic results or the theoretically determined minimum energy conformation of the free molecule. (Of course, neither the solid state conformation nor the calculated vapor-phase conformation is necessarily the correct receptor-bound conformation).

(2) Many compounds exist in active form as charged species (e.g. amines as cations). Since the electrostatic potential of charged molecules is completely dominated by the net charge, the detailed differences between molecules is overwhelmed. In order to bring out information it is necessary to employ a neutral system. One can use either the neutral species (e.g., for amines the unprotonated base) or the charged species with a counter-charged group placed nearby. The maps from both schemes are very similar[5,10,12]. Such cancellation of charge is not unreasonable: it is likely that the charged groups of drugs react with counter-charged groups on the receptor as the primary step. The rest of the molecule is then effectively neutralized and the specific interactions take place for the neutral molecules.

Electrostatic Fingerprints

The use of electrostatic potentials reported here differs in two respects from most other research in this field:

(1) Our electrostatic potential maps are to be regarded purely as an analytical chemistry tool--just as a biochemist views chromatography. IR and NMR spectra are often employed as molecular fingerprints and electrostatic potential maps are another, three dimensional, version of this concept. We are not concerned with underlying biochemical mechanisms nor with the biological consequences of substituent effects on a parent compound.

(2) We are attempting to compare widely differing molecular species--a specific class of plant opiates (e.g. morphine and derivatives) with a naturally occurring brain peptide (enkephalin). It is worth noting that this comparison of disparate molecular entities closely parallels a general problem faced in contemporary pharmaceutical research strategy. The design of drugs most frequently starts with information about a naturally occurring molecule known to strongly interact with a target site of interest and produce a pharmacological

effect. The synthetic organic molecules which are then devised to effect a similar action at the target site are often quite different from the biological models. In our enkephalin example we are using detailed structural information about a known active extraneous molecule (morphine) as a model against which we match various conformational hypotheses for a larger endogenous biochemical molecule (Met-enkephalin). A general property of electrostatic potentials is of special significance here: different atoms with different local geometries can yield the same electrostatic potential, thus the same drug action. The combined action of several atoms together is not at all apparent from a ball-and-stick model, but is an automatic result of electrostatic potentials.

A central problem in the use of this approach is: How does one select the appropriate common features between the biological model and the synthetic analogue? The only answer is systematic cataloguing of many examples, but the availability of a fundamental and powerful analytical technique for carrying out the task may possibly provide a major advance in drug design.

Enkephalins

The existence of individual sites on nerve cells which serve as opiate receptors has been supported by the discovery of Hughes et al.[14] of endogenous peptides with narcotic agonist activity. The smallest of these naturally occurring peptides are the enkephalins: Met-enkephalin (Tyr-Gly-Gly-Phe-Met) and Leu-enkephalin (Tyr-Gly-Gly-Phe-Leu). The enkephalins bind to opiate receptors in the central nervous system and produce shortlived analgesic effects. (See Miller and Cuatrecasas[15] for a comprehensive review.) The conformation of the enkephalin at the receptor site is undetermined. The extreme flexibility of the molecule due to its short length and its internal glycine residues allows for the possibility of many low energy conformers. Several research workers have proposed enkephalin conformations. The approaches have involved (i) spectroscopic analysis of enkephalin in solution[16-20], (ii) crystallographic studies[18,21,22], (iii) theoretical energy calculations of isolated enkephalin[23-28], (iv) secondary structure analysis to determine which backbone conformations are consistent with the activity of various substituted enkephalins[29], and (v) model-building studies where stick or space-filling models of enkephalins are folded to overlap the spatial structure of rigid opiates[30-32].

Gorin et al.[33] have reviewed the strengths and weaknesses of various conformational proposals. It appears that a combination of approaches (iv) and (v)

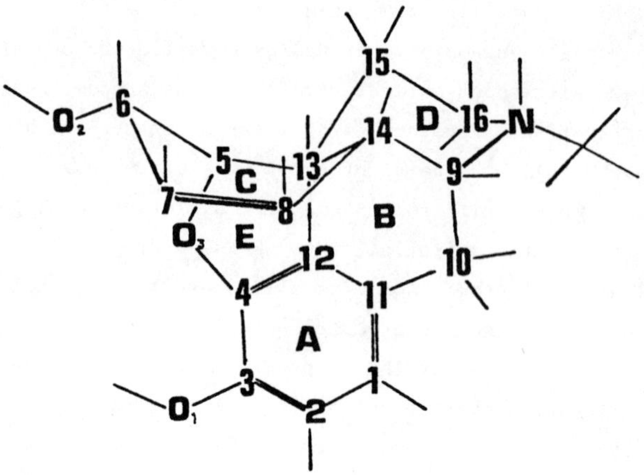

Fig. 1. Schematic representation of morphine skeleton. (Modified after Lowe et al.[10])

is most likely to produce the correct conformation. It should be noted that any proposed conformation must be compatible with data on active structural enkephalin analogs.

Figure 1 schematically represents the skeleton of morphine and derivatives. In structural comparison of enkephalin with opiates it is generally assumed that the enkephalin Tyr phenol ring corresponds to the A ring of the opiate, and the N-terminus to the quaternary N atom. The ring, nitrogen, and connecting carbons are collectively known as the tyramine moiety. There is no unanimous agreement as to the correspondence of the other groups.

In this contribution we discuss the comparison of the electrostatic potential field of morphine with that of three proposed conformers of Met-enkephalin: the model-built conformers of Gorin and Marshall,[31] the energy minimized conformer of Isogai et al.[27] and a selected energy minimized conformer of Momany.[26] Gorin and Marshall's proposal is based on topographical comparison. It superimposes the tyramine moiety of enkephalin and morphine and further overlaps atoms of Phe 4 ring with C5 and C6 of morphine. This model is the tetrapeptide Tyr-Gly-Gly-Phe, the smallest enkephalin fragment exhibiting activity. They claim the conformer is consistent with nearly all data on analogs. The model of Isogai et al. (number 7 in their paper) is the lowest energy conformer by an empirical force-field calculation. Spatial overlap with morphine is slight. Momany calculated the energies of a number of active substituted enkephalins and found one conformation (VIC in his paper) which was likely to be close to the active one. This structure has some overlap with morphine, but while taking into account the activity data on some analogs, is incompatible with data on certain others.

METHODS

We have employed the point charge model to produce the electrostatic potential maps of morphine and some enkephalin conformers. In this model the charge on a given atom is represented by a point charge mounted at its nuclear position. We have been able to show for small molecule analogs of amino acids that the electrostatic potential field around such a point charge model mimics that calculated directly from the molecular wavefunction for regions outside the van der Waals envelope[3,34]. This procedure minimizes the computational cost. Ab initio atomic charges for morphine were obtained from the calculations of Popkie et al.[35]. The charges for amino acid residues are from the library of Hayes and Kollman[36]. The qualitative features of the potential maps are independent of ab initio basis set for both wavefunction and point charge treatments. Semiempirical methods, however, do not adequately represent the potential around aromatic groups[8].

Morphine and enkephalins were treated as neutral molecules for the reasons discussed in the previous section. Morphine geometry was taken from crystallography[37]. Enkephalin geometry was constructed using standard amino acid bond lengths and angles. Dihedral angles describing the conformation of enkaphalin were taken from the three conformation proposals cited above and are listed in Table 1.

A schematic representation of the opiate receptors has been proposed in the literature[38]. Three essential features have been suggested which are disposed approximately as shown in Figure 2:

A. A flat portion onto which the aromatic ring of opiates (or Tyr from enkephalin) can "stack" by van der Waals forces. A hydrophilic group is probably associated with this site, since polar substituents on the aromatic portion of the opiates appears important.

B. A cavity complementary to the $C_{15}-C_{16}$ ridge of the piperidine D ring.

C. An anionic site to interact with the quaternary nitrogen.

TABLE 1

DIHEDRAL ANGLES FOR PROPOSED ENKEPHALIN CONFORMATIONS

Angle (°)		Gorin and Marshall	Isogai et al. No. 7	Momany VIC
Tyr	ϕ	-60[a]	-84	-56
	ψ	129	155	82
	ω	180	-176	-178
	χ^1	-106	-174	-61
	χ^2	-163	82	-75
	χ^6	125[b]	-147	-178
Gly	ϕ	160	-159	69
	ψ	-87	100	-127
	ω	180	173	180
Gly	ϕ	-118	74	-65
	ψ	98	-100	-55
	ω	180	175	177
Phe	ϕ	-87	-85	-64
	ψ	60[a]	-41	114
	ω	--	-179	-174
	χ^1	-87	-179	177
	χ^2	-56	74	-109
Met	ϕ	--	-165	49
	ψ	--	124	56
	χ^1	--	-174	-62
	χ^2	--	57	-176
	χ^3	--	-178	177
	χ^4	--	60	58

a Angles we have assumed because the value was not given in the original work.
b Value taken from the corresponding atoms of morphine.

295

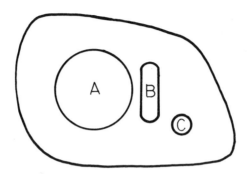

Fig.2. Main features of opiate receptor. A. Flat surface for aromatic ring.
     B. Cavity for C_{15}–C_{16}. C. Anionic site for binding quaternary nitrogen.
     (Modified after Lowe et al.[10])

   Some receptor schemes require another flat hydrophobic site for the aromatic
F ring which is present in some opiates more potent than morphine.

   Given the importance of the substituted aromatic ring, and the probability
that it binds roughly parallel to the receptor surface, we have constructed our
electrostatic potential maps for planes parallel to that of the aromatic ring.
Sections A are 2 Å toward the center of gravity of the morphine/enkephalin
molecule (above the ring). Sections B are taken through the ring. Sections
C are 2 Å away from the main body of the molecule, i.e. toward the receptor
(below the ring). Most important interactions with the receptor probably take
place within the defined volume.

RESULTS AND DISCUSSION

   Isopotential contours of morphine and enkephalin conformers are shown in
Figure 3 through 6. The van der Waals envelope of each conformer is outlined
and the positions of the phenol rings and the quaternary nitrogen are indicated.
Solid contour lines (in kcal) represent repulsive (to a positive charge)
potentials; dotted lines, attractive potentials. The potential field around
morphine (Figure 3) is characterized by two lobes of negative potential, corresponding to the phenolic oxygen (O1) and furan oxygen (O3). Neutral morphine
shows a negative potential region around what corresponds to the N lone pair.
Regions of negative potential around the aromatic group above and below the

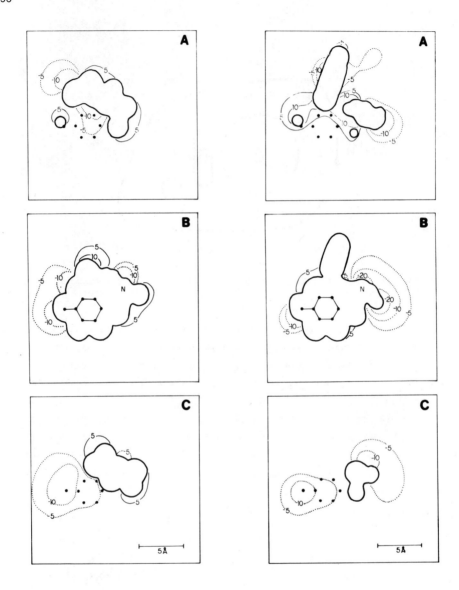

Fig. 3. Electrostatic isopotential contour map for morphine. See text for explanation.

Fig. 4. Electrostatic isopotential map for conformer of Gorin and Marshall.

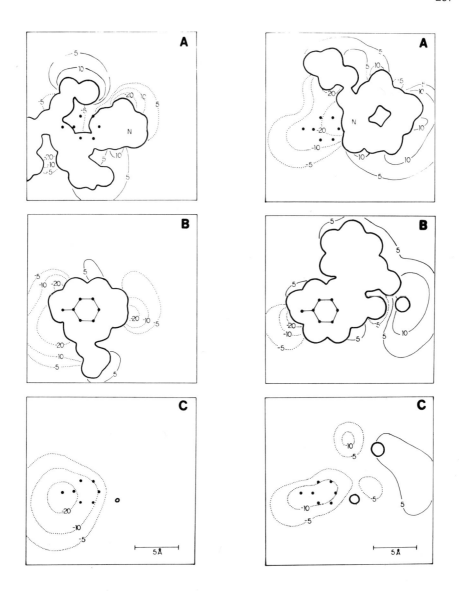

Fig. 5. Electrostatic isopotential
        map for conformer No. 7
        of Isogai et al.

Fig. 6. Electrostatic isopotential
        map for conformer VIC of
        Momany.

plane correspond to the influence of the pi electrons. (These regions appear in all conformers.) Our results agree with other <u>ab</u> <u>initio</u> studies on morphine[1].

In making comparisons we must keep in mind that morphine only accidently fits the enkephalin receptor, and not the reverse. Therefore, at best, morphine gives a minimal picture of the receptor. If the enkephalin approaches morphine in potential field and/or shape of van der Waals envelope, this could be considered a sufficient condition for binding. However, it would certainly not be <u>necessary</u> to match every feature.

The Gorin and Marshall conformer, (Figure 4) as mapped in the phenol plane shows a negative potential around the hydroxyl oxygen similar to that around O1 of morphine. However there is no region corresponding to that around O3. Above the plane there is some correspondence of the negative aromatic region of Phe 4 with that of O3. An additional region near the N lone pair is due to the carbonyl oxygen of Tyr 1. This broad region has some slight analogy to the O3 region of morphine. If the Phe 4 ring were removed, a small positive region would appear immediately above the van der Waals surface at the top of Section B and a small negative region immediately to the left, thereby creating a map with considerable similarity to morphine. The reversed sign of the potential around N (immediately to the right of the van der Waals surface in Section B) remains as an unresolved conflict, however.

The conformer of Isogai <u>et</u> <u>al</u>. shows a greatly increased area of negative potential in the phenol plane. This might resemble the area around O1 and O2 of morphine. A negative region to the right of the molecule has no counterpart to morphine. It is not surprising that the Isogai potential field does not show correspondence to that of morphine since there is no steric overlap.

Momany's conformer places the Phe 4 ring in the plane of Tyr 1. The pi negative region appears in section C near the pi region of Tyr. The N lone pair contributes to the region in Section A.

We are currently producing conformations which more nearly mimic the potential field of opiates and finding which of these are consistent with the stereochemical properties of enkephalin derivatives. We also plan to investigate a more potent narcotic such as PET or oripavine to expand our ideas of the opiate pharmacophore. It is our belief that the electrostatic potential fingerprint is a new and potentially valuable tool in elucidating the receptor-bound conformations of enkephalins.

ACKNOWLEDGEMENT
     The financial assistance of the NIH, Grant GM 26462-01, is gratefully acknowledged.

REFERENCES

1. Petrongolo, C. (1978) Gazz. Chim.Ital., 108, 445-478.
2. Scrocco, E. and Tomasi, J. (1978) Adv. Quant. Chem., 11, 116-193.
3. Sheridan, R. P. (1979) Ph.D. thesis, Princeton University.
4. Pullman, A. and Berthod, H. (1978) Theor. Chim. Acta, 48, 269-277.
5. Weinstein, H., Maayani, S., Srebrenik, S., Cohen, S., and Sokolovsky, M. (1973) Molec.Pharm., 9, 820-834.
6. Weinstein, H., Srebrenik, S., Maayani, S. and Sokolovsky, M. (1977) J. theor. Biol., 64, 295-309.
7. Petrongolo, C., Macchia, F., and Martinelli, A. (1977) J. Med. Chem., 20, 1645-1653.
8. Petrongolo, C., Preston, H.J.T., and Kaufman, J.J. (1978) Int. J. Quant. Chem., 13, 457-468.
9. Breon, T. L., Petersen, H., Jr., and Paruta, A. N. (1978) J. Pharm. Sci., 67, 73-80.
10. Loew, G. H., Berkowitz, D., Weinstein, H., and Srebrenik, S. (1974) in Molecular and Quantum Pharmacology, Bergmann, E. D. and Pullman, B., eds., B. Reidel, Boston, pp. 355-389.
11. Politzer, P. and Daiker, K. C. (1977) Int. J. Quant. Chem. QBS4, 317.
12. Weinstein, H., Chou, D., Kang, S., Johnson, C. L., Green, J.P. (1976) Int. J. Quant. Chem. QBS3, 135-150.
13. Kaufman, J. J., Popkie, H. E., and Preston, H. J. T. (1978) Int. J. Quant. Chem. QBS5, 201-218.
14. Hughes, J., Smith, T. W., Kosterlitz, H. W., Fothergill, L. H., Morgan, B.A., Morris, H. (1975) Nature, 258, 577-579.
15. Miller, R. J. and Cuatrecasas, P. (1978) Vitamins and Hormones, 36, 297-382.
16. Stimson, E. R., Meinwald, Y. C., and Scheraga, H. A. (1979) Biochemistry, 18, 1661-1671.
17. Spirtes, M. A., Schwartz, R. W., Mattice, W. L., and Coy, D. H. (1978) Biochem. Biophys. Res. Comm., 81, 602-608.
18. Fournie Zaluski, M. C., Prange, T., Pascard, C., and Roques, B. P. (1977) Biochem. Biophys. Res. Comm., 79, 1199-1206.
19. Jones, C. R., Garsky, V. and Gibbons, W. A. (1977) Biochem. Biophys. Res. Comm., 76, 619-625.
20. Roques, B. P., Garbay-Jaureguiberry, C., Oberlin, R., Anteunis, M., and Lala, A. K. (1976) Nature, 262, 778-779.
21. Smith, G. D. and Griffin, J. F. (1978) Science, 199, 1214-1216.
22. Carson, W. M. and Hackert, M. L. (1978) Acta. Cryst., B34, 1275-1280.
23. Balodis, Y. Y., Nikiforovich, G. V., Grinsteine, I. V., Vegner, R. E., and Chipens, G. I. (1978) FEBS Lett., 86, 239-242.
24. Loew, G. H. and Burt, S. K. (1978) Proc. Nat. Acad. Sci. USA, 75, 7-11.
25. Momany, F. A. and Aubuchon, J. R. (1978) Biopolymers, 17, 2609-2615.
26. Momany, F.A. (1977) Biochem. Biophys. Res. Comm., 75, 1098-1103.
27. Isogai, Y., Némethy, G., and Scheraga, H. A. (1977) Proc. Nat. Acad. Sci. USA, 74, 414-418.
28. DeCoen, J. L., Humblet, C., and Koch, M.H.J. (1977) FEBS Lett., 73, 38-42.
29. Beddell, C., Chang, K.-J., Cuatrecasas, P., Clark, R. B., Lowe, L. A., Miller, R. J., and Wilkinson, S. (1977) Br. J. Pharmacol., 61, 351-356.
30. Clarke, F. H., Jaggi, H., and Lovell,R.A.(1978) J. Med. Chem., 21, 600-606.
31. Gorin, F. A. and Marshall, G. R. (1977) Proc. Nat. Acad. Sci. USA, 74, 5179-5183.
32. Bradbury, A.F., Smyth, D. G., and Snell, C. R., (1976) Nature, 260, 165-166.

33. Gorin, F. A., Balasubramanian, T. M., Barry, C. D., and Marshall, G. R., (1978) J. Supramol. Structure, 9, 27-39.
34. Bonaccorsi, R., Petrongolo, C., Scrocco, E., and Tomasi, J. (1971) Theor. Chim. Acta, 20, 331-342.
35. Popkie, H. E., Koski, W. S., and Kaufman, J. J. (1976) J. Amer. Chem Soc., 98, 1342-1345.
36. Hayes, D. M. and Kollman, P. A. (1976) J. Amer. Chem. Soc., 98, 3335-3345.
37. Gylbert, L. (1973) Acta. Cryst. B 29, 1630-1635.
38. Beckett, A. H., and Casy, A. F. (1965) Prog. Med. Chem., 4, 171-218.

DISCUSSION

G. DAVID SMITH (Medical Foundation of Buffalo, Inc., Buffalo, NY; invited comments): The use of electrostatic potentials should prove to be very useful in correlating the binding of various drug molecules to their receptors, and, more importantly, to permit the receptor site to be mapped by comparing the potentials of a large number of active as well as inactive analogues. This is particularly true if the molecule under consideration has little or no conformational flexibility. However, if the molecule happens to be a flexible one, the choice of which conformer to consider is critical.

The opiate receptor provides just such an example. Several crystal structures have been reported for the very rigid agonist, morphine,[1-3] permitting the calculation of the electrostatic potential which is seen by the receptor. However, as Sheridan et al. point out,[4] "morphine only accidently fits the enkephalin receptor, and not the reverse". Thus, it may not be necessary to impose the conformation of the "tyramine" moiety of morphine on the tyrosine side chain of the endogenous opiate, enkephalin, as so many studies have done. Rather, it may be the positioning of the nitrogen and hydroxy groups which is relevant for activity. The fact the [Phe][1] - enkephalin is inactive[5] suggests that the hydrophilic interaction of the hydroxy group is far more important than any "stacking" of an aromatic ring on a flat surface of the receptor. It is also clear that morphine possesses other features which are necessary for binding since tyramine is inactive; in addition to the C15-C16 ridge of the piperidine D ring, it has also been suggested that the C ring is involved in binding to the receptor.[6] Since the D-[Ala][2] analogues of enkephalin have been found to be quite active,[7] models which cannot accommodate a D configuration at residue 2 are not relevant at the receptor site. This is in accord with the finding that the model proposed by Isogai et al.[8] shows neither correspondence to the potential field nor steric overlap to that of morphine.

Many conformations have been proposed on the basis of spectral and energy minimization studies, and three of these models[8-10] were used in the calcula-

tions described.[4] It would be of considerable interest to perform similar
calculations upon the X-ray crystallographically observed conformation,[11] the
only unambiguously demonstrated low energy form of enkephalin, or upon the
tetrapeptide[12] which comprises residues 1 through 4. A type I' beta bend,
centered on the two glycine residues, is observed in the solid state structure
of [Leu][5]-enkephalin[11] (Figure 1) and is further stabilized by two anti-
parallel intramolecular hydrogen bonds between tyrosine and phenylalanine.
Since the fifth residue is not involved in intramolecular hydrogen bonds, it

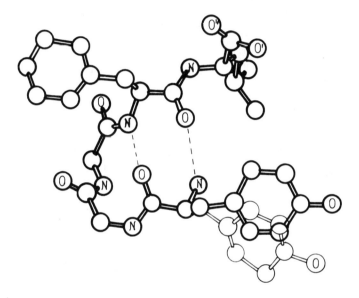

Figure 1.

is possible to alter this residue (to Met, for example) and not change the
backbone conformation. One can even imagine removing this residue without
seriously perturbing the backbone. In fact, a type I' beta bend, centered on
the two glycines and stabilized by a single intramolecular hydrogen bond, is
observed in the crystal structure of the tetrapeptide,[12] the smallest enkephalin fragment which is active.

EDITOR's comments: It is of interest that a dipeptidyl carboxypeptidase,
one of the two recognized types of enkephalinases, which are known to inactivate endogenous brain opiates, was recently found to be identical with a
membrane-bound angiotensin-converting enzyme in rat and rabbit brain tissues.[13]
The enkephalinase activity is very sensitive to inhibition by captopril

(SQ 14,225), the specific angiotensin-converting enzyme inhibitor discussed by
Dr. Ondetti.[14]

REFERENCES

1. Bye, E. (1976) Acta Chem. Scand. B30, 549-554.
2. Gylbert, L. (1973) Acta Cryst. B29, 1630-1635.
3. Mackay, M. and Hodgkin, D.C. (1955) J. Chem. Soc. 3261-3267.
4. Sheridan, R.P., Brantley, S.L. and Allen, L.C. (1979) this volume.
5. Frederickson, R.C.A., Nickander, R., Smithwick, E.L., Shuman, R. and
   Norris, F.H. (1976) in Opiates and Endogenous Opioid Peptides, Elsevier,
   Amsterdam, pp. 239-246.
6. Childers, S.R., Creese, I., Snowman, A.M. and Snyder, S.H. (1979)
   Eur. J. Pharmacol. 55, 11-18.
7. Roemer, D., Buescher, H.H., Hill, R.C., Pless, J., Bauer, W., Cardinaux, F.
   Closse, A., Hauser, D. and Huguenin, R. (1977) Nature, 268, 547-549.
8. Isogai, Y., Némethy, G. and Scheraga, H.A. (1977) Proc. Nat. Acad. Sci.
   USA, 74, 414-418.
9. Momany, F.A. (1977) Biochem. Biophys. Res. Comm. 75, 1098-1103.
10. Gorin, F.A. and Marshall, G.R. (1977) Proc. Nat. Acad. Sci. USA, 74,
    5179-5183.
11. Smith, G.D. and Griffin, J.F. (1978) Science, 199, 1214-1216.
12. Fournie Zaluski, M.C., Prange, T., Pascard, C. and Roques, B.P. (1977)
    Biochem. Biophys. Res. Comm. 79, 1199-1206.
13. Benuck, M. and Marks, N. (1979) Biochem. Biophys. Res. Comm. 88, 215-221.
14. Ondetti, M.A., Cushman, D.W., Sabo, E.F. and Cheung, H.S. (1979) this
    volume.

303

Author Index

Subject Index